behavior
and brain
electrical
activity

behavior and brain electrical activity

Edited by
neil burch
and
h. l. altshuler

Texas Research Institute of Mental Sciences
Texas Medical Center
Houston, Texas

plenum press·new york and london

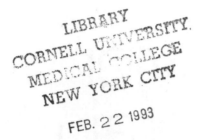
Library of Congress Catalog Card Number 75-24841
ISBN 0-306-30868-1

Proceedings of the Seventh Annual Symposium on Behavior and Brain Electrical
Activity held at the Texas Research Institute of Mental Sciences, Texas
Medical Center, Houston, Texas, November 28-30, 1973

© 1975 Plenum Press, New York
A Division of Plenum Publishing Corporation
227 West 17th Street, New York, N.Y. 10011

United Kingdom edition published by Plenum Press, London
A Division of Plenum Publishing Company, Ltd.
Davis House (4th Floor), 8 Scrubs Lane, Harlesden, London, NW10 6SE, England

Printed in the United States of America

contributors

W. Ross Adey, M.D.
Professor of Anatomy and Physiology and Member, Brain Research Institute, University of California—Los Angeles School of Medicine, Los Angeles, California

H.L. Altshuler, Ph.D.
Chief, Neuropsychopharmacology Research Section, Texas Research Institute of Mental Sciences; Assistant Professor of Pharmacology, Baylor College of Medicine, Houston, Texas

Edward C. Beck, Ph.D.
Director of Neuropsychology Laboratory, Veterans Administration Hospital; Chairman, Division of Medical Psychology, University of Utah, Salt Lake City, Utah

*Reginald G. Bickford, M.D., F.R.C.P.
Professor of Neurosciences and Director, EEG Laboratory, University of California School of Medicine at San Diego, La Jolla, California

Edward Bixler, Ph.D.
Sleep Research and Treatment Facility and Department of Psychiatry, Pennsylvania State University, Milton S. Hershey Medical Center, Hershey, Pennsylvania

Cletis R. Booher, B.S.E.E.
Bioengineering Systems Division, National Aeronautics and Space Administration, Lyndon B. Johnson Space Center, Houston, Texas

*session chairman

Neil R. Burch, M.D.
> Head, Research Division and Chief, Psychophysiology Research Section, Texas Research Institute of Mental Sciences; Associate Professor of Psychiatry, Baylor College of Medicine, Houston, Texas

Enoch Callaway, III, M.D.
> Chief of Research, Langley Porter Neuropsychiatric Institute; Department of Psychiatry, University of California Medical Center, San Francisco, California

Lawrence C. Cowden, A.S.E.T.
> Department of Psychiatry, University of Oklahoma Health Sciences Center, Oklahoma City, Oklahoma

Milton R. DeLucchi, Ph.D.
> Assistant, Neurophysiology Service, The Methodist Hospital; Assistant Professor of Physiology, Baylor College of Medicine, Houston, Texas

Robert E. Dustman, Ph.D.
> Neuropsychology Laboratory, Veterans Administration Hospital; Division of Medical Psychology, University of Utah, Salt Lake City, Utah

*Robert J. Ellingson, Ph.D., M.D.
> Professor of Medical Psychology and Neurology and Director of Research, Nebraska Psychiatric Institute, Omaha, Nebraska

Frank R. Ervin, M.D.
> Professor of Psychiatry, University of California—Los Angeles Center for the Health Sciences, Los Angeles, California

*William S. Fields, M.D.
> Professor and Director, Program in Neurology, The University of Texas School of Medicine at Houston, Houston, Texas

James D. Frost, Jr., M.D.
> Associate Chief, Neurophysiology Service, The Methodist Hospital; Professor of Physiology, Baylor College of Medicine, Houston, Texas

Alan S. Gevins, B.S.
> Co-director, EEG Systems Group, Langley Porter Neuropsychiatric Institute, San Francisco; Director, Advanced Digital Intelligence, Berkeley, California

*session chairman

E. Roy John, Ph.D.
   Professor and Director, Brain Research Laboratories, Department of
   Psychiatry, New York Medical College, New York, New York

Laverne C. Johnson, Ph.D.
   Head, Psychophysiology Division, Navy Medical Neuropsychiatric
   Research Unit, San Diego, California

Anthony Kales, M.D.
   Chairman, Department of Psychiatry and Director, Sleep Research and
   Treatment Facility, Pennsylvania State University, Milton S. Hershey
   Medical Center, Hershey, Pennsylvania

Peter Kellaway, A.M., Ph.D.
   Professor of Physiology, Baylor College of Medicine; Chief of Neurophysiology, The Methodist Hospital; Director, Blue Bird Clinic Research Unit, Houston, Texas

Eva King Killam, Ph.D.
   Professor of Pharmacology, University of California School of Medicine, Davis, California

Keith F. Killam, Ph.D.
   Professor and Chairman, Department of Pharmacology, University of
   California School of Medicine, Davis, California

John R. Knott, Ph.D.
   Professor and Head, Division of Electroencephalography and Clinical
   Neurophysiology, University of Iowa and Iowa Security Medical Facil-
   ity, Iowa City, Iowa

Romulo T. Lara, M.D.
   Department of Psychiatry, Division of Electroencephalography, University of Iowa and Iowa Security Medical Facility, Iowa City, Iowa

Lawrence E. Larsen, M.D., MAJ, MC
   Assistant Professor of Physiology, Baylor College of Medicine, Houston,
   Texas. Dr. Larsen is now with the Department of Microwave Research,
   Walter Reed Army Institute of Research, Washington, D.C.

Boyd K. Lester, M.D.
   Professor of Psychiatry, University of Oklahoma Health Sciences

Center, Oklahoma City, Oklahoma

*Donald B. Lindsley, Ph.D.
    Professor, Departments of Psychology, Physiology, and Psychiatry,
    University of California, Los Angeles, California

Robert E. Litman, M.D.
    Adjunct Professor of Psychiatry, University of California—Los Angeles
    School of Medicine; Co-director, Suicide Prevention Center and Insti-
    tute for Studies of Self-Destructive Behavior, Los Angeles, California

Walter D. Obrist, Ph.D.
    Professor of Medical Psychology, Duke University Medical Center,
    Durham, North Carolina

Jon F. Peters, M.S.
    Department of Psychiatry, Division of Electroencephalography, Univer-
    sity of Iowa and Iowa Security Medical Facility, Iowa City, Iowa

Merl D. Robinson, M.D.
    Department of Psychiatry, Division of Electroencephalography, Univer-
    sity of Iowa and Iowa Security Medical Facility, Iowa City, Iowa

Orvis H. Rundell, M.S.
    Department of Psychiatry, University of Oklahoma Health Sciences
    Center, Oklahoma City, Oklahoma

Joseph G. Salamy, Ph.D.
    Life Sciences Division, Technology, Inc., Houston, Texas

Bernard Saltzberg, Ph.D.
    Professor of Biomathematics, Department of Psychiatry and Neurology,
    Tulane University School of Medicine, New Orleans, Louisiana

Charles Shagass, M.D.
    Professor of Psychiatry, Eastern Pennsylvania Psychiatric Institute and
    Temple University Medical Center, Philadelphia, Pennsylvania

Daniel E. Sheer, Ph.D.
    Professor of Psychology, University of Houston, Houston, Texas

*session chairman

Harold W. Shipton, C. Eng., F.I.E.R.E.
  Professor and Director, Bioengineering Resource Facility, University of
  Iowa College of Medicine, Iowa City, Iowa

William H. Shumate, Ph.D.
  Neurophysiology Section, National Aeronautics and Space Administration, Lyndon B. Johnson Space Center, Houston, Texas

Jack R. Smith, Ph.D.
  Professor of Electrical Engineering and Psychiatry, University of Florida, Gainesville, Florida

Robert W. Thatcher, Ph.D.
  Brain Research Laboratories, Department of Psychiatry, New York
  Medical College, New York, New York

Richard D. Walter, M.D.
  Professor of Neurology and Psychiatry, University of California—Los
  Angeles Center for the Health Sciences, The Neuropsychiatric Institute,
  Los Angeles, California

*W. Grey Walter, Sc.D., M.D.
  Burden Neurological Institute, Bristol, England

Elliot D. Weitzman, M.D.
  Professor and Chairman, Department of Neurology, Montefiore Hospi-
  tal and Medical Center and The Albert Einstein College of Medicine,
  Bronx, New York

Louis Jolyon West, M.D.
  Professor and Chairman, Department of Psychiatry, University of
  California—Los Angeles School of Medicine, Los Angeles, California

Harold L. Williams, Ph.D.
  Professor of Psychology, University of Minnesota, Minneapolis, Minnesota

*Robert L. Williams, M.D., D.C.
  Irene Ellwood Professor and Chairman of Psychiatry, Baylor College of
  Medicine, Houston, Texas

*session chairman

Charles L. Yeager, M.D., Ph.D.
    Professor of Psychiatry in Residence, University of California; Director,
    EEG Laboratory, Langley Porter Neuropsychiatric Institute, San Fran-
    cisco, California

foreword

This volume is dedicated to the faith that the future will offer hard quantitative measures of the human thought process and affect-emotional system. The symposium from which this volume issues was an opportunity for us to invite a number of our friends to help in collecting some of the current contributions to this belief.

The participants and topics weave a mosaic of the future. The selection was made in an attempt to project into the future what is most important in the present and in the relatively recent past in terms of generating hard data of the elusive cognitive-affect systems.

We regret, because of editorial constraints, that we have not been able to include some of the outstanding contributions offered by our various chairmen. In particular, we are sorry that this volume does not reflect the thoughts of Robert Williams, R.J. Ellingson, William Fields, and especially those of our esteemed grand marshal, W. Grey Walter.

This volume deals initially with the electroencephalographic measurement of sleep profiles as such profiles may be used to measure the stresses of special environments and special patient populations. Of particular interest is the correlation of sleep profiles with basic endocrine functions. We expect the measurement of sleep profiles to become more of a routine clinical examination in the next few years, as our understanding of this fascinating state of consciousness increases in terms of how it is influenced by real life stresses and disease processes.

Hard quantitative measurement of brain electrical activity is dealt with in a set of papers introduced by a discussion on selecting optimum signal parameters. The forlorn cry of "How do I best analyze my data?" is familiar to all students of analog signals. This section attempts a partial answer in terms of both conceptualization and hardware systems.

Initial state and change of state in brain activity as a function of drug effects, biofeedback effects, and impressed electrical fields is considered in a series of contributions. We would call special attention to W. Ross Adey's paper as a tour de force of neurophysiological understanding at multiple levels. Changes in brain electrical activity with maturation and disease processes are presented by leading scientists in these important areas. The normative standards in human growth and maturation and the deviation from these standards induced by disease and pathology will be the most important measures in psychiatry of the future.

The final section analyzes the behavioral pattern of violence and aggression in the context of sociological concern. This is an area of immense importance fraught with more than just the difficulties attendant on all scientific endeavor. The issue of individual human privacy, free and informed consent, and the needs of society in relation to the rights of the individual all require proper resolution before we can reaffirm that the proper study of mankind is man. Scientists endeavoring to understand and to ameliorate human violence are themselves in jeopardy from social forces desiring to abolish all research in this area rather than to arrive at a reasonable balance between the needs of the present and the needs of the future.

With great pride we asked our friends to gather, friends who represent that cadre of the scientific community dedicated to quantitative measurement and better understanding of the magic of human thought and human feeling.

Neil R. Burch, M.D.
and
H.L. Altshuler, Ph.D.

acknowledgments

We are grateful to Abbott Laboratories, Ciba-Geigy Corporation, George and Mary Josephine Hamman Foundation, Hoffmann-LaRoche, Inc., The Lanier Foundation, Merck & Company, Inc., and Wyeth Laboratories for their generous financial support.

If the cause of justice were to be served, Meredith Riddell might well appear as senior editor of this volume. The extent of her editorial contribution has been immeasurable and, under the watchful supervision of Lore Feldman, has been highly professional.

contents

☐ **Sleep Profiles and Behavior**

☐ **Measurement and Analysis of Electrical Activity**

☐ **Change of State**

Drug Effects

Feedback Effects

Contents

behavior
and brain
electrical
activity

the effect of total, partial, and stage sleep deprivation on eeg patterns and performance

Laverne C. Johnson, Ph.D.

Navy Medical Neuropsychiatric Research Unit
San Diego, California

Less than 20 years ago, few scientists would have considered sleep an appropriate topic for a symposium concerning behavior and brain electrical activity. Though some investigators had studied brain electrical activity during sleep (Loomis, Harvey, and Hobart 1937), sleep was hardly conceived as a fruitful period for behavioral research. Sleep was regarded as a quiet period, even referred to as a state of unconsciousness. We are now aware of the richness of sleep behavior, and perhaps in no other area are brain electrical activity and behavior so closely coupled as in a person going from awake to the drowsy period of stage 1, then on to sleep identified by the brain's unique signature, sleep spindles and bursts of K-complexes. The sleep spindles and large-amplitude delta rhythms of stages 2, 3, and 4 (nonREM sleep) periodically give way to the low-voltage electroencephalographic (EEG) activity with associated rapid eye movements (REMs) reflecting the characteristic 90-100 minute cycle of REM-nonREM sleep. This cycle and the unique behavioral and physiological activity associated with each phase are tracked nightly in laboratories throughout the world by means of electroencephalographic recordings of brain electrical activity. Not only is this electrical activity of the sleeping brain a universal human phenomenon, but comparable activity is also present in nonhuman species. Clearly sleep is an excellent area to study the relation between brain electrical activity and behavior.

With the loss of all sleep (total sleep deprivation), reduction of usual

1

total sleep time (partial sleep loss), or denial of certain stages of sleep (sleep-stage deprivation), there are changes in both behavior and EEG activity during sleep. It is perhaps obvious that if it were not for the well-defined and stable patterns of sleep stages and EEG activity, we would not be able to excise selected stages from a night of sleep.

In the late fifties and sixties, there were dramatic reports detailing the behavioral, EEG, and psychological changes following prolonged periods of wakefulness: 200 hours (Brauchi and West 1959); 205 hours (Kollar et al. 1969); 220 hours (Luby et al. 1960); and the most heroic effort, 264 hours without sleep, by a 17-year-old male (Johnson, Slye, and Dement 1965; Gulevich, Dement, and Johnson 1966). As subsequent studies cast doubt on the earlier beliefs that sleep deprivation could be used to produce a model psychosis and as prolonged wakefulness studies were stressful for both subject and researcher, interest in sleep-loss studies of long duration was brief. As the sixties drew to a close, interest in total sleep loss of any duration waned as interest in partial sleep loss and selective stage deprivation increased. Review articles on total sleep loss replaced new research reports (Johnson 1969, Webb 1969, Naitoh 1969, Naitoh and Townsend 1970, Colquhoun 1972). Since the area of total sleep deprivation is not now an area of active research interest and since it has been so well covered with generally consistent conclusions, after a brief review of total sleep loss I shall devote most of my presentation to partial sleep loss and selective stage deprivation where most of the research is now focused.

EEG Changes Following Total Sleep Loss

Total sleep loss is invariably followed by a decrease in percentage of waking alpha activity and an increase in percentage of delta and theta. In a detailed quantitative analysis of EEG spectra in four subjects during 205 hours of wakefulness, Naitoh, Pasnau, and Kollar (1971) noted that up to 60 hours of wakefulness, alpha occupied 60 to 70 percent of total EEG activity; delta, 14 to 20 percent; theta 11 to 14 percent; and there was a small amount of beta. Beyond 100 hours of sleep loss, delta increased to 31 to 44 percent; theta to 20 to 33 percent, with a concomitant decrease in percentage of alpha. Naitoh, Pasnau, and Kollar (1971) reported virtually no change in EEG beta activity during the 205 hours of sleep loss. The decrease in alpha abundance tended to stabilize after the 100-hour period, and, with additional sleep loss, the four subjects tended to regain some alpha but its abundance never approached the pre-sleep loss level.

Naitoh et al. (1969) observed that after about 115 hours of sleep loss, closing of the eyes failed to generate alpha activity. Johnson, Slye, and Dement (1965) reported that after 249 hours of sleep loss their subject showed no EEG response to eyes opening and closing. External stimuli did not produce alpha enhancement nor any autonomic indications of an orienting response.

Another EEG response that decreases and finally disappears with sleep loss is the surface-negative slow potential (CNV) associated with an expectancy to respond. Naitoh, Johnson, and Lubin (1971) used a 4.5-second period between the warning stimulus S1 and the imperative stimulus S2 to study the CNV under baseline, total sleep deprivation, and recovery conditions in eight subjects. The S1 (warning stimulus) was a click; the S2 (imperative stimulus) was a set of photoflashes. During baseline all subjects developed the CNV between S1 and S2. One night of sleep loss decreased CNV amplitude, and two nights of sleep loss abolished the CNV. Figure 1 illustrates the response from a single subject, and Figure 2 the average response for all eight subjects of the study. Only those CNV trials with a background EEG indicating a waking state and with a reaction time of less than a second were used in this analysis. The results thus were not due to sleepiness but rather to sleep loss.

The low-voltage EEG pattern with decreased alpha is also seen in activated and alert subjects. Malmo and Surwillo (1960) and Tyler, Goodman, and Rothman (1947) have interpreted the decrease in alpha abundance following sleep loss as indicating increased activation. Armington and Mitnick (1959), Johnson, Slye, and Dement (1965), and Naitoh et al. (1969) interpret the EEG changes as a shift toward drowsiness with increasing lapses or transient periods of brief sleep, sometimes called microsleep, as sleep loss progresses. With prolonged sleep loss, however, there seems to be a decrease in responsiveness. As noted earlier, alpha enhancement after eye closure or an arousal stimulus is lost, and the expected orienting response is not present for either EEG or autonomic activity (Johnson, Slye, and Dement 1965). When the subject is allowed to go to sleep, both EEG and autonomic responses reappear after only a few minutes of stage 2 sleep, raising the question of whether the sleep responses reflect the potency of the recovery function of sleep or whether the responses reflect the involvement of different response mechanisms with the change in state.

EEG Activity During Sleep

On the first recovery night after sleep loss, there is invariably an increase in slow-wave sleep (stages 3 and 4) over that present before deprivation (Berger and Oswald 1962; Williams et al. 1964; Gulevich, Dement, and Johnson 1966). REM sleep usually stays at pre-sleep loss levels or decreases on the first recovery night. If an increase in REM sleep occurs, it is usually seen on the second recovery night. A quantitative analysis shows that the increase in slow-wave sleep (SWS) is due to both an earlier entry into SWS and longer duration of the SWS periods (Figure 3). Most of the increase in SWS occurs during the first four hours of sleep with no marked changes in the delta cycles.

Performance Changes

Beginning with the detailed studies conducted at Walter Reed Army Institute of Research by Harold Williams and his colleagues (Williams, Lubin, and Goodnow 1959), the performance decrement following sleep loss has been well-defined and a consistent pattern has emerged (Williams et al. 1962; Williams et al. 1964; Williams, Kearney, and Lubin 1965; Williams, Gieseking, and Lubin 1966; Williams and Williams 1966; Williams and Lubin 1967). The Walter Reed group confirmed earlier reports that the primary

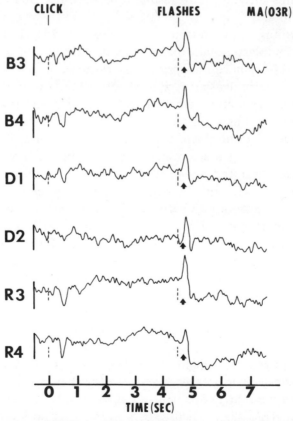

Figure 1. Disappearance of CNV (surface-negative slow potential) for single subject during total sleep deprivation (D1-D2) with return following recovery sleep (R3-R4). Average reaction time for each CNV is shown by arrow. (From Johnson et al. 1972)

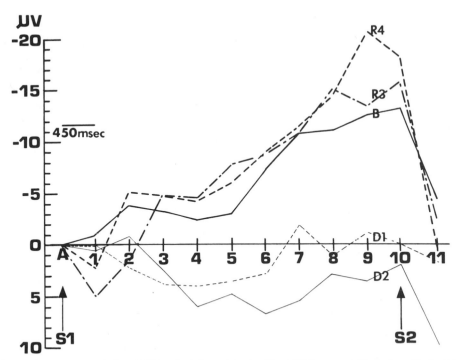

Figure 2. Average of the CNVs of eight subjects. The CNVs were adjusted so that all had same starting point at the time of S1. (From Naitoh, Johnson, and Lubin 1971)

impairment during sleep loss takes the form of lapses; the subject is unable to maintain efficient behavior and increasingly shows short periods when performance falters or stops. Figure 4 illustrates an example of a lapse in functioning in a serial counting and auditory vigilance task following one night without sleep. With the cessation of responses on the counting task, there is a decrease in alpha activity, appearance of vertex sharp waves in the C_z-A_2 lead, decrease in heart rate, increase in finger pulse amplitude, and the respiration becomes shallow (Naitoh and Townsend 1970).

Wilkinson (1961) has reported that repeated loss of total sleep increased the effects of such sleep loss on performance, and he has questioned whether one can build up a tolerance to repeated experiences of sleep loss. There are some techniques, however, that can be used to reduce the performance decrement. Alerting factors such as massive sensory stimulation, feedback of information as to quality of performance, and frequent task changes help to reduce the frequency and duration of lapses. Lubin (1967), in a summary presentation of the Walter Reed studies, noted that in self-paced tasks sleep loss is easier to resist than in experimenter-paced tasks, that in shorter tasks subjects are more resistant to sleep loss than in longer tasks, and that in performing complex tasks with high interest they are less im-

paired than in doing simple, repetitive tasks. In newly acquired skills and
tasks that rely upon short-term memory the subjects are less resistant to the
effects of total sleep loss.

For most performance total sleep loss interacts with the circadian
rhythms. Wilkinson (1972) demonstrated that, with a decrease in total sleep
time, the decline in task performance is greatest for the morning tests and
least in the evening. This interaction was greatest when total sleep time was
decreased to two hours or less for two or more nights.

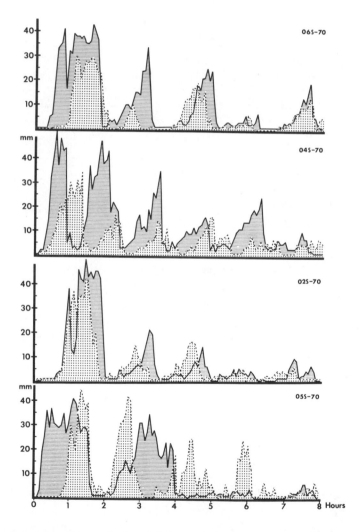

Figure 3. Analog computer analysis of delta activity (1-3 Hz) before sleep loss, dotted histograms, and that following 60 hours of wakefulness plus two additional nights of stage 4 deprivation. The recovery sleep delta profiles for REM-deprived subjects were the same as those for stage 4-deprived subjects.

While the lapse hypothesis explains most performance decrements following sleep loss, especially vigilance-requiring tasks or tasks requiring motor performance, it does not adequately account for all types of performance decrement, especially that seen in tasks involving memory. In their exploration of memory deficits following sleep loss, Williams, Gieseking, and Lubin (1966) studied immediate recall of word lists. Since the subject was required to write down each word immediately after its presentation, they concluded the deficit was not caused by failure of sensory registration that would occur during a lapse. Sleep loss seems to cause difficulties in formation of the memory trace. This hypothesis was tested and supported in a subsequent study (Williams and Williams 1966).

Buck and Gibbs (1972) have also questioned whether the lapse hypothesis is adequate to explain sleep-loss performance decrement in tasks with a high degree of uncertainty as posited by Williams, Kearney, and Lubin (1965). Buck and Gibbs (1972) prefer to emphasize change in information-processing capability rather than the tendency to take periods of microsleep, though they admit the two explanations are not necessarily incompatible.

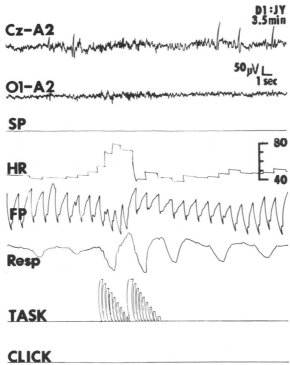

Figure 4. Auditory vigilance and continuous task performances 3½ minutes after task onset following one night of sleep loss. Note associated autonomic arousal with EEG appearance of alpha and counting responses. (From Naitoh and Townsend 1970)

Behavioral Response

While the importance of personality factor in determining sleep-loss effects is not clearly defined (Corcoran 1962, Wilkinson 1969), the behavioral observations of subjects during prolonged sleep loss indicate a common occurrence of visual and, to a much lesser extent, auditory hallucinations. The earlier view (West et al. 1962, Luby and Gottlieb 1966) that prolonged sleep deprivation results in a psychotic state that persists after deprivation has ceased has not been supported by the follow-up studies of Johnson (1969) and by the studies of Kollar and his colleagues (Pasnau et al. 1968) at the University of California at Los Angeles.

In studies in which florid psychotic behavior accompanied sleep deprivation, some predisposition of the subject seemed evident (Brauchi and West 1959; Bliss, Clark, and West 1959; Luby et al. 1960). Post-sleep deprivation psychoses were not seen by Gulevich, Dement, and Johnson (1966) or by Kollar et al. (1969). Each subject's response to sleep loss depends upon his age, physical condition, the stability of his mental health, expectations of those around him, whether drugs or stimulants are used to maintain wakefulness, and the support he receives from his environment.

Partial Sleep Loss

How much sleep does a person need? Many people, intentionally or not, have shortened their sleep for brief periods, but it is not known whether habitual sleep times can be reduced permanently. If such reduction is possible, how will this be reflected in sleep patterns and awake behavior?

When a person's usual sleep regimen is restricted over a 24-hour period, partial sleep loss occurs. The important reference point is restriction of the usual sleep regimen and not the amount of sleep obtained. Jones and Oswald (1968) reported on two cases who slept only about 3 hours in each 24 hours with no sleep-loss complaints. A more extreme example is the report of a 70-year-old woman who slept on the average of one hour each night with no daytime naps and was reported to be alert, competent, with no need or desire for more sleep (Meddis, Pearson, and Langford 1973). How did these subjects come by their ability to tolerate these short sleep regimens?

Studies of partial sleep loss have traditionally involved abrupt restriction of usual total sleep time (Webb 1969, Naitoh 1969). I will review these studies before discussing the more recent attempts to change the usual sleep regimen by a gradual, progressive restriction of sleep.

EEG Changes

The EEG changes reported during partial sleep loss have been those associated with sleep. Our initial inspection of awake EEG changes indicated no changes in the awake spectra. The sleep findings were highly consistent (Webb and Agnew 1965; Sampson 1965; Webb and Agnew, in press). When total sleep time was reduced, there was no reduction in SWS, stages 3 and 4, and often a slight increase when sleep was reduced to five or fewer hours. Webb and Agnew (in press) noted that the increase in stage 4 was greatest during the first week of a 60-day period at 5½ hours. As the restricted regime continued, there was an adaptation and a return to baseline stage 4 levels. Though there was no decrease in SWS, there was a stage 4 rebound, above baseline, on the first recovery night.

In partial sleep loss, the end of the night, in which most REM sleep occurs, is chopped off. Since the precedence of SWS over REM in the course of the night seems to be extremely stable, a decrease in total REM time is to be expected. Webb and Agnew (in press) reported that REM sleep consistently decreased. There is, however, an earlier onset of REM sleep as partial sleep loss continues which helps to minimize the REM deficit, but REM sleep never replaces SWS in order of appearance, regardless of severity or duration of restriction.* Time in stage 2 also decreases during sleep loss, and there is usually a decrease in stage 1, the transition from awake to stage 2.

Performance Changes Following Abrupt and Brief Periods of Sleep Restriction

Interest in effects of sleep length on cognitive and motor responses, especially on memory, dates back to the early 1900s (Smith 1916; Moore, Jenkins, and Barker 1922; Robinson and Richardson-Robinson 1922; Laird and Wheeler 1926; Laslett 1928; Freeman 1932; Omwake 1932; Van Ormer 1932). The results of these early studies varied and no consistent effects of reduced sleep could be inferred.

With the resurgence of sleep research based upon EEG monitoring of sleep stages, R.T. Wilkinson, W.B. Webb, and H.W. Agnew have contributed most of the work on partial sleep loss (Webb and Agnew 1965; Wilkinson, Edwards, and Haines 1966; Wilkinson 1969; Hamilton, Wilkinson, and Edwards 1972; Webb and Agnew, in press). Reduced sleep studies have also been published by Dement and Greenberg (1966) and by Sampson (1965).

---

*In research begun since the symposium, 1-hour naps are being permitted every 3 hours over a 40-hour period; REM-onset sleep has been observed in some of these naps. None of the 14 subjects studied have a history or symptoms of narcolepsy.

The daily length of sleep allowed varied from 2½ hours over three days (Sampson 1965) to 5½ hours over 60 days (Webb and Agnew, in press). In an earlier study, Webb and Agnew (1965) permitted 3 hours of sleep per day over eight days while Dement and Greenberg (1966) allowed their subjects 4 hours of daily sleep for three or six days. Wilkinson, Edwards, and Haines (1966) permitted either 1, 2, 3, 4, or 5 hours over two days, while the Hamilton, Wilkinson, and Edwards (1972) sleep schedule allowed either 7½, 6, or 4 hours of sleep for four consecutive days.

Even though most of these post-1930 studies have carefully monitored EEG indices of sleep, used a larger variety of tasks and a larger number of subjects for longer periods of time, the effects of partial sleep loss on performance have been no more consistent from study to study than the pre-1930 studies.

In their first study Webb and Agnew (1965) found no uniform or consistent changes in their eight subjects allowed only 3 hours of sleep per day for eight consecutive days. Only after the seventh and eighth days were decrements noticed on a paced addition test, on a vigilance task in which the subject listened to tape-recorded letters and pressed a button each time he heard the letter "x", and on a vigilance task in which the subject pressed a signal button each time a red light was flashed on one of the five positions in a pentagon.

In their recent study Webb and Agnew (in press) curtailed the daily sleep time of 16 young adults from 7½ to 8 hours to 5½ hours for 60 days. Performance tests used were the Williams Word Memory Test (Williams and Williams 1966; Williams, Gieseking, and Lubin 1966), the Wilkinson Addition Test (Wilkinson 1969), and the Wilkinson Auditory Vigilance Task (Wilkinson 1969). The only significant decrease in performance was a slight but steady decline in correct detections on the auditory vigilance task. Webb and Agnew attributed this decrement to a decline in the subjects' willingness to perform the task rather than to a decline in their vigilance due to sleep loss. The subjects' sleep-onset latencies decreased during the first week, then stabilized. Getting up in the morning was reported to be difficult during the entire 60 days though it was most difficult during the first week. Feelings of drowsiness also were most frequently reported during the first week. There were no significant changes in mood or affect during the study.

Wilkinson, Edwards, and Haines (1966), employing the Wilkinson Vigilance and Addition Tasks, had six subjects work a full day for two successive days in each of six successive weeks. On each of the nights before the two test days, the subjects were allowed 0, 1, 2, 3, 5, or 7½ hours of sleep, varied according to the week of testing. Five hours of sleep resulted in a performance decrement on the second reduced-sleep day but not on the first. Less than 5 hours of sleep on a single night impaired vigilance performance; when sleep was reduced to less than 3 hours, performance on the addition task was impaired.

In an extension of the Wilkinson, Edwards, and Haines (1966) study, Hamilton, Wilkinson, and Edwards (1972) examined performance following 7½, 6, and 4 hours of sleep per night for four days. The vigilance and addition tasks were again used, and a digit-span test added. There was a significant decrease in correct detections and number of sums completed when sleep was reduced to 4 hours. The effect of partial sleep loss was found to be cumulative over the four-day period. In contrast, the subjects' performance on the digit-span test was above baseline values when they were allowed only 4 hours of sleep.

Sampson (1966) found a significant performance decrement in six subjects whose sleep was reduced to 2½ hours for three consecutive nights. His tasks were digit span and a complex serial subtraction task.

Wilkinson believes that when partial sleep-loss studies yield negative results, the tests used are too short and the experimental paradigm does not provide for tests scheduled as a part of a workday. Taking a more positive view, Webb and Agnew (in press) conclude that stable sleepers accustomed to 7 to 8 hours of sleep per night can maintain 5 to 6 hours of sleep per night for as long as two months, with little or no decrement in performance from such a reduction.

Gradual Sleep Reduction

Although most subjects continue to function with minimal impairment during an abruptly induced restricted sleep regimen, they return to their usual sleep schedule when the imposition is removed. They do not adapt to, nor do they prefer to continue, their restricted sleep diet longer than necessary. Many, however, do sleep about 6 hours and some, as in the cases noted above, sleep 3 hours or less. How did these short sleepers achieve their restricted sleep regimen? There are no data on any problems they encountered in achieving their sleep reduction or on the time period required before their reduced sleep time became stabilized. Hartmann et al. (1971) report significant differences in life styles and psychological traits between short and long sleepers, but Webb and Friel (1971) could find no differences. Hartmann et al. found short sleepers efficient, hard-working, and somewhat hypomanic.

To learn whether sleep length could be decreased without the usual sleep-loss effects and whether the shorter sleep regimen would be preferred once achieved, a gradual sleep-reduction study was carried out for two subjects by Johnson and MacLeod (1973). Gordon Globus and Joyce Friedmann, University of California, Irvine (UCI), reduced sleep gradually for four subjects with 7½- to 8-hour baseline sleep regimens. We are collaborating with the UCI investigators in this latter study.

In the Johnson and MacLeod study, two young adults (one male and one female) reduced their total sleep time by 30 minutes every two weeks from an initial 7½ hours to 4 hours. The 4-hour regimen was maintained for three weeks and then ad libitum sleep was permitted. A third subject resigned from the study during the 4½-hour regimen. He reported that he found it too difficult to force himself to get up after his summer job terminated and there was nothing to do. The daily sleep and nap logs of the other two subjects reflected similar difficulty in maintaining the restricted sleep schedule when their sleep was reduced below 6 hours.

As in the abrupt sleep-restriction studies, the EEG sleep records at 5½ hours indicated earlier onset of REM sleep. There were no other noticeable changes on this recording. At 4 hours, there was a marked increase in stages 3 and 4 with a decrease in stage 2 and REM sleep. The sleep characteristics for the two subjects who completed the study are presented in Table 1. Mood and performance showed changes beginning at 5½ hours, but these changes were not marked or consistent. An eight-month follow-up report indicated that both subjects had maintained a sleep schedule 1 to 2 hours below their previous baselines.

In the current study with Globus and Friedmann, data from four subjects (two couples) have been collected. Couples were chosen to insure that there would be support available during the shorter sleep periods; they could apply the electrodes to each other and provide at least one other person willing to stay up. In addition to measuring mood and performance changes during each sleep regimen, EEG sleep recordings were obtained three nights a week in the subjects' homes. These data were obtained by a small tape-recording unit developed by Jim Humphrey of the UCI laboratory. One EEG and two electro-oculogram (EOG) channels were recorded from all subjects on quarter-inch tape for later rerecording on a strip chart and on FM tape for sleep-stage scoring and computer analysis.

The performance data included the Wilkinson Auditory Vigilance and Addition Tasks and a modified Williams Word Memory Task. Daily sleep logs, nap logs, and the Stanford Sleepiness Scale (Hoddes et al. 1973) were completed upon awakening. The Profile of Mood States (POMS) (McNair, Lorr, and Droppleman 1971) was completed on the evenings of the EEG recording. These data were collected during a baseline month, during gradual sleep reduction, and during a six-month ad lib sleep follow-up period.

More details will be published by Globus et al. when all the ad lib sleep data on these four subjects are obtained and after another year of data collection on four more subjects is completed. The results discussed here, therefore, must be viewed as preliminary.

TABLE 1. Sleep Characteristics for Two Subjects

	Baseline		5½		4		Recovery	
	Min	%	Min	%	Min	%	Min	%
Subject 1								
TST	479		306		227		354	
TWT	44	8	19	5	13	5	27	7
Stage 1	44 (7)	9	18 (15)	6	24	11	31 (20)	9
REM	71 (0)	15	39 (22)	13	22	10	44 (24)	13
Stage 2	263 (122)	56	163 (118)	53	86	38	215 (114)	61
Stage 3	16 (8)	3	30 (13)	10	20	8	12 (8)	4
Stage 4	80 (68)	17	54 (54)	18	75	33	52 (52)	15
Time to REM	225		110		207		146	
Time to stage 4	54		43		24		46	
No. stage changes	54 (23)		32 (25)		30		47 (32)	
No. movements	50 (26)		28 (23)		20		24 (14)	
Subject 2								
TST	469		327		239		300	
TWT	2	1	0	0	2	1	1	3
Stage 1	16 (7)	4	9 (0)	3	2	1	9 (4)	3
REM	105 (31)	23	68 (37)	21	30	13	84 (36)	28
Stage 2	227 (123)	49	164 (123)	50	104	43	160 (114)	53
Stage 3	24 (13)	5	26 (21)	8	21	9	11 (11)	4
Stage 4	90 (72)	19	59 (37)	18	82	34	35 (35)	12
Time to REM	135		73		76		60	
Time to stage 4	14		21		12		29	
No. stage changes	49 (27)		37 (32)		31		24 (20)	
No. movements	75 (27)		49 (31)		36		51 (42)	

Note—The numbers in parentheses are for the first 4 hours of sleep so that a comparison of comparable sleep times can be made over all periods. Results for baseline, 5½, and 4 hours are the averages over two nights.

Over a period of seven months, two of our married subjects (BS and SS) reduced their sleep from 8 hours to an average of 5 hours while the second, our unmarried, couple (JP and PM) reduced their sleep from 8 hours to 4½ hours over an eight-month period. Like the subjects studied by Johnson and MacLeod, these subjects reduced their sleep time by going to bed later.

Sleep times were obtained from the daily sleep-log cards in addition to the EEG recordings. In other studies, total sleep times from the EEG and sleep logs were shown to be comparable (Naitoh, Johnson, and Austin 1971; Townsend, Johnson, and Muzet 1973). In Figure 5 are the sleep times from the EEG data for the four subjects during sleep reduction and from sleep-log data for the first four months of ad lib sleep. Six-month ad lib data, obtained after preparation of Figure 5, indicated that all four subjects were sleeping between 5 to 6½ hours during the fifth month and all subjects were still 1 to 2½ hours below their baseline levels at six months. Subjects BS and SS reported total sleep times of near 6 hours for the fifth and sixth months. While all four subjects' ad lib sleep was less than 8 hours, the initial amounts of ad lib sleep differed for each subject and there was also a difference in sleep time between the two couples. Subjects BS and SS initially required more ad lib sleep than JP and PM. The initial rise in ad lib total sleep time for BS and SS probably reflected the accumulated fatigue that appeared to have been greater for BS and SS than for JP and PM. The findings that BS

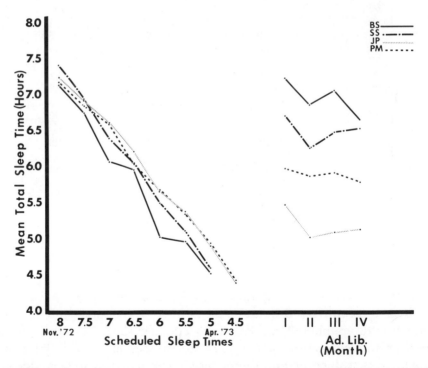

Figure 5. Total sleep times during gradual sleep reduction and ad lib sleep. During gradual sleep reduction, sleep times were computed from EEG recordings. Ad lib sleep times were obtained from sleep logs.

and SS reported higher fatigue ratings, felt less rested, and terminated their sleep reduction earlier indicate that sleep reduction was more difficult for them. With more sleep these feelings decreased and they again reduced their total sleep time. If the six-month data persist, they indicate that all four subjects were eventually able to adjust to reduced total sleep times 1 to 2½ hours below their usual 8 hours. Similar sleep reductions after eight months of ad lib sleep were reported by the two subjects studied by Johnson and MacLeod.

All of the subjects reported they discontinued reducing their sleep time because they felt more fatigued and had less vigor and did not feel rested in the morning (Figure 6), and the feeling of need for more sleep became too intense (Figure 7). Neither of the male subjects reported significant changes in their graduate course work (BS and JP) due to reduced sleep, nor did the two women (SS and PM) feel that the sleep loss caused problems in their jobs. Performance on the Wilkinson addition test and Williams word memory test did not show any decrement. There was some decrement on the Wilkinson Auditory Vigilance Task, but the analysis of this task is incomplete. The POMS scales showed no consistent changes over the sleep-reduction period in confusion, anxiety, tension, depression, and anger, but there was an increase in the fatigue scale score with a decrease in the vigor scale score.

It was not obvious performance decrement but feelings of fatigue that appeared to set the lower limits for their sleep time. The fatigue was probably due, in part, to the extra effort necessary to maintain an effective level of performance.

It was noted above that ad lib data obtained at five and six months indicated that the total sleep time for BS and SS had decreased to near 6 hours. Subjective ratings during the fifth and sixth ad lib months also indicated that their ratings as to need for more sleep, and how rested they felt upon arising, had returned to baseline values when they were obtaining 8 hours of sleep.

Hartmann has indicated that short and long sleepers differ with respect to energy level and life style. On the POMS, JP and PM had much higher vigor scores throughout the study than the other two subjects. The overall POMS total mood disturbance score also differed from the study's onset for the two couples. BS had a score of 44 and SS's score was 47, while JP's score was a -19 and PM's score was -16. A high score reflects greater mood disturbance and, in these subjects, a high score was associated with a felt need for more sleep regardless of duration and with initially longer ad lib sleep. These differences in vigor and mood may have been a factor in how difficult it was for each subject to reduce his sleep, but since at six months all four subjects have reduced their sleep, these factors may not be decisive for determining ultimate sleep time. Webb (personal communication) believes "that long and short sleepers are like tall and short people, i.e., all are expressing natural inherent conditions which can influence behavior indirectly rather than directly."

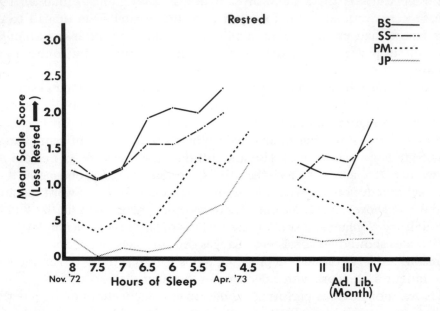

Figure 6. Ratings as to feeling of being rested after morning awakening during gradual sleep reduction.

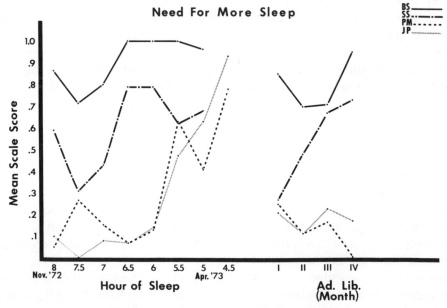

Figure 7. Ratings as to need for more sleep.

EEG Sleep Changes

The sleep changes during gradual sleep reduction for these four subjects were very similar to those reported by Jones and Oswald (1968) for their 3-hour sleepers, those reported by Webb and Agnew (in press) during abrupt sleep restriction, and those reported by Johnson and MacLeod (1973) for their two subjects during gradual sleep reduction. In our four subjects, as sleep decreased from 8 to 5 hours, the minutes spent in stage 1 and stage 3 did not change, there was an increase in minutes of stage 4 as the sleep decreased from 7½ to 6½ hours, then no further increase; stage REM decreased during the entire period as did the minutes spent in stage 2 (Figure 8). Of all the stages, the largest decrease was for time spent in stage 2. When time spent in each stage was converted to percentage of total sleep time, the pattern was the same for all stages but REM. REM percentage showed essentially no change during sleep reduction (Figure 9). The stability of REM percentage was due to the progressively earlier onset of the first REM period as sleep time was reduced (Figure 10). The latencies to the other sleep stages did not consistently change with sleep reduction.

When only the first 5 hours of sleep were analyzed for all sleep regimens (Figure 11), the results indicated that relative to the first 5 hours when total sleep time was 8, 7½, and 7 hours, there was more stage 4 and REM and less stage 2 when the total sleep time was 5 hours. Although REM moves forward, total REM time at 5 hours never equaled that obtained during 8 hours of sleep, but the amount of stage 4 obtained when total sleep time was 5 hours exceeded that obtained during an entire 8-hour night.

Although its significance is still unknown, this study joins a growing list indicating that SWS will not be denied (Dement and Greenberg 1966; Agnew, Webb, and Williams 1967; Empson and Clarke 1970; Berger et al. 1971; Johnson and MacLeod 1973). Whether total sleep time is decreased abruptly through imposition of a curtailed sleep regimen or reduced gradually over months or shortened by self-selection, the amount of stage 4 does not decrease. To the contrary, if the reduction is severe (for example, total sleep time is 3 to 4 hours), stage 4 time may increase. REM sleep time in all instances decreases.

Hartmann et al. (1971) in their report on self-selected long and short sleepers advance the hypothesis that there is "a relatively constant requirement for SWS and a requirement for D sleep [REM sleep] that is related to the individual's personality and life style" [p. 1001]. For Hartmann et al., the sleep regimen one selects is related to his need for REM sleep even though numerous studies have failed to support the earlier assertions that REM sleep is closely related to awake performance or psychological functioning. The results of the several sleep-reduction studies suggest that

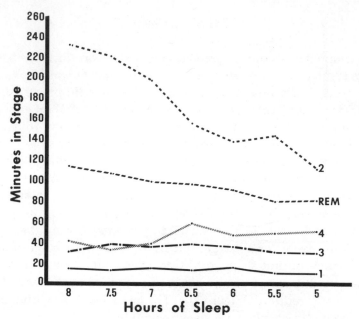

Figure 8. Time spent in stage 1 and sleep stages 2, 3, 4, and REM during gradual sleep reduction.

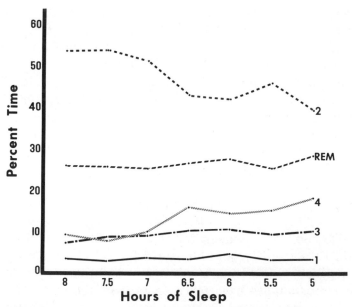

Figure 9. Percentage of time spent in stage 1 and sleep stages 2, 3, 4, and REM during gradual sleep reduction.

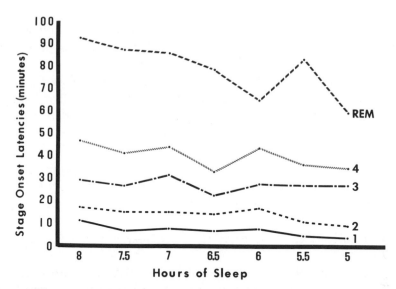

Figure 10. Stage onset latencies during gradual sleep reduction.

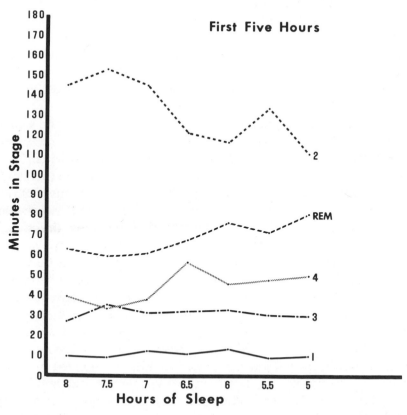

Figure 11. Minutes in various stages obtained during first 5 hours of sleep regardless of total sleep time.

amount of REM sleep is a result of, not the cause of, shortened sleep. In all instances, regardless of how total sleep time is reduced, there is a reduction of REM sleep time.

We believe that the nature of sleep patterns offers a more parsimonious explanation than do differences in psychological factors. The biologically determined cycles of sleep insure the appearance of SWS before REM. When sleep is reduced, REM sleep will be chopped off. Webb and Friel (1971) draw the obvious conclusion that there is a point at which shortening of the total time available for sleep will result in REM restriction. While the type of sleep one gets is determined primarily by the length of sleep, the total sleep time may be influenced by psychological factors.

Sleep-Stage Deprivation

Dement (1960) reported that five nights of REM deprivation resulted in "psychological disturbances such as anxiety, irritability, and difficulty in concentrating." [p. 1707] Fisher and Dement (1963) warned that REM deprivation, and thus dream deprivation, would lead to "a great intensification of the pressure of instinctual drives toward discharge, eventual eruption of the dream cycle into the waking state and the development of hallucinations, delusions and other psychotic symptoms." [p. 1164] In 1965, Dement stated that he no longer believed that REM sleep occurs in order to satisfy a need for the experience of dreaming.

The first two statements reflect the initial enthusiasm and belief that REM sleep provided a unique psychological function closely related to dreaming, while the last statement reflects the failure of subsequent research to support these expectations of REM sleep. Snyder (1963), Kales et al. (1964), Sampson (1965, 1966), Agnew, Webb, and Williams (1967), and Chernik (1972) all failed to find significant effects of REM deprivation on awake behavior. Prolonged deprivation of REM sleep by drugs has also caused no obvious changes in awake behavior in nonpsychotic patients.

From the beginning, there have been fewer expectations that nonREM sleep, stages 2, 3, and 4, would prove important for waking behavior. The fact that Agnew, Webb, and Williams (1967) found no consistent significant performance differences between REM-deprived and stage 4-deprived subjects was not helpful to those wishing to push studies of stage 4 sleep. Agnew, Webb, and Williams (1967), however, did report some psychological differences between six REM-deprived and six stage 4-deprived subjects. The stage 4-deprived subjects displayed more hypochondriacal and depressive reactions while the REM-deprived subjects showed increased irritability and emotional lability. These differences were small and not significant, however, and they need to be replicated, but they offer some support to the findings by Clemes and Dement (1967). Based upon psychological test findings, Clemes and Dement reported an increase in "need and feeling intensity and certain ego functions" based upon responses to the Holtzman Inkblot Test. Mood check lists, however, showed no difference between the REM-deprived and nonREM awakening nights for their six subjects.

We now know that dreaming occurs in some form in all stages of sleep and that REM deprivation does not prevent dreams or cause marked changes in awake behavior. We still do not know, however, what functions are served by the different sleep stages, and the question of whether each sleep stage meets a unique need is still unanswered. Although each new study offers little support for a unique need hypothesis, most researchers would probably still support Wilse Webb's statement, "I do find it difficult to reject a belief in the functional difference between Stage 4 and Stage REM sleep" (Webb 1972, p. 129). My colleagues and I are no exception. Instead of continuing to search for psychological correlates of stage deprivation, however, we have focused on the recuperative value of sleep. In our first sleep-stage-deprivation experiment, we asked, What are the relative recuperative values of REM and stage 4 sleep after total sleep deprivation? In a second experiment, the procedure was reversed to determine whether deprivation of REM or stage 4 sleep before total sleep loss would potentiate the sleep-loss effects.

In Experiment 1 (Lubin et al. 1974), performance measures on addition, memory, and vigilance tasks, measures of affect and mood, and indices of autonomic and central nervous system activity were obtained from 16 Navy enlisted men, ages 17 to 21. After four baseline days, 12 subjects were totally sleep-deprived for two nights. Total sleep deprivation was followed by either (1) uninterrupted recovery sleep for five nights (the control group, N = 4); (2) two nights of REM deprivation and then three nights of uninterrupted recovery sleep (this REM-deprived group was allowed all nonREM sleep, N = 4); or (3) two nights of stage 4 sleep deprivation and then three nights of uninterrupted sleep (this group was allowed all stages of sleep but stage 4, N = 4). Four subjects were not deprived of any sleep and served as a second control group for test practice effects.

Stage 4-deprived subjects were aroused when the EEG indicated stage 3 sleep. At the first appearance of a stage 1 EEG pattern with rapid eye movements, subjects to be deprived of stage REM were aroused. The remaining four subjects were allowed about 8 hours of uninterrupted sleep every night during the two-week period. Both uninterrupted and interrupted recovery sleep were limited to the period between 10 p.m. and 6 a.m. A rebound effect for both REM and SWS was present for the appropriate groups on the first night of uninterrupted sleep, indicating that the selective sleep-stage deprivation was effective.

Performance on a serial counting task, the Wilkinson addition test,

auditory vigilance, X cross-out test, Williams immediate word-recall test, and
a serial addition test (plus 7) deteriorated significantly during total sleep loss.
Fewer signals were detected on the vigilance task, fewer additions were
attempted, fewer words were scanned on the cross-out test, and fewer words
were recalled in the memory test. Accuracy in all tasks tended to decrease as
sleep loss increased. Our non-sleep-deprived control subjects showed some
practice effect on most of the tests.

    All sleep-deprived subjects improved after the first night of recovery
sleep, but there was no significant difference in the amount of recovery for
the three kinds of recovery sleep. Performance on the auditory vigilance task
presented in Figure 12 is representative of all the tasks. Similar results were
obtained on mood scales. After two nights without sleep, subjects, not un-

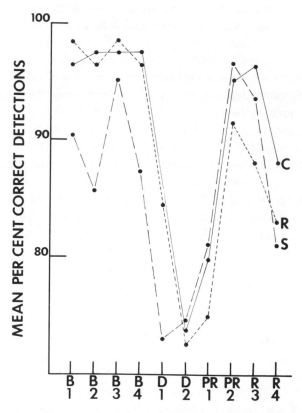

*Figure 12. Performance on the auditory vigilance task during four baseline days (B1, B2,
B3, B4), during total sleep deprivation (D1 and D2), during deprivation of stage REM for
R group, stage 4 for S group (PR1 and PR2), and during uninterrupted recovery sleep (R3
and R4). The control (C) group was not sleep stage-deprived.*

expectedly, were more fatigued, depressed, and hostile, and less energetic, happy, and friendly. As with the performance tasks, the return to the pre-deprivation psychological states was the same for all subjects regardless of the type of recovery sleep (Johnson et al. 1972). Our measures of autonomic and central nervous system activity also showed no significant differences between the REM- and stage 4-deprived groups.

The results from our first stage-deprivation study did not support the belief that stage REM or stage 4 has unique recuperative value. Following sleep loss, the amount rather than the type of sleep seems to be the most important factor.

Still not ready to abandon the idea that deprivation of stage REM or stage 4 would have unique, deleterious effects, we hypothesized in our next study that deprivation of either of these two stages of sleep might lessen the person's ability to tolerate the stress of total sleep loss and perhaps other stressors. Although we were now cautious enough not to predict overtly which stage deprivation would be more debilitating, we covertly expected the subjects deprived of stage 4 to show the most decrement following total sleep loss (Johnson et al. 1974).

Fourteen Navy enlisted men, ages 18 to 21, participated in this study. After three nights of baseline sleep, seven subjects were deprived of REM sleep and seven were deprived of stage 4 sleep for three nights. Next, both groups were deprived of total sleep for one night and finally allowed two nights of recovery sleep. Sleep-stage deprivation was produced by arousing the subjects as in the first experiment.

The physiological and performance measures obtained in Experiment 1 were recorded again, but other tests were added to obtain measures of both long-term and short-term memory, measures of reading speed and comprehension, and additional ratings of affect for feelings of happiness, anger, fear, depression, and arousal. A Rorschach measure of conceptual consistency, conformity, and looseness was also included (McReynolds 1954).

Three nights of REM and stage 4 deprivation produced minimal changes in our subjects, and the changes present were similar for both groups. Following the night of total sleep loss, the expected decrement in the tests was evident and, again, the decrement was the same for both groups. Prior deprivation of stage REM or of stage 4 did not potentiate the effect of total sleep loss. An example of these results for the Wilkinson addition test is shown in Figure 13.

EEG Changes

The EEG changes during stage deprivation have offered support to the conception of sleep stages as need states. With each successive night of stage

REM or stage 4 deprivation, subjects strive to overcome the stage restrictions and barriers by increasing the number of attempts to obtain the deprived stage. More arousals are required to deprive stage REM or stage 4 with each successive night of deprivation. In further support of the need hypothesis is the rebound or increase in the deprived stage during recovery sleep. There

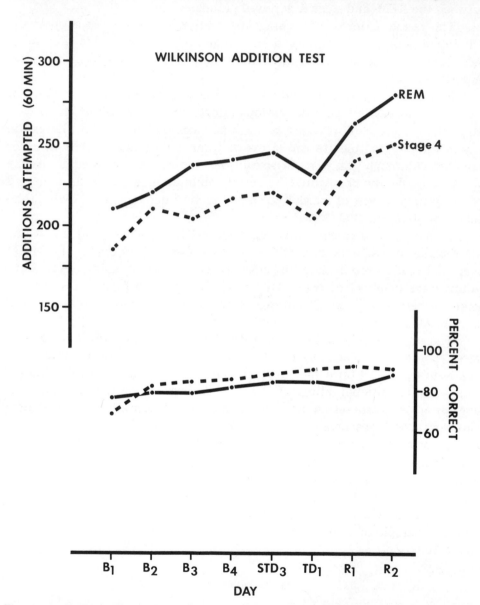

Figure 13. Performance on the Wilkinson addition test during baseline (B1, B2, B3, B4) following three nights of stage REM or stage 4 deprivation (STD3), following one night of total sleep loss (TD1), and following recovery sleep (R1 and R2).

seems to be a need to "replace" that which was denied. The increase in attempts to obtain the deprived stage and the rebound phenomena have been consistent findings for stage 4 deprivation, but the REM rebound phenomenon is not as universal as was once believed (Cartwright, Monroe, and Palmer 1967). Data in our laboratory (Moses et al., in press) are consistent with those of Cartwright, Monroe, and Palmer in finding that not all subjects show a REM rebound.

As one would expect from the distribution of sleep stages throughout the night, most arousals for stage 4 deprivation occur during the first half of the night while most arousals for REM deprivation occur during the last half. Because he found it required more arousals to deprive subjects of stage 4 than of REM, Webb (1969) inferred a stronger tendency for stage 4 than stage REM. In our stage-deprivation studies, we found no difference in number of arousals required for REM and stage 4 deprivation when the subjects were not sleep-deprived. Following two nights of total sleep loss, however, deprivation of stage 4 required a significantly larger number of arousals than were necessary to prevent subjects from obtaining stage REM following sleep loss.

During stage-deprivation nights, there is an increase in stage 2 during stage 4 deprivation and an increase in stage 1 on REM-deprivation nights. The explanations for the increases in the two sleep stages are simply the results of either stage 4 or REM deprivation per se. When aroused from stage 4, the subject goes to stage 2 or awakens and then goes back to stage 2. As long as he stays in stage 2, he is not aroused.

When the REM-deprived subject is aroused, he awakes and then goes back to stage 1. The frequent awakenings thus lead to an increase in stage 1 and, in some instances, as in our Experiment 2, a decrease in total sleep time for the REM-deprived subjects.

As with partial sleep-loss studies, there have been no studies reporting EEG changes in the awake records of sleep stage-deprived subjects.

A Point of View

While the pattern of performance decrement depends on several variables, it is obvious from numerous studies that human beings cannot function effectively without sleep. Sleep, however, can be shortened without serious disruption of waking activities, and humans perform quite well without entering into all stages of sleep or with only limited amounts of each stage. In other papers (Johnson et al. 1972, Johnson 1973), I raised the question of abandoning the concept of stages of sleep and again thinking of sleep as a single state. The 1973 paper rejected that alternative. From our sleep stage-deprivation results, one could argue that recovery sleep is unitary with respect to its recuperative function, but that the various physiological and biochemical measures obtained during sleep clearly indicate that sleep is not a single state. In the 1972 and 1973 papers, however, an alternative to the concept of five separate sleep stages was offered. Our computer analysis of EEG activity supports those who divide sleep into two types, REM and nonREM. I, however, would include only stages 2, 3, and 4 as nonREM sleep. I support the position of Snyder and Scott (1972) and Agnew and Webb (1972) that the appearance of the first spindle should be used to identify sleep onset. Stage 1 is viewed as a transition period between wakefulness and sleep. Coherent EEG activity in the 12- to 14-Hz range was found only during sleep stages 2, 3, and 4. Sleep sigma spindles appear to be an EEG rhythm that uniquely separates stages 2, 3, and 4 from REM, stage 1, and awake. The 1973 article further suggested that since stage REM is more like waking than sleep stages 2, 3, and 4, more attention should be given to the awake-like qualities of REM sleep. In view of the negative results of our attempts to use stages of sleep as indices of satisfactory sleep, our increasing interest in the stability of the REM-nonREM cycle as a more fruitful measure of sleep behavior was discussed in both the 1972 and 1973 papers.

For many sleep researchers, the study of sleep is a means by which they hope to gain a better understanding of waking behavior. To date, however, we can predict more confidently how waking activities will influence sleep behavior than how changes in sleep will affect awake behavior. As we shift our attention away from dreams and psychological needs to other aspects of sleeping and waking, and as we realize that sleep is not the slow delta waves and perhaps not even the 12- to 14-Hz spindles on our EEGs, perhaps the hoped-for correlation between awake and asleep behavior will be realized.

Acknowledgments

This work was supported in part by Department of the Navy, Bureau of Medicine and Surgery, under Work Unit MF12.524.0049008DA5G; by National Science Foundation Grants GB-6008 and GB-14829 to the California State University, San Diego, Foundation; and by National Institute of Mental Health research grant 45-1469 to Dr. Gordon G. Globus, University of California, Irvine. The opinions and assertions contained herein are the private ones of the author and are not to be construed as official or as reflecting the views of the Navy Department.

References

Agnew, H.W., Jr., and Webb, W.B. 1972. Measurement of sleep onset by EEG criteria. *American Journal of EEG Technology* 12:127.

Agnew, H.W., Jr., Webb, W.B., and Williams, R.L. 1967. Comparison of stage four and 1-REM sleep deprivation. *Percept. Mot. Skills* 24:851.

Armington, J.C., and Mitnick, L.L. 1959. Electroencephalogram and sleep deprivation. *J. Appl. Physiol.* 14:247.

Berger, R.J., and Oswald, I. 1962. Effects of sleep deprivation on behaviour, subsequent sleep, and dreaming. *J. Ment. Sci.* 108:457.

Berger, R.J., Walker, J.M., Scott, T.D., Magnuson, L.J., and Pollack, S.L. 1971. Diurnal and nocturnal sleep stage patterns following sleep deprivation. *Psychonomic Science* 23:273.

Bliss, E.L., Clark, L.D., and West, C.D. 1959. Studies of sleep deprivation—Relationship to schizophrenia. *Arch. Neurol. Psychiatry* 81:348.

Brauchi, J.T., and West, L.J. 1959. Sleep deprivation. *JAMA* 171:11.

Buck, L., and Gibbs, C.B. 1972. Sleep loss and information processing. In W.P. Colquhoun (ed.), *Aspects of Human Efficiency*, p. 47. London: English Universities Press.

Cartwright, R.D., Monroe, L.J., and Palmer, C. 1967. Individual differences in response to REM deprivation. *Arch. Gen. Psychiatry* 16:297.

Chernik, D.A. 1972. Effect of REM sleep deprivation on learning and recall by humans. *Percept. Mot. Skills* 34:283.

Clemes, S.R., and Dement, W.C. 1967. Effect of REM sleep deprivation on psychological functioning. *J. Nerv. Ment. Dis.* 144:485.

Colquhoun, W.P. (ed.) 1972. *Aspects of Human Efficiency*. London: English Universities Press.

Corcoran, D.W.J. 1962. Individual differences after loss of sleep. Unpublished doctoral dissertation, University of Cambridge, Cambridge. England.

Dement, W. 1960. The effect of dream deprivation. *Science* 131:1705.

Dement, W.C. 1965. Recent studies on the biological role of rapid eye movement sleep. *Am. J. Psychiatry* 122:404.

Dement, W., and Greenberg, S. 1966. Changes in total amount of stage four sleep as a function of partial sleep deprivation. *Electroencephalogr. Clin. Neurophysiol.* 20:523.

Empson, J.A.C., and Clarke, P.R.F. 1970. Rapid eye movements and remembering. *Nature* 227:287.

Fisher, C., and Dement, W.C. 1963. Studies on the psychopathology of sleep and dreams. *Am. J. Psychiatry* 119:1160.

Freeman, G.L. 1932. Compensatory reinforcements of muscular tension subsequent to sleep loss. *J. Exp. Psychol.* 15:267.

Gulevich, G., Dement, W., and Johnson, L. 1966. Psychiatric and EEG observations on a case of prolonged (264 hours) wakefulness. *Arch. Gen. Psychiatry* 15:29.

Hamilton, P., Wilkinson, R.T., and Edwards, R.S. 1972. A study of four days partial sleep deprivation. In W.P. Colquhoun (ed.), *Aspects of Human Efficiency*, p. 101. London: English Universities Press.

Hartmann, E., Baekeland, F., Zwilling, G., and Hoy, P. 1971. Sleep need: How much sleep and what kind? *Am. J. Psychiatry* 127:1001.

Hoddes, E., Zarcone, V., Smythe. H., Phillips, R., and Dement, W.C. 1973. Quantification of sleepiness: A new approach. *Psychophysiology* 10:431.

Johnson, L.C. 1969. Psychological and physiological changes following total sleep deprivation. In A. Kales (ed.), *Sleep: Physiology & Pathology,* p. 206. Philadelphia: Lippincott.

Johnson, L.C. 1973. Are stages of sleep related to waking behavior? *Am. Sci.* 61:326.

Johnson, L.C., and MacLeod, W.L. 1973. Sleep and awake behavior during gradual sleep reduction. *Percept. Mot. Skills* 36:87.

Johnson, L., Naitoh, P., Lubin, A., and Moses, J. 1972. Sleep stages and performance. In W.P. Colquhoun (ed.), *Aspects of Human Efficiency,* p. 81. London: English Universities Press.

Johnson, L.C., Naitoh, P., Moses, J.M., and Lubin, A. 1974. Interaction of REM deprivation and stage 4 deprivation with total sleep loss: Experiment 2. *Psychophysiology* 11:147.

Johnson, L.C., Slye, E.S., and Dement, W. 1965. Electroencephalographic and autonomic activity during and after prolonged sleep deprivation. *Psychosom. Med.* 27:415.

Jones, H.S., and Oswald, I. 1968. Two cases of healthy insomnia. *Electroencephalogr. Clin. Neurophysiol.* 24:378.

Kales, A., Hoedemaker, F.S., Jacobson, A., and Lichtenstein, E.L. 1964. Dream deprivation: An experimental reappraisal. *Nature* 204:1337.

Kollar, E.J., Pasnau, R.D., Rubin, R.T., Naitoh, P., Slater, G.G., and Kales, A. 1969. Psychological, psychophysiological, and biochemical correlates of prolonged sleep deprivation. *Am. J. Psychiatry* 126:488.

Laird, D.A., and Wheeler, W. 1926. What it costs to lose sleep. *Indust. Psychol.* 1:694.

Laslett, H.R. 1928. Experiments on the effects of the loss of sleep. *J. Exp. Psychol.* 11:370.

Loomis, A.L., Harvey, E.N., and Hobart, G.A. III. 1937. Cerebral states during sleep, as studied by human brain potentials. *J. Exp. Psychol.* 21:127.

Lubin, A. 1967. Performance under sleep loss and fatigue. In S.S. Kety, E.V. Evarts, and H.L. Williams (eds.), *Sleep and Altered States of Consciousness,* p. 506. Baltimore: Williams & Wilkins.

Lubin, A., Moses, J.M., Johnson, L.C., and Naitoh, P. 1974. The recuperative effects of REM sleep and stage 4 sleep on human performance after complete sleep loss: Experiment 1. *Psychophysiology* 11:133.

Luby, E.D., Frohman, C.E., Grisell, J.L., Lenzo, J.E., and Gottlieb, J.S. 1960. Sleep deprivation: Effects on behavior, thinking, motor performance, and biological energy transfer system. *Psychosom. Med.* 22:182.

Luby, E.D., and Gottlieb, J.S. 1966. Sleep deprivation. In S. Arieti (ed.), *American Handbook of Psychiatry,* vol. 3, p. 406. New York: Basic Books.

Malmo, R.B., and Surwillo, W.W. 1960. Sleep deprivation: Changes in performance and physiological indicants of activation. *Psychol. Monogr.* 74 (15, Whole No. 502).

McNair, D.M., Lorr, M., and Droppleman, L.F. 1971 *Profile of Mood States.* San Diego, Calif.: Educational and Industrial Testing Service.

McReynolds, P. 1954. Rorschach concept evaluation technique. *J. Project. Techn.* 18:60.

Meddis, R., Pearson, A.J.D., and Langford, G. 1973. An extreme case of healthy insomnia. *Electroencephalogr. Clin. Neurophysiol.* 35:213.

Moore, L.M., Jenkins, M., and Barker, L. 1922. Relation of number of hours of sleep to muscular efficiency. *Am. J. Physiol.* 59:471.

Moses, J.M., Johnson, L.C., Naitoh, P., and Lubin, A. Sleep stage deprivation and total sleep loss: Effects on sleep behavior. *Psychophysiology*, (in press).

Naitoh, P. 1969. Sleep loss and its effects on performance. *Navy Medical Neuropsychiatric Research Unit*, San Diego, Calif., Report No. 68-3.

Naitoh, P., Johnson, L.C., and Austin, M. 1971. Aquanaut sleep patterns during Tektite I: A 60-day habitation under hyperbaric nitrogen saturation. *Aerosp. Med.* 42:69.

Naitoh, P., Johnson, L.C., and Lubin, A. 1971. Modification of surface negative slow potential (CNV) in the human brain after total sleep loss. *Electroencephalogr. Clin. Neurophysiol.* 30:17.

Naitoh, P., Kales, A., Kollar, E.J., Smith, J.C., and Jacobson, A. 1969. Electroencephalographic activity after prolonged sleep loss. *Electroencephalogr. Clin. Neurophysiol.* 27:2.

Naitoh, P., Pasnau, R.O., and Kollar, E.J. 1971. Psychophysiological changes after prolonged deprivation of sleep. *Biol. Psychiatry* 3:309.

Naitoh, P., and Townsend, R.E. 1970. The role of sleep deprivation research in human factors. *Human Factors* 12:575.

Omwake, K.T. 1932. Effect of varying periods of sleep on nervous stability. *J. Appl. Psychol.* 16:623.

Pasnau, R.O., Naitoh, P., Stier, S., and Kollar, E.J. 1968. The psychological effects of 205 hours of sleep deprivation. *Arch. Gen. Psychiatry* 18:496.

Robinson, E.S., and Richardson-Robinson, F. 1922. Effects of loss of sleep. II. *J. Exp. Psychol.* 5:93.

Sampson, H. 1965. Deprivation of dreaming sleep by two methods. I. Compensatory REM time. *Arch. Gen. Psychiatry* 13:79.

Sampson, H. 1966. Psychological effects of deprivation of dreaming sleep. *J. Nerv. Ment. Dis.* 143:305.

Smith, M.A. 1916. A contribution to the study of fatigue. *Br. J. Psychol.* 8:327.

Snyder, F. 1963. The new biology of dreaming. *Arch. Gen. Psychiatry* 8:381.

Snyder, F., and Scott, J. 1972. The psychophysiology of sleep. In N.S. Greenfield and R.A. Sternbach (eds.), *Handbook of Psychophysiology*, p. 645. New York: Holt, Rinehart & Winston.

Townsend, R.E., Johnson, L.C., and Muzet, A. 1973. Effects of long term exposure to tone pulse noise on human sleep. *Psychophysiology* 10:369.

Tyler, D.B., Goodman, J., and Rothman, T. 1947. The effect of experimental insomnia on the rate of potential changes in the brain. *Am. J. Physiol.* 149:185.

Van Ormer, E.B. 1932. Retention after intervals of sleep and waking. *Arch. Psychol.* 49:5.

Webb, W.B. 1969. Partial and differential sleep deprivation. In A. Kales (ed.), *Sleep: Physiology & Pathology*, p. 221. Philadelphia: Lippincott.

Webb, W.B. 1972. General discussion, Proceedings of NATO Scientific Affairs Division Conference, Strasbourg, France, July 13-17, 1970. In W.P. Colquhoun (ed.), *Aspects of Human Efficiency*, p. 129. London: English Universities Press.

Webb, W.B., and Agnew, H.W., Jr. 1965. Sleep: Effects of a restricted regime. *Science* 150:1745.

Webb, W.B., and Agnew, H.W., Jr. The effects of a chronic limitation of sleep length. *Psychophysiology*, (in press).

Webb, W.B., and Friel, J. 1971. Sleep stage and personality characteristics of "natural" long and short sleepers. *Science* 171:587.

West, L.J., Janszen, H.H., Lester, B.K., and Cornelisöon, F.S. 1962. The psychosis of sleep deprivation. *Ann. N.Y. Acad. Sci.* 96:66.

Wilkinson, R.T. 1961. Interaction of lack of sleep with knowledge of results, repeated testing, and individual differences. *J. Exp. Psychol.* 62:263.

Wilkinson, R.T. 1969. Sleep deprivation: Performance tests for partial and selective sleep deprivation. In L.E. Abt and B.F. Riess (eds.), *Progress in Clinical Psychology*, vol. 8. *Dreams and Dreaming*, p. 28. New York: Grune & Stratton.

Wilkinson, R.T. 1972. Sleep deprivation—eight questions. In W.P. Colquhoun (ed.), *Aspects of Human Efficiency*, p. 25. London: English Universities Press.

Wilkinson, R.T., Edwards, R.S., and Haines, E. 1966. Performance following a night of reduced sleep. *Psychonomic Science* 5:471.

Williams, H.L., Gieseking, C.F., and Lubin, A. 1966. Some effects of sleep loss on memory. *Percept. Mot. Skills* 23:1287.

Williams, H.L., Granda, A.M., Jones, R.C., Lubin, A., and Armington, J.C. 1962. EEG frequency and finger pulse volume as predictors of reaction time during sleep loss. *Electroencephalogr. Clin. Neurophysiol.* 14:64.

Williams, H.L., Hammack, J.T., Daly, R.L., Dement, W.C., and Lubin, A. 1964. Responses to auditory stimulation, sleep loss and the EEG stages of sleep. *Electroencephalogr. Clin. Neurophysiol.* 16:269.

Williams, H.L., Kearney, O.F., and Lubin, A. 1965. Signal uncertainty and sleep loss. *J. Exp. Psychol.* 69:401.

Williams, H.L., and Lubin, A. 1967. Speeded addition and sleep loss. *J. Exp. Psychol.* 73:313.

Williams, H.L., Lubin, A., and Goodnow, J.J. 1959. Impaired performance with acute sleep loss. *Psychol. Monogr.* 73 (14, Whole No. 484).

Williams, H.L., and Williams, C.L. 1966. Nocturnal EEG profiles and performance. *Psychophysiology* 3:164.

sleep characteristics during the 28- and 59-day skylab missions

James D. Frost, Jr., M.D.[1]
Neurophysiology Service
The Methodist Hospital and
Department of Physiology,
Baylor College of Medicine
Houston, Texas

William H. Shumate, Ph.D.
Neurophysiology Section
National Aeronautics and
Space Administration
Lyndon B. Johnson Space Center
Houston, Texas

Joseph G. Salamy, Ph.D.[2]
Life Sciences Division
Technology, Inc.
Houston, Texas

Cletis R. Booher, B.S.E.E.
Bioengineering Systems Division
National Aeronautics and
Space Administration
Lyndon B. Johnson Space Center
Houston, Texas

In the early days of manned space flight, there was much speculation about the possible adverse effects of this novel environment upon sleep (Berry 1970). Ideas ranged from insomnia, or inability to sleep, through narcolepsy, which is associated with sleep at inappropriate times, to severe disturbances of sleep quality, such as alterations in the stage characteristics.

It soon became apparent, especially during the Gemini program, that fairly long-duration space flight was not associated with any catastrophic alteration of sleeping behavior. Men could sleep in space and, at least some-

[1]Supported in part by Contract NAS 9-12974 from the National Aeronautics and Space Administration.

[2]Supported in part by Contract NAS 9-13291 from the National Aeronautics and Space Administration.

times, did so fairly well. On the other hand, in the Gemini and Apollo programs it also became clear that subjective reports of insomnia were frequent. Crew fatigue was a problem in some instances and apparently led to performance decrements. On several occasions, these difficulties resulted in the use of drugs, including hypnotics to promote sleep and amphetamines to increase alertness following sleep loss.

In spite of these obvious sleeping problems, very little objective information was attained prior to Skylab. Such information is obtained only by continuous EEG monitoring, and the problems associated with data acquisition and analysis in space are considerable. The only previous attempt to examine the EEG during the United States' series of space flights was carried out on the Gemini 7 mission in 1965 (Maulsby 1966; Maulsby and Kellaway 1966; Adey, Kado, and Walter 1967; Burch et al. 1971). Technical difficulties at that time limited recording to the first two sleep periods, thereby eliminating the possibility of an adequate analysis of adaptation to the weightless environment. Consequently, the purpose of the sleep-monitoring experiment developed for the Skylab missions was to obtain the first truly objective evaluations of man's ability to sleep during extended space travel.

General Features

The Skylab orbiting laboratory provides an opportunity to study the effectiveness of man working in a weightless environment for prolonged periods of time. The three-man crews carry out a wide variety of research projects covering the physical and biomedical sciences. The size of the laboratory is comparable to that of a moderate-sized house (12,763 ft^3 working volume), with adequate space and facilities for working, recreation, eating, and sleep. The crews follow a 24-hour schedule based on Central Standard Time, to which they are accustomed on the ground, although at the approximate 270 mile altitude, Skylab circles Earth every 93 minutes.

Each astronaut has his own sleeping compartment, equipped with a sleep-restraint system similar in appearance and function to a sleeping bag. All crew members have the same rest period, typically eight hours, scheduled between 10 p.m. and 6 a.m.

Sleep, thus far, has been studied on two Skylab astronauts, one during the first, or 28-day, mission and one during the second, or 59-day, mission.

Methods

General

The apparatus designed for this experiment provides a complete system for analyzing sleep during space flight and includes data-acquisition hardware, onboard-analysis circuitry, and real-time telemetry. In the course of Skylab missions, a crew member's sleep status is monitored throughout selected eight-hour rest periods. The onboard analyzer automatically provides sleep-stage information and transmits it to Mission Control, where a profile of sleep stage versus time is accumulated. Analog data (electroencephalogram, or EEG; electrooculogram, or EOG; and head-motion signals) are also preserved by onboard magnetic-tape recorders to allow detailed visual and computer postflight analysis when the tapes are returned.

The hardware (Figure 1) consists of three basic units: the recording cap, the preamplifier/accelerometer assembly, and the control-panel assembly. The equipment and methodology have been discussed in detail in a previous publication (Frost et al. 1974) and will be reviewed only briefly below.

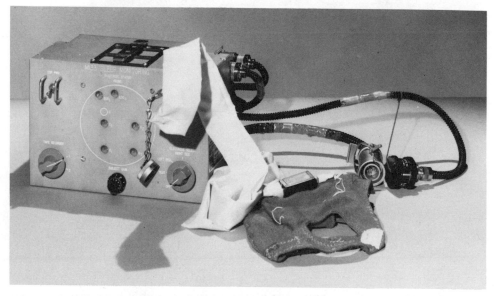

Figure 1. Skylab sleep-monitoring experiment. **Left:** *control-panel assembly.* **Lower right:** *recording cap with preamplifier/accelerometer attached.*

Cap Assembly

The recording cap, as shown in Figure 2, is constructed from an elastic-type fabric that stretches to conform to the subject's head. Sponge-type electrodes are attached to the inside of the cap material in positions necessary for acquisition of EEG and EOG signals, and these are joined by wires

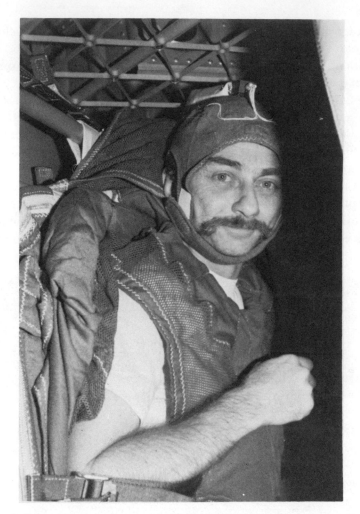

Figure 2. Scientist pilot astronaut from the 59-day mission in his sleeping bag.

to a miniature electrical connector at the vertex, which allows rapid linkage with the preamplifier/accelerometer assembly. The cap contains seven electrodes, arranged such that four (left and right central positions, C_1 and C_2; and left and right occipital positions, O_1 and O_2) provide a composite EEG channel (C_1 and C_2 paired together and referred to O_1 and O_2 paired); two provide one EOG channel (one electrode lateral to, and one above, the left eye); while the seventh electrode serves as a ground.

The caps are stored in a ready-to-use condition (that is, the electrodes are prefilled with conductive electrolyte gel), and the donning procedure requires only a few minutes of the subject's time before going to bed. Each cap is used only once, and the used cap is discarded at the end of each sleep period after the preamplifier/accelerometer assembly is disconnected.

Preamplifier/Accelerometer Assembly

This small, lightweight unit is mounted on the recording cap and contains EEG and EOG preamplifiers (gain of approximately 6), electroshock-protection circuitry, and dual-axis accelerometers for detecting motion of the subject's head in both the lateral (side-to-side) and vertical (up-down) axes. The amplified signals pass through a cable to the control-panel assembly, which provides final amplification.

The preamplifier/accelerometer assembly is quickly attached to the cap at the vertex of the head by a velcro patch, and electrical continuity with the electrodes is established by an electrical connector.

Control-Panel Assembly

The control-panel assembly is mounted on the wall of the subject's sleeping compartment so that it is within easy reach. Circuitry within this unit performs automatic electrode testing, final signal amplification, and real-time data analysis, and provides outputs to the analog tape recorders.

Automatic testing of each electrode is accomplished immediately after the subject dons the recording cap, just before he begins the sleep period. The front panel, readily visible to the subject in his sleeping bag, contains a number of indicator lamps arranged in a configuration simulating the position of the recording electrodes on the head. When the test circuit is activated by the crewman, a small current (≈ 10 μA) passes through the single ground electrode to each of the recording electrodes in succession. Interelectrode resistance is determined, and if a given electrode is in proper scalp contact (resistance 50,000 Ω or less), the lamp corresponding to that electrode is illuminated. Improper contact is corrected when the subject rocks the electrode from side to side to position the tip through the hair.

During the sleep period, EEG, EOG, and head-motion signals are monitored continuously. After final amplification within the control-panel assembly, the signals are routed to data-analysis circuitry and to analog magnetic-tape recorders. The analog recording system consists of two recording units, each capable of preserving up to 150 hours of data. At the conclusion of each Skylab mission, the onboard analog data tapes are returned by the crew. These data are then analyzed by conventional visual scoring techniques after playback onto a graphic recorder.

During the monitoring sessions the data-analysis circuitry within the control-panel assembly supplies sleep-stage information to observers in Mission Control in a near real-time fashion. The EEG, EOG, and head-motion signals are processed onboard in real time. EEG alone is used to determine stages awake, 1, 2, 3, and 4 of sleep. EEG and EOG signals differentiate stage REM (rapid eye movement). The EEG and accelerometer outputs delineate periods that are likely to be contaminated by artifactual signals and exclude these from consideration by the analysis section.

The EEG-analysis scheme uses the decline in frequency and the general increase in amplitude seen as an individual progresses from the awake state to stage 4 sleep, and consequently the criteria used are very similar to those of visual scoring techniques. The single EEG channel is initially filtered to limit further consideration to activity in the 0.7 to 13 Hz range. The filtered signal then enters an amplitude-weighted frequency-meter circuit whose output is a varying dc level, highest when the input signal is intermediate in amplitude and high in frequency, and lowest when the input is high in amplitude and low in frequency.

This signal is consequently proportional to sleep state in the awake to stage 4 range, with the awake state associated with the highest output value. A series of comparator circuits senses this voltage and compares it to previously determined voltage ranges, each range corresponding to one of the clinical sleep stages. Thus, while the EEG-analysis output remains within the range specified for a particular sleep stage, a constant indication of that stage is supplied to the final output logic of the system.

The EEG-analysis circuitry does not differentiate stage REM, and it is typically classified as either stage 1 or 2 by this circuitry, due to its similarity in frequency and amplitude. Additional circuitry observes the single EOG channel, and events that resemble rapid eye motion are detected. Provision has been made to recognize and exclude from further consideration certain EEG events (for example, K-complexes) which may appear in the EOG channel and mimic true eye movements. Other circuits use EEG and head-motion signals to prevent signals with high probability of artifactual contamination from influencing the EEG and EOG sleep-determination circuits. Outputs from the EEG, EOG, and artifact-detection circuitry are combined in the final output logic of the analysis scheme so that a single output value representing one of the possible sleep states is supplied to the spacecraft telemetry at all times. Stage REM is indicated if periods of rapid eye movement are present coincidentally with an EEG-section output characteristic of either stage 1 or 2. REM indications occurring during other stages are ignored, and the EEG-section output alone is accepted.

The output of the analysis circuitry thus continuously indicates the presence of one of seven possible states: awake; stages 1 through 4 and REM of sleep; or stage 0, indicating the absence of adequate data. This output, essentially a three-bit code, is telemetered to Mission Control in a real-time fashion as the spacecraft passes over tracking stations. Between tracking stations, the digital signals are recorded onboard and then transmitted at a high rate during a subsequent tracking-station pass.

Ground-Based Data Processing

Data-processing equipment in the Mission Control Center collates the incoming data from various tracking stations around the world and preserves the time relationships so that a complete tabulation of sleep stage versus elapsed time eventually evolves. This listing is then reprocessed by a second computer system to obtain a data format suitable for interpretation. A compact graphic plot (Figure 3) is generated, showing the complete profile of sleep stage versus time over the course of an entire sleep period. A printed statistical summary of the all-night data is also supplied, which indicates the total sleep time, sleep latency, number of arousals, absolute and percentage of time occupied by each sleep stage, and other detailed sleep parameters.

At the conclusion of each Skylab mission, the analog data tapes recorded onboard during each sleep session are returned by the crew. These data are then analyzed by conventional visual scoring techniques (Rechtschaffen and Kales 1968) after playback onto a graphic recorder. These same data will also be suitable for other forms of computer analysis directed toward both sleep and more general observations of EEG characteristics.

The experiment thus provides a means of on-line, near real-time evaluation of sleep during the mission and a capability for more detailed postflight analysis of sleep characteristics.

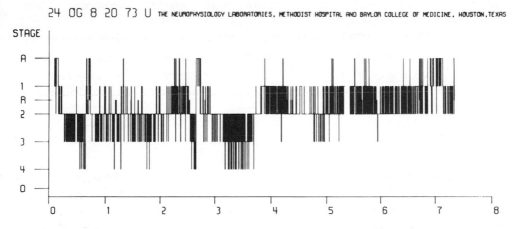

Figure 3. Computer-generated sleep plot for the scientist pilot astronaut on day 24 of the 59-day mission.

Experiment Design

During each Skylab flight one crew member participated in these sleep-monitoring activities. Preflight baseline data were obtained on the subjects during three consecutive nights of sleep monitoring, using portable apparatus functionally identical to the onboard flight hardware. The crewman for the 28-day mission was studied in his own home two months before launch, while the subject of the 59-day mission was monitored in the preflight quarantine facility two weeks before the launch. In addition, a standard clinical electroencephalogram was performed on each subject before the flight, thus permitting precise EEG amplitude determinations for calibration of the flight hardware.

Inflight monitoring was accomplished during 12 selected nights of the 28-day mission (nights 5, 6, 7, 10, 11, 15, 17, 19, 21, 24, 25, and 26) and during 20 nights of the 59-day mission (nights 7, 8, 9, 12, 15, 18, 21, 24, 27, 29, 33, 36, 39, 42, 45, 48, 52, 55, 56, and 57). Although it would have been desirable to obtain data during the first few inflight days, operational factors associated with the activation and function of various spacecraft systems prevented such recordings.

Crew bedtime was usually 10 p.m., with the scheduled sleep period terminating at 6 a.m., although occasional deviations from this schedule were necessitated by work requirements not associated with the sleep-monitoring experiment. Also, during the last week of each mission, sleeping schedules were adjusted forward by a total of four hours (that is, bedtime usually was 6 p.m.). An adjustment of two hours was made on days 20 and 22 of the 28-day mission, and there was a similar change of two hours on days 51 and 53 of the 59-day mission. These schedule alterations were necessitated by the activities associated with splashdown and recovery operations, which required earlier awakening on the final days of the mission.

After return to Earth, postflight baseline studies were carried out on each sleep-monitoring participant. Following the 28-day mission, recordings were done on nights 4, 6, and 8, while in the case of the 59-day mission, monitoring was done on the second, fourth, and sixth nights following splashdown.

Operational Factors

Immediately after the launch of the Skylab Orbital Workshop, a portion of the solar heat shield was lost. The resultant period of elevated temperatures in the workshop before the arrival of the first crew created two problems for the sleep-monitoring activities scheduled for the first (28-day) mission. Some of the recording-cap electrodes were partially dehydrated, and as a result most of the data were lost during one scheduled recording night. In addition, the analog tape-recording system was damaged, and following return of the tapes at the end of the mission, it was determined that only two nights were successfully recorded.

The recording-cap problem was resolved after a few days by the discovery that a number of caps stored in a cooler location onboard the spacecraft had not been severely damaged. These caps were the ones intended for use on future flights, but they were used instead for the remaining nights of the first mission.

For the second manned Skylab mission (59 days), the crew took a repair kit that permitted the sleep subject to refurbish the damaged recording caps by injecting supplementary electrolyte gel before use. Additionally, repair of the recording system was attempted prior to the first night of recording. These steps generally were successful, although one additional night was lost because of recording-cap problems, and six nights of tape-recorded data were lost near the end of the mission when the recording system again failed. A significant data loss also occurred on two other nights of the 28-day mission and on one other night of the 59-day mission, stemming from ground-based problems in the tracking and data-processing system.

In spite of the unforeseen problems, however, successful near real-time monitoring was accomplished on 9 of the 12 attempted recording nights during the 28-day mission and on 18 of the 20 nights attempted on the 59-day mission. Postflight return of the analog tapes permitted visual confirmation of the results on 2 of the 9 nights of the 28-day mission and on 12 of the 18 nights of the 59-day mission.

Statistical Analysis

The results described below represent the best available estimates of the various sleep parameters. When possible, the results presented are those obtained by visual analysis of the tape-recorded EEG, EOG, and head-motion signals, since this method is considered the most reliable and least influenced by various artifactual components that occasionally mix with such signals. When this was not possible because recorded data were lost on several nights, the results of onboard automatic analysis have been used after application of certain corrective factors. The corrections were based on past performance of the system and on correlation of the inflight results with those of visual analysis for the nights on which both types of information were available.

The uncorrected results of automatic analysis consistently underestimate stage REM sleep. This occurs because the criteria for continuous stage REM indication used by the automatic system include the occurrence of at least one detectable rapid eye motion per 30-second time epoch. If such an eye motion does not occur, the output will revert to stage 1 or 2, as determined by EEG criteria alone. In most individuals, true stage REM sometimes occurs for periods longer than 30 seconds in the absence of eye motion of sufficient amplitude to be detected by the automatic circuitry. Typically, then, the automatic system's output during a continuous stage REM period is a fluctuation between stages 1, REM, and 2. Such periods usually are readily identified by inspection of the plotted sleep profile. When the automatic data are modified by the assignment to stage REM of all time within such a period, the overall results are significantly enhanced. Such modification introduces an element of subjectivity into otherwise objective data; however, we believe this is justified in this case, since past experience has confirmed its validity.

Other than eliminating certain obviously artifactual sections of data (for example, sections near the start of each sleep period associated with cap-donning and electrode-testing procedures), the REM-modification step was the only corrective factor instituted during the inflight portions of the Skylab missions.

After the 59-day mission, we compared the results of corrected inflight analysis with those of visual analysis of the taped data for 11 of the first 12 recording nights. The average (mean) error of automatic analysis based upon visually determined total rest-period time was as follows: total rest-period time, +1 percent; total sleep time, +4 percent; sleep latency, -0.3 percent. The average (mean) error of automatic analysis in sleep-stage determination (as compared to the same visually determined parameter) was as follows: stage 1, +5.6 percent; stage 2, -0.4 percent; stage 3, -10.6 percent; stage 4, -0.7 percent; stage REM, +6.1 percent.

In most cases, then, automatic analysis gave satisfactory estimates of the actual value. The worst case, percent of stage 3 sleep, was apparently a result of the particular subject's sleeping pattern, in which a large proportion of the misclassified epochs were borderline in terms of stage 2 versus stage 3. The underestimation was consistent throughout all 11 comparison nights. The stage REM overestimation, on the other hand, was not consistent and appeared to result solely from the inherent limitations of the automatic-analysis scheme in detecting this stage and in rejecting certain artifacts.

Regression analysis, after correlation of automatic and visual results, provided a means for further modifying the results of automatic analysis for those six nights of the 59-day mission unconfirmed by visual analysis (that is, nights 42, 45, 48, 52, 56, and 57, for which the analog tape data were lost).

As noted above, the overall correlation between visual and automatic results for stage REM percentage was low and consequently could not be used for reliable prediction of the remaining six values. However, it was determined that stage REM values below 20 percent, as indicated by automatic analysis, were better correlated with visual results; consequently, regression analysis for this stage was based upon correlations of only 6 of the 11 nights (discarding nights 7, 8, 9, 12, and 29). Corrected REM values were thus predicted for 5 of the 6 remaining nights, discarding the value (30.4 percent) for day 48, which exceeded 20 percent.

These statistical maneuvers provided a consistent means for utilizing all the available information. The values obtained are included in the results presented below and were subjected to further statistical analysis along with the visual-analysis results, although it was determined that the overall significance of the results was the same, whether or not these values were included.

Finally, for each mission, preflight, inflight, and postflight conditions for each parameter were treated by an analysis of variance. A posteriori comparisons were made in cases where the overall F test reached conventional levels of statistical significance ($p < 0.05$).

In summary, with respect to the results outlined below, of the 9 nights recorded during the 28-day mission, only the first 2 are based upon visual analysis. The remainder are based upon automatic analysis as modified inflight with respect to stage REM. For the 59-day mission, the results of the first 12 nights are based upon visual analysis, while the last 6 are automatic results modified both inflight in terms of REM period and postflight by the application of corrective factors based on visual/automatic comparison on the first 12 nights.

Results

Sleep Latency

Sleep latency is defined here as the amount of time elapsed from the onset of the sleep period (that is, bedtime) until the first appearance of stage 2 sleep. The sleep-latency characteristics observed during the first two Skylab missions are summarized in Figure 4. Average inflight, preflight, and postflight figures are indicated in Table 1. Sleep latency varied considerably during the 28-day mission (Figure 4A), ranging from a low value of 3.6 minutes on day 21 to a maximum of 45 minutes on day 19. Day 19 was, however, the only instance in which the latency exceeded the preflight values, and, in fact, the average inflight value of 18 minutes represents a decrease of 20 minutes as compared to the preflight average of 37.8 minutes. Postflight values were all relatively low but well within the inflight range. Statistically, the inflight and postflight latencies were less than the preflight

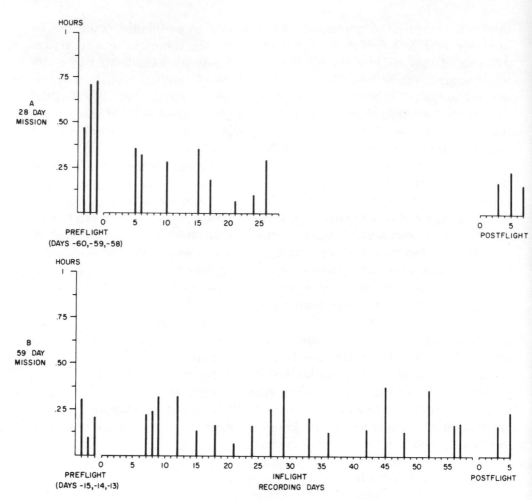

Figure 4. Sleep-latency characteristics from the 28-day and 59-day missions.

TABLE 1.
Average Nightly Values of Selected Sleep Characteristics

28-Day Mission				59-Day Mission		
Preflight	Inflight	Postflight	Sleep Characteristics	Preflight	Inflight	Postflight
7.8	6.9	8.9	total rest time (hr)	7.5	7.32	7.8
6.9	6.0	8.5	total sleep time (hr)	6.4	6.31	6.6
0.84	0.72	0.38	total awake time (hr)	1.10	1.01	1.19
37.8	18.0	11.4	sleep latency (min)	12.0	12.6	9.6
5.3	6.0	5.1	stage 1%	8.8	8.9	10.2
54.8	43.4	56.6	stage 2%	56.3	59.7	57.8
14.8	16.0	12.2	stage 3%	17.4	17.5	10.1
2.9	16.7	1.1	stage 4%	2.8	1.4	0.4
22.2	17.9	25.0	stage REM%	14.7	12.1	21.6

values ($p<0.01$).

The relatively high preflight value, compared to either inflight or post-flight results, apparently is explainable at least in part by a difference in the subject's routine rather than by direct influence of the environment. This individual regularly spent a few minutes reading in bed before falling asleep during the preflight studies in his own home, but he did not continue this practice either during the flight or in the postflight period.

No statistically significant changes in sleep latency were noted during the 59-day mission, as indicated in Figure 4B, although on several days the values were somewhat above the preflight average of 12 minutes. This para-meter ranged from a low of 4 minutes on day 21 to a maximum of 24 minutes on day 45. A somewhat cyclic fluctuation of sleep latency was seen, with maxima near days 10, 29, 45, and 53. The inflight average value (12.6 minutes), however, was almost exactly the same as the preflight value. The postflight latencies, averaging 9.6 minutes, are only slightly less than either the pre- or inflight measurements.

In general, then, there was no evidence in either mission of unusual difficulty falling asleep.

Sleep Time

A commonly used measure of sleep adequacy is the total sleep time obtained in a given sleep period (that is, total rest-period time minus total time spent awake). Figure 5 illustrates the total rest-period length, the total sleep time, and the total awake time for each Skylab recording night and for the pre- and postflight baseline studies.

In the 28-day mission, there was a reduction of total sleep time (solid bars, Figure 5A) throughout the inflight period as compared to the pre- and postflight studies. Postflight, total sleep time was significantly greater than the pre- and inflight values ($p<0.05$ and 0.01, respectively). As indicated in Table 1, the inflight average of 6.0 hours is almost one hour less than the preflight value of 6.9 hours and more than 2 hours less than the postflight average (8.5 hours). This decrease in sleep time, however, was due not to an unusual amount of time spent in the awake state (Figure 5A, dashed portion of bars) but instead to a reduction in the total rest-period time itself (total height of bars, Figure 5A). The subject thus slept quite well on most nights while he was in bed; however, he did not spend as much time in bed as he did during studies either before or after the mission.

The postflight average value for total rest-period time (8.9 hours) was significantly higher than the inflight average ($p<0.01$) but did not differ significantly from the preflight value.

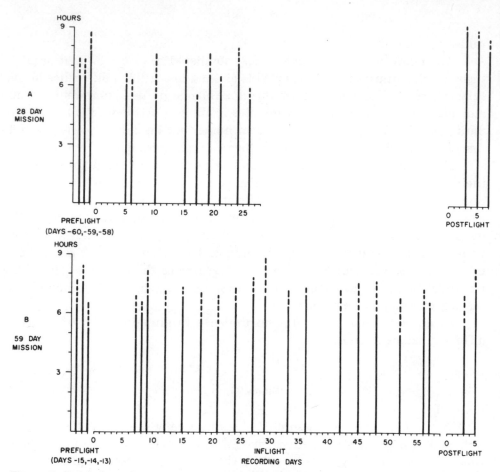

Figure 5. Total sleep time versus total awake time. **A:** *28-day mission.* **B:** *59-day mission.*
Solid lines: *total sleep time.* **Dashed lines:** *total awake time.* **Total height of bars:** *total
sleep-period time.*

No significant changes in the total sleep-total rest characteristics were
obtained during the 59-day mission, as shown graphically in Figure 5B. The
total rest time (overall height of bars, Figure 5B), which averaged 7.3 hours
inflight (Table 1), was only slightly lower than either the preflight average of
7.5 hours or the postflight value of 7.8 hours. In terms of total sleep time
(solid bars, Figure 5B), although there was considerable fluctuation, only
one day (52) was below the range established during the preflight series, and
the subject obtained in excess of 5 hours of sleep on all other nights. The
inflight average value of 6.3 hours (Table 1) is nearly the same as the preflight average (6.4 hours) and slightly lower than the postflight results (average, 6.6 hours).

The above results suggest that obtaining adequate sleep is not a problem
inherent in space flight.

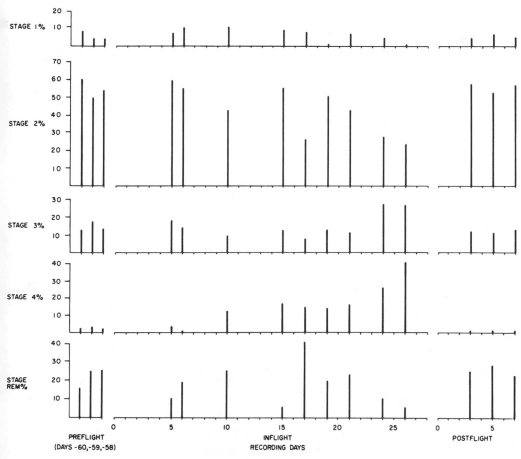

Figure 6. Sleep-stage characteristics from the 28-day mission.

Stage Characteristics

Sleep-stage characteristics for the two missions, expressed as percentages of the total sleep time for each recording night, are illustrated in Figures 6 and 7. Average percentage figures for the various stages in the preflight, inflight, and postflight periods are listed in Table 1.

If the average values are considered, stages 1, 2, 3, and REM were not significantly altered during the inflight period of the 28-day mission. Stage 1 occupied 5.3 percent of the total sleep time preflight and averaged 6.0 percent inflight and 5.1 percent postflight. The day-to-day inflight characteristics (Figure 6) show considerable fluctuation in stage 1 percent, with a tendency toward slightly decreased values in the latter portions of the flight (days 19 through 26). Stage 3, averaging 14.8 percent in the preflight period, rose slightly to an average of 16.0 percent inflight and dropped to 12.2 percent postflight. As seen in Figure 6, a small increase in the stage 3 percent average was largely a result of moderate increases in this stage on days 24 and 26 at the end of the mission. Stage REM decreased only slightly from a 22.2 percent preflight average to 17.9 percent inflight, although again there was considerable variation throughout the flight, with some tendency toward a more marked decrease near the end of the mission. The postflight stage REM average (25.0 percent) was somewhat higher than either the pre- or inflight values, but it did not attain statistical significance.

Fairly clear-cut changes were seen in stage 2 and stage 4 percentages. In both cases, the most obvious alterations were seen in the last few days of the flight. Stage 2 dropped from an average of 54.8 percent preflight to 43.4 percent inflight, returning to 56.6 percent postflight. These differences, however, were not significant. Similarly, stage 4 rose from 2.9 percent preflight to 16.7 percent inflight, then dropped significantly ($p<0.05$) postflight to 1.1 percent.

Thus, the 28-day mission was characterized by increased percentages of stages 3 and 4 and corresponding decreases of stages REM, 1, and 2, with the alterations confined primarily to the last few days of the flight.

Sleep-stage features for the 59-day mission are illustrated in Figure 7, and average values are tabulated in Table 1. Stage 1, averaging 8.8 percent preflight, showed considerable variation inflight but averaged almost the same (8.9 percent). The postflight average value of 10.2 percent was only slightly above the inflight result. Stage 2 remained fairly consistent throughout (preflight, 56.3 percent; inflight, 59.7 percent; postflight 57.8 percent), although there was a decrease during the final days of the flight (days 56 and 57). Thus, neither stage 1 nor stage 2 changed significantly. Stage 3 was similar inflight (17.5 percent) and preflight (17.4 percent) and also exhibited a change near the termination of the flight, tending to increase slightly. The postflight average of 10.1 percent, however, was significantly lower ($p<0.01$) than either the pre- or inflight values. This subject showed very little stage 4 sleep in his preflight study (2.8 percent), and this parameter decreased significantly ($p<0.05$) inflight (1.4 percent) and postflight (0.4 percent) ($p<0.05$). Stage REM showed the greatest alteration, dropping from 14.7 percent during the preflight baseline series to 12.1 percent inflight and then rising significantly ($p<0.01$) to 21.6 percent postflight. This postflight increase in REM was also significantly greater than the preflight value ($p<0.05$). The REM decrease seen inflight was most prominent in the final phase of the study (days 52, 56, and 57).

Thus, the 28- and 59-day missions were, in terms of altered sleep-stage features, similar in only three respects: (1) both subjects showed a decrease in stage REM percentage near the final portion of the flights and likewise showed an increase in stage REM postflight; (2) both showed postflight decreases in stage 3 and little inflight change in this stage; (3) both showed

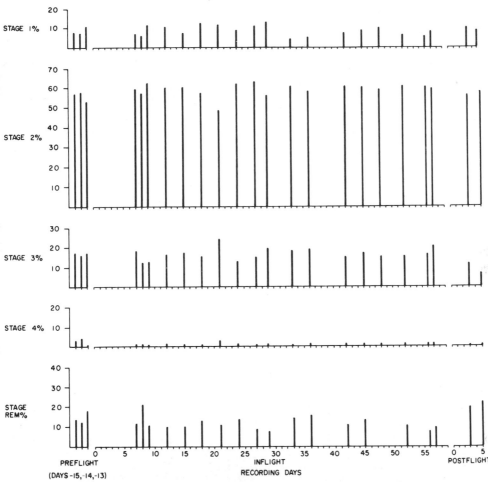

Figure 7. Sleep-stage characteristics from the 59-day mission.

small postflight decreases in stage 4 percentage as compared to preflight studies, although they differed with respect to inflight stage 4 characteristics. The two flights differed in that (1) inflight reduction in stage 2 was not seen during the 59-day mission as it was on the 28-day mission, and (2) an increase in inflight stage 4 percentage was seen only during the 28-day mission, and this measure decreased slightly during the 59-day mission.

REM Latency

REM latency is defined as the elapsed time from sleep onset (that is, the first appearance of stage 2 sleep) until the onset of the first stage REM period of the night. Compared to preflight values, this measure was shortened during the postflight period of both missions. During the 28-day mission, the REM latency averaged 1.5 hours preflight and 1.1 hours postflight, or a decrease of 24 minutes. Although substantial, this decrease was not statistically significant. The phenomenon was more apparent during the 59-day mission, as illustrated in Figure 8 which includes only data based upon visual analysis. In the preflight baseline period, the values ranged from 1.6 to 2.2 hours, with an average latency of 1.9 hours. The inflight values showed considerable fluctuation, but the average of 2.1 hours was not significantly different compared to the preflight results. In the postflight period, however, the latency dropped to 0.9 hours, which represented a decrease of 1 hour below the preflight findings. This postflight REM latency was significantly ($p<0.01$) less than both pre- and inflight values.

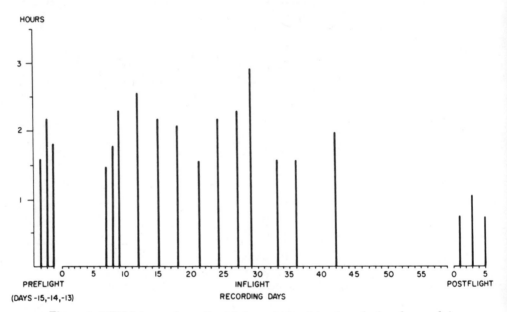

Figure 8. REM latency from the 59-day mission (visual-analysis values only).

Discussion

Preliminary analysis of the data obtained during the first two Skylab missions suggests that prolonged space flight and the accompanying weightless state are not associated with major changes in sleep characteristics. In addition, the alterations observed in sleep patterns were not of the type which might be associated with significant degradation of performance capability. These conclusions are somewhat surprising in view of the numerous subjective reports of sleep difficulty occurring during the Gemini and Apollo programs which led to the suspicion that weightlessness itself might in some way seriously disrupt the normal sleep-wakefulness mechanisms.

Before Skylab, it had been suspected that the greatly altered sensory input to the central nervous system associated with the zero-g state might interfere with sleep onset even though a crewman might adapt rapidly with respect to waking activities. Thus, we might have expected to see a prolongation of the sleep-latency measure and perhaps long periods of wakefulness following arousals from sleep. The results, however, showed that in neither the 28- nor the 59-day mission was sleep latency significantly elevated above preflight levels, nor was there evidence of consistently increased amounts of time spent awake during the night.

The results thus indicate that during space flight it is possible to obtain adequate amounts of sleep during regularly scheduled eight-hour rest periods. While some reduction in total sleep time was observed on the 28-day mission, this was the result of a voluntary (on the part of the subject) reduction of the rest-period time to accommodate a heavy work load. During the 59-day mission, the subject maintained a total rest and total sleep-time profile very similar to his preflight baseline. Sleep quality, as reflected in sleep-stage characteristics, was also studied, and while changes were seen on both flights, they were not of great magnitude and were not all necessarily related to the weightless environment. Thus, the decrease in stage REM percentage seen near the end of both missions is more likely a result of the changed pattern of activities associated with preparation for return to Earth, including alterations of sleep schedules, than it is a result of space flight as such. Individual variations were also evident. For example, the increase of stage 4 percentage observed during the 28-day mission was not repeated during the 59-day mission; instead, this measure dropped slightly.

Changes in sleep-stage characteristics were somewhat more consistent between the subjects with respect to the postflight findings. Postflight, both showed an increase in stage REM percentage, a decrease in stage 3 percentage, and a small decrease in stage 4 percentage, as compared to preflight studies. The increases in stage REM percentage are worthy of consideration, since such findings are typical of the rebound effect seen after periods of relative deprivation of stage REM. It is possible that significant REM deprivation did occur during the terminal portions of these flights, as suggested by the decline seen in REM percentage on the last recording nights of each mission. This situation cannot be assessed fully, however, since recording was not accomplished during the last two nights of each mission.

The shortening of REM latency observed postflight on both missions (achieving statistical significance on the 59-day mission) was an unexpected finding. A shortening of REM latency is another manifestation of a prior period of REM deprivation, although, for the reasons mentioned above, it is not possible to assess thoroughly this aspect with respect to the Skylab studies.

A factor arguing against a prior period of REM deprivation as the causative agent of the REM percentage increase and latency decrease seen postflight is that no lessening of the effect was evident even on the sixth night after recovery of the 59-day mission nor after the eighth night following the 28-day mission recovery. Nor can the postflight REM changes be reasonably attributed to alterations in the astronauts' sleep schedules (that is, the four-hour advance in bedtime during the last week of each mission). Shortening of REM latency has been associated with delaying sleep periods by four hours, but is has not been reported with comparable advances in sleep onset. In addition, delaying sleep periods has been found to increase REM percentage, while advancing sleep periods *decreased* REM percentage (Taub and Berger 1973).

It is therefore possible that decreased REM latency and increased REM percentage represent a true influence of the reinstated one-*g* condition, and that it signifies a basic alteration in the sleep-wakefulness mechanism of the central nervous system.

One of the current theories concerning the function of sleep, especially of the REM stage, centers on evidence that a role in the organization of memory may be subserved (Gaarder 1966; see also reviews by Greenberg 1970, and Dewan 1970). In particular, it has been suggested that REM may be involved in a consolidation or reprogramming of short-term memory into a more permanent or long-term form. It might be predicted, then, that activities associated with acquisition of new motor skills and coordinated motor activity are associated with increased need for stage REM.

Zimmerman, Stoyva, and Metcalf (1970) found that during adaptation to an inverted visual field, REM time increased. Likewise, reinverting the visual field back to normal was also accompanied by an increase in REM-sleep amount. An analogous situation may occur in adjusting to the weightless state. The withdrawal of gravitational cues and decreased proprioceptive and vestibular inputs place a considerable burden upon the visual system as the sole means of maintaining spatial orientation. The return to Earth following a mission would likewise require psychophysiological reorganization appropriate to one-*g* conditions. Thus, one might hypothesize that during adaptation to zero-*g* or readaptation to one-*g*, increase in REM time would be observed. On both missions, REM percentage increased in the postflight period relative to pre- and inflight conditions. However, inflight values were generally lower than preflight values and therefore do not support the expectation that adaptation to zero-*g* would be accompanied by increased REM percentage. This hypothesis cannot, however, be ruled out completely, because no sleep data were obtained before day 5 of the 28-day mission and day 7 of the 59-day mission. Thus, pertinent changes could have been missed. Evidence that adaptation to weightlessness occurred within the first five to seven days is indicated by the absence of motion-sickness symptoms after this time, although they had been present earlier. The final Skylab flight should help clarify these findings.

The objective information provided by these two Skylab crewmen was supplemented by subjective reports of sleep quality provided by the other astronauts participating in the missions. Although on occasional nights they reported poor sleep, over the long run they felt that they had obtained adequate sleep and that no real problem existed in this area.

The two participants in these studies showed considerable individual variation in their sleep patterns, as reflected in the recorded results. The subject of the 28-day mission showed the most classical sleep profile in his preflight baseline studies, with well-defined cycles, relatively few arousals, and fairly typical stage characteristics. The astronaut monitored during the 59-day mission exhibited poorly defined cycles, had frequent arousals, averaged less sleep per night, and had a relatively low percentage of stage REM. In both cases, however, the same basic sleep pattern persisted during the missions, thereby maintaining the individual differences noted preflight.

Based on the results of these first two Skylab experiments, it seems that the sleep problems encountered during earlier space flights were not a result of the zero-g environment itself. The Apollo and Gemini series of space flights differed considerably from Skylab, even though atmospheric and gravitational factors were essentially identical in all cases. With respect to sleep, the most significant difference is probably the size of the spacecraft, or, more specifically, the working volume. At $12,763$ ft^3, the Skylab living area provides adequate room for separate eating, exercising, working, and sleeping areas. With about three percent of this volume for the Apollo and less than one percent for the Gemini spacecraft, all tasks were made more difficult, and the sense of confinement was undoubtedly an adverse factor. The Skylab routine is, in most respects, comparable to ground-based, everyday activity. The sleeping-bag arrangement and individual sleeping compartments are a considerable improvement over the prior spacecraft and minimize interference with sleep caused by activity of other crewmen. While there is undoubtedly a higher level of danger in all space flights than there is in typical everyday activity on the ground, this element seems to be minimized in Skylab by the establishment of a daily routine, and this itself probably contributes to improved sleeping conditions.

Summary and Conclusions

Sleep was monitored successfully by objective means during two relatively long-duration orbital space flights. The subject of the 28-day mission showed a voluntary decrease in his total sleep time, a decrease in sleep latency, a slight increase in the percentage of sleep occupied by stage 4, and a decrease in stage 2. The 59-day mission results showed that the crewman had no significant alteration in his total sleep time or sleep latency, but stage 3 decreased significantly postflight, and stage 4 showed a significant decrease during and following the flight. The subjects of both flights showed a decrease of stage REM near the termination of their missions and increases of REM in the postflight periods. In the 59-day mission, this effect was significant compared with pre- and inflight conditions. Significant shortening of REM latency was also observed in the postflight period of the 59-day mission, and a similar trend appeared following the 28-day mission as well.

The alterations of sleeping patterns observed inflight were considered insignificant in terms of any possible adverse effect upon performance capability. In general, we conclude that these results indicate that it is possible to obtain sleep of adequate quantity and quality during the long periods of weightlessness and confinement which are typical of space flight.

References

Adey, W.R., Kado, R.T., and Walter, D.O. 1967. Computer analysis of EEG data from Gemini flight GT-7. *Aerosp. Med.* 38:345.

Berry, C. 1970. Summary of medical experience in the Apollo 7 through 11 manned space flights. *Aerosp. Med.* 41:500.

Burch, N.R., Dossett, R.G., Vorderman, A.L., and Boyd, K.L. 1971. Period analysis of an electroencephalogram from an orbiting command pilot. In J.F. Lindsay and J.C. Townsend (eds.), *Biomedical Research and Computer Application in Manned Space Flight*, NASA SP-5078, p. 117. Washington, D.C.: Technology Utilization Office, NASA.

Dewan, E.M. 1970. The programing (p) hypothesis for REM sleep. In E. Hartmann (ed.), *Sleep and Dreaming*, p. 295. Boston: Little, Brown.

Frost, J.D., Jr., Shumate, W.H., Booher, C.R., and DeLucchi, M.R. 1974. Skylab sleep monitoring experiment: methodology and initial results. In A. Graybiel (ed.), *Proceedings of the Fifth International Symposium on Basic Environmental Problems of Man in Space*, to be published in *Astronautica Acta* (in press).

Gaarder, K. 1966. A conceptual model of sleep. *Arch. Gen. Psychiatry* 14:253.

Greenberg, R. 1970. Dreaming and memory. In E. Hartmann (ed.), *Sleep and Dreaming*, p. 258. Boston: Little, Brown.

Maulsby, R.L. 1966. Electroencephalogram during orbital flight. *Aerosp. Med.* 37:1022.

Maulsby, R.L., and Kellaway, P. 1966. Electroencephalogram during orbital flight: evaluation of depth of sleep. In *Proceedings of the Second Annual Biomedical Research Conference*, p. 77. Houston: NASA, Manned Spacecraft Center.

Rechtschaffen, A., and Kales, A. (eds.) 1968. *A Manual of Standardized Terminology, Techniques and Scoring System for Sleep Stages of Human Subjects.* Washington, D.C.: Public Health Service, U.S. Govt. Printing Office.

Taub, J.M., and Berger, R.J. 1973. Sleep stage patterns associated with acute shifts in the sleep-wakefulness cycle. *Electroencephalogr. Clin. Neurophysiol.* 35:613.

Zimmerman, J., Stoyva, J., and Metcalf, D. 1970. Distorted visual feedback and augmented REM sleep. *Psychophysiology* 7:298.

alcohol and sleep in the chronic alcoholic

Boyd K. Lester, M.D.
Orvis H. Rundell, M.S.
Lawrence C. Cowden, A.S.E.T.

University of Oklahoma Health Sciences Center
Oklahoma City, Oklahoma

Harold L. Williams, Ph.D.

University of Minnesota
Minneapolis, Minnesota

The purposes of this study were to compare physiological sleep profiles of sober chronic alcoholics with those of age-matched normal control subjects, and to examine the effects of two days of drinking on the sleep of the alcoholic patients.[1]

Extreme disturbance of sleep in the chronic alcoholic, especially during acute alcoholic psychoses, was recognized many years ago; but Gross and his colleagues (Gross et al. 1966, Gross and Goodenough 1968, Gross et al. 1972) were apparently the first to undertake systematic studies of sleep in these patients. Reviewing the clinical histories of a group of chronic alcoholic patients who suffered acute alcoholic psychoses, they noted that periods of heavy drinking were frequently associated with insomnia. Some patients reported that they could get to sleep only after consuming large quan-

---

[1] Some of these data were presented in *Alcohol Intoxication and Withdrawal* (pp. 261-277), edited by Milton M. Gross, Plenum Press, New York, 1973.

tities of alcohol, but that continued drinking caused further disruption of sleep. Quantitative studies of sleep during delirium tremens and alcoholic hallucinosis by Gross and his co-workers (1966) and by Greenberg and Pearlman (1967) revealed considerable fragmentation of sleep and, for most patients, total absence of high-voltage stage 4 sleep. Mello and Mendelson (1970) observed that both ingestion and withdrawal of alcohol were usually accompanied by sleep disruption. Johnson, Burdick, and Smith (1970) and Johnson (1972), using electroencephalographic (EEG) measures, confirmed this observation and found almost no slow-wave sleep (stages 3 and 4) in 33- to 45-year-old alcoholics who first drank and were then withdrawn from alcohol during 12 days of hospitalization. In that study, sleep disruption, manifested by frequent awakenings, frequent changes of EEG stage, and frequent body movements, was somewhat greater during the initial two-day period of heavy drinking than at the end of the subsequent ten-day withdrawal period. Total stage REM, which was depressed during the drinking phase, reached normal levels toward the end of hospitalization. This increase in stage REM resulted specifically from a decrease in latency to the first REM epoch and in the time between REM periods, rather than from increased duration of REM episodes. Although absent in most patients during heavy drinking, stage 3 showed some recovery by the tenth withdrawal night, but stage 4 remained totally absent in nine of the fourteen patients. Allen and his colleagues (1971) also examined the effects of prolonged intoxication and withdrawal in chronic alcoholics, noting profound disturbance of stage REM and slow-wave sleep as well as disturbances in sleep rhythmicity.

The alterations caused by alcohol consumption in the sleep patterns of alcoholics resemble in certain aspects those found in intoxicated normal subjects. For example, Gross et al. (1966), Gross and Goodenough (1968), Gross et al. (1973), and Johnson, Burdick, and Smith (1970) reported the suppression of stage REM and increased latency to REM onset found by others after alcohol ingestion in normal subjects (Gresham, Webb, and Williams 1963; Yules, Freedman, and Chandler 1966; Rundell et al. 1972). Moreover, as in normal subjects (Rundell et al. 1972), alcohol apparently reduced the density of such phasic events of sleep as nonspecific electrodermal responses, sigma spindles, and K-complexes (Gross and Goodenough 1968; Johnson, Burdick, and Smith 1970). However, the sedative effects associated with alcohol in normal subjects (Rundell et al. 1972) were not invariably found in alcoholics. For example, neither sleep-onset latency nor latency of slow-wave sleep was reduced by alcohol in Johnson's patients. With four to six days of heavy drinking, Gross's patients showed biphasic trends for slow-wave sleep, that is, enhancement over the first few days of drinking, followed by suppression (Gross et al. 1973).

Interpretation of these altered sleep patterns in intoxicated and sober chronic alcoholics is complicated by the possible influence on sleep patterns of factors other than alcoholism. For example, Johnson's patients were received from a city jail; all were unemployed and their nutritional history was unknown; most were in early stages of withdrawal from heavy drinking; and a high percentage had suffered delirium tremens. Head injuries, various brain syndromes, malnutrition, or chronic psychosis, any of which might be present in the history of the "skid-row" alcoholic, could have contributed to their disordered sleep (Feinberg 1969; Lester, Chanes, and Condit 1969; Snyder 1969; Meltzer et al. 1970; Hawkins 1970). Interpretation is further complicated by the fact that normal aging is associated with diminished ability to sustain sleep and with gradual loss of high-voltage, slow-wave sleep (Feinberg, Koresko, and Hellen 1967; Kahn and Fisher 1969). Thus it should be informative to compare the sleep patterns of sober chronic alcholics with those of age-matched controls.

For those reasons we studied a more "middle-class" group of alcoholics, nearly all of whom, at hospitalization, had been continuously employed in their primary occupations for several months to several years. Each patient, matched in age with a normal control, had been dry for at least three weeks before the sleep studies; each was in good clinical health with good nutritional status and with no evidence of gross liver damage, brain damage, or gross psychopathology. As will be seen, our results with this lower-middle to middle-class sample of "healthy" chronic alcoholics strengthen previous conclusions (reviewed above) that chronic abuse of alcohol per se causes systematic changes in sleep.

Method

Subjects. Twenty male alcoholic patients were selected from volunteers on an experimental alcoholic-treatment ward at Central State Hospital, Norman, Oklahoma. The ward was operated by personnel of the Oklahoma Center for Alcohol-Related Studies. Each patient met the criteria of alcoholism recommended by the Alcoholism Sub-Committee of the Expert Committee on Mental Health of the World Health Organization (1952). At the first sleep session all had been hospitalized, dry, and drug-free for at least three weeks. Their mean age was 39 years (range 24 to 55), and their average education was 11.1 years (range 8 to 19). Eighteen were employed in their primary occupations at the time of hospitalization, the number of months on the most recent job ranging from 1 to 408 (median = 34.5). For the employed patients, 2 were unskilled, 13 were semiskilled, and 3 were skilled (or semiprofessional) workers. Twelve were divorced. They had histories of heavy drinking ranging from 3 to 30 years (median=10.5). Three of the patients reported having had convulsions, and 7 at least one episode of delirium tremens; none reported significant head injuries. At hospitalization, none of the patients had physical, neurological, or laboratory evidence of brain damage or of gross liver damage, and none had histories of mental illness.

Each alcoholic patient was matched within five years of age with a male control subject drawn either from a group of normal men who had volunteered for a longitudinal study of cardiac insufficiency (N = 13), or from students and faculty in the University of Oklahoma Medical School (N = 7). Seven controls were moderate social drinkers in that they consumed alcoholic beverages at occasional evening social events. The remaining 13 were totally abstinent. None were on drugs or prescription medication at the time of the study. The mean age for the controls was 41 years (range 24 to 56), and their mean education was 14.4 years (range 8 to 20). Nineteen of the controls were employed in their primary occupations which varied from unskilled trades (N = 1), semiskilled (N = 6), skilled (N = 5), to semiprofessional and professional (N = 4), and student (N = 3). Five were divorced.

Procedure. After at least three weeks of drug-free sobriety, each alcoholic patient slept in the laboratory for one adaptation night (data discarded) and two successive baseline sessions. One week later, each patient then imbibed alcohol on a controlled drinking schedule for two consecutive days. Beginning at 1300 hours, and at each hour thereafter until 2100 hours, the patient was given a choice of zero, one, or two drinks consisting of 95 percent ethyl alcohol mixed (1:4) with ginger ale. The actual amount of alcohol administered was covertly adjusted to produce an average hourly blood-alcohol concentration (BAC) of about 150 mg/100 ml (Stephenson Breathalyzer). Sleep sessions (beginning at 2200 hours) were run after each of the two drinking days and for two consecutive recovery nights thereafter. A final baseline session occurred one week after the second recovery night.[2] Total bedtime for each sleep session was eight hours. During the drinking days the patients were offered and usually ate three meals at the usual times.

The control subjects slept in the laboratory for three sessions, the first of which was not recorded. Bedtime was eight hours beginning at 2200 hours.

Measures. The following physiological measures were taken on all 40 subjects: (1) Continuous EEG recorded on a Grass Model 6 electroencephalograph from symmetrical C_4/A_1 and C_3/A_2 placements, using a time constant of 0.1 seconds; (2) submental electromyogram (EMG); and (3) left and right electrooculogram (EOG) from lateral electrode placements at the outer

---

[2] During drinking days the patient's behavior was rated and performance assessed in various tasks and social situations. These data will be reported elsewhere.

canthi of the eyes, each referenced to Fpz.

In addition to the above measures, three autonomic variables were monitored continuously (Grass Model 7 polygraph) on ten subjects in each group: (1) Spontaneous galvanic skin responses (GSR) were recorded with silver-silver chloride electrodes from the palmar surface of the left-hand middle finger (active site) referenced to the inner surface of the lower left arm. GSR activity was amplified by a GSR amplifier (Bio-Physical Research Instruments) with an eight-second time constant; (2) heart rate was monitored with a modified lead II electrocardiographic (EKG) placement; and (3) respiration was obtained by strapping a mercury-filled strain gauge across the solar plexus.

Quantitative analysis. The EEG stages of sleep were classified by visual inspection using the criteria recommended by Rechtschaffen and Kales (1968). Each 20 seconds of record was scored independently by two experienced scorers with overall agreement of 87 percent, disagreements being resolved by the senior investigator (BKL). The EEG tracings were evaluated for the following variables: (1) Percentages of the stages of sleep; (2) latency of onset of sleep (first sigma spindle of stage 2); (3) latency of onset of stage REM (first rapid eye movement); (4) times from REM offsets to REM onsets; (5) duration of REM episodes; (6) number of brief arousals (our term for movement arousals defined in the Rechtschaffen and Kales manual (1968)); (7) number of changes of stage; (8) sigma spindle frequency in stage 2 sleep; and (9) rapid eye movements during stage REM.

The latter two variables (spindles and rapid eye movements) were evaluated for 15 one-minute epochs of stage 2 or stage REM, randomly selected from the first four hours and, again, from the last four hours of each night. Similarly for the autonomic events, 15 one-minute epochs were randomly chosen from the first and last four hours of each night in sleep stages 2, REM, and slow-wave (stages 3 and/or 4) and in waking. Sleep spindle bursts (12- to 14-Hz sigma activity) of at least 0.5-second duration were counted and expressed as bursts per minute. Cardiorespiratory events were likewise counted and are reported in rates per minute. Frequency per minute of nonspecific GSR responses was measured by counting the number of responses greater than 100 ohms. Rapid eye movement density during stage REM was expressed as the number of 10-second epochs per minute containing rapid eye movements.

Using one-way analyses of variance, mean scores on each measure in the alcoholic sample were compared across the two predrinking baseline and the two recovery sessions that followed alcohol ingestion. Since no consistent differences were found, scores from the four sessions were averaged to form a single baseline score. Similarly, since none of the comparisons between the two sessions in the control group reached statistical significance, scores from nights two and three were also averaged for that group. Average baseline scores for the two groups were compared using two-tailed t-tests for correlated means, backed up by the Wilcoxin signed-ranks test. Data from the baseline, the two alcohol and final recovery sessions were then compared (t-test and Wilcoxin) within the alcoholic sample.

Results

Baseline Differences Between Alcoholics and Controls

EEG stages of sleep. In general, the alcoholic patients had significantly higher percentages of stage 1 and stage REM than controls and significantly less stage 3.[3] They did not differ from controls on total time awake, percentage of stage 2, or percentage of stage 4, though the latter stage tended to be greater in controls than in patients.

Table 1 shows the means and standard deviations for percentages of wakefulness and the stages of sleep in alcoholics and controls. The absence of a significant difference in percentage of stage 4 between the two groups is noteworthy because previous studies have reported absence of stage 4 to be a cardinal symptom in chronic alcoholics.

The data in Table 2, categorized by age, clarify this finding. Among the older subjects (age 40 to 56), neither the alcoholics nor the matched controls had much stage 4 sleep. Six of the ten controls and seven of the ten alcoholics had no 20-second epochs which could be classified as stage 4 sleep by the Rechtschaffen-Kales (1968) criteria. On the other hand, among the younger subjects (age 24 to 39), eight of the ten controls, but only four of the ten alcoholics, had some stage 4 sleep. The difference in percentage of stage 4 between younger alcoholics and controls was significant, whereas the difference for older alcoholics and matched controls was not. These trends resulted in a significant interaction between the effects of alcoholism and age. The Pearson correlation coefficients between age and percentage of stage 4 were -0.59 ($p<.01$) in the controls and -0.05 (NS) in the alcoholics. None of the other stages of sleep showed systematic age effects, but older controls were awake significantly longer than younger controls.

The amounts of stage 4 were lower on average in both alcoholics and controls than in young normal adults studied by Rundell et al. (1972), and lower than those usually reported by others for comparable age groups. Our younger and older controls averaged 4.3 and 1.2 percent stage 4, respectively; whereas Webb and Agnew (1968) reported 10 percent stage 4 in 30-

---

[3] Unless otherwise specified, "significant" means 0.05 level or better, t-test, and Wilcoxin signed-ranks tests (two-tailed).

TABLE 1.

Stages of Sleep (percentage)

		Controls	Alcoholics
Awake*	$\overline{X}$	10.7	10.1
	s	7.5	5.2
Stage 1	$\overline{X}$	5.4	10.5
	s	2.9	4.1
Stage 2	$\overline{X}$	61.9	58.1
	s	7.9	5.0
Stage 3	$\overline{X}$	9.4	4.2
	s	4.1	4.4
Stage 4	$\overline{X}$	2.8	1.1
	s	3.8	2.6
REM	$\overline{X}$	20.5	26.1
	s	4.3	3.2

*Means and standard deviations for awake are based
on percentage of total bedtime. All other entries
are percentages of total sleep with waking excluded.

TABLE 2.

Stage of Sleep by Age

		Younger Subjects (Age 24-39)		Older Subjects (Age 40-56)	
		Controls**	Alcoholics**	Controls	Alcoholics
Awake*	$\overline{X}$	7.8	9.3	13.7	11.0
	s	4.0	5.2	9.0	5.4
Stage 1	$\overline{X}$	5.2	10.2	5.6	10.7
	s	2.4	3.6	3.5	4.7
Stage 2	$\overline{X}$	60.9	57.8	62.8	58.3
	s	9.2	3.3	6.9	6.4
Stage 3	$\overline{X}$	9.4	4.9	9.4	3.5
	s	3.5	3.3	4.8	5.3
Stage 4	$\overline{X}$	4.3	0.6	1.2	1.6
	s	4.1	1.1	2.9	3.5
REM	$\overline{X}$	20.2	26.4	20.9	25.9
	s	5.7	3.5	2.5	3.1

*Means and standard deviations for awake are based on percentage of total bedtime. All
other entries are percentages of total sleep excluding waking.

**Means in each column are based on N = 10.

to 39-year-old normals and 3 percent in 50- to 59-year-olds. Feinberg (1969) reported 7 percent stage 4 in a sample of normals ranging in age from 65 to 96. However, the overall average in our alcoholic sample (Table 1) of 1.1 percent is very close to the 0.8 percent stage 4 reported by Johnson, Burdick, and Smith (1970). The differences between our statistics on normal subjects and those in the literature probably result from our use of the rather rigorous amplitude criteria specified for stage 4 in the Rechtschaffen-Kales manual (1968).

The latter suggestion raises an interesting question. Do the low amounts of stage 4 found both with aging and with chronic alcoholism result from loss of frequencies in the delta band (0.5 to 4 Hz), or of reduced amplitude of delta activity, or both?

Figure 1 illustrates the results of independent quantitative analysis of delta periodicity and EEG amplitude over the first six hours of the night in a 27-year-old alcoholic and his age-matched control.[4] Both subjects show two well-defined peaks in density of delta periodic activity (Delta Index) shortly after the first and second hours of sleep. However, for the alcholic patient, the average EEG amplitude function is markedly depressed at these same peaks of delta frequency activity.

Figure 2 shows similar time functions for a 52-year-old alcoholic and his matched control. Again, the alcoholic's EEG amplitude function appears markedly depressed compared to the control subject at the peaks of delta periodicity. At this writing, quantitative EEG analyses are not yet completed for all subjects, so that the results shown above must be regarded with caution. However, the trends do suggest that alcoholic patients may generate sufficient activity in the delta frequency band to qualify as stage 4 sleep, although the voltage does not reach the Rechtschaffen-Kales criterion for that classification. Nothing in the analyses illustrated in Figures 1 and 2 indicates whether aging affects the two EEG parameters differentially.

Other sleep measures and sleep quality. The data shown in Table 3 indicate that alcoholics had about three times as many brief arousals during the night ($p<.001$) as controls, as well as more frequent changes of stage ($p<.01$) and longer latencies to sleep onset. The latter difference between alcoholics and controls was not quite significant at the 0.05 level. As Table 3 shows, the higher percentage of stage REM found in the alcoholic patients (Table 1) was not due to increased duration of REM episodes. REM episodes

---

[4] Average delta periodicity was obtained with a modified Biodata period analyzer (Burch and Childers 1963) which coded the EEG signal into square-wave trains and classified their periods into frequency bands. The Delta Index, expressed as the percentage of time delta activity was present, was averaged over five-minute epochs. Amplitude data were obtained over the same five-minute epochs by a reset integrator and are expressed as mean microvolts (peak to peak).

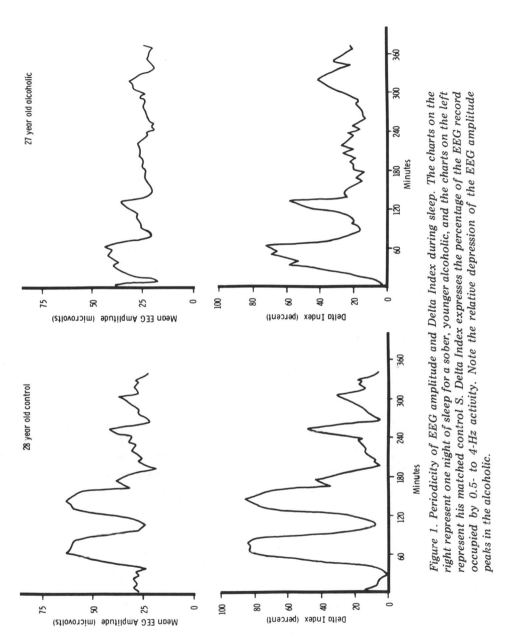

Figure 1. Periodicity of EEG amplitude and Delta Index during sleep. The charts on the right represent one night of sleep for a sober, younger alcoholic, and the charts on the left represent his matched control S. Delta Index expresses the percentage of the EEG record occupied by 0.5- to 4-Hz activity. Note the relative depression of the EEG amplitude peaks in the alcoholic.

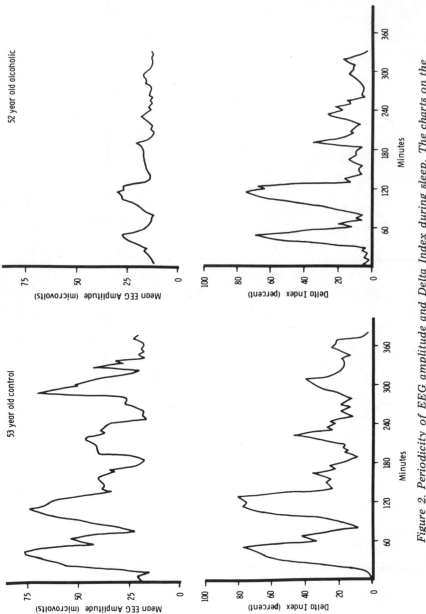

Figure 2. Periodicity of EEG amplitude and Delta Index during sleep. The charts on the right represent one night of sleep for a sober, older alcoholic, and those on the left represent his age-matched control. Delta Index expresses the percentage of the EEG record occupied by 0.5- to 4-Hz activity. Note the relative depression of the EEG amplitude peaks in the alcoholic.

were significantly shorter and more frequently disrupted in the alcoholics. None of the measures reported in Table 3 were influenced by age, either in alcoholic patients or controls.

Figure 3 shows the average distribution of time intervals from REM offset to REM onset for alcoholics and controls on baseline nights. Note that in each group the distribution is bimodal. With time intervals on the abscissa, the modes to the left of 12 minutes represent the proportions of intervals which we classified as REM disruptions, whereas the modes to the right (between 60 and 90 minutes) represent the basic period of the REM-to-REM cycle. The mode for that cycle is about 15 minutes shorter in the alcoholics than in the controls, and the difference between corresponding means is statistically significant. The latency of onset of the first REM episode was also significantly shorter in alcoholics than in controls, averaging 64 minutes (SD = 4.2) and 102 minutes (SD = 6.1) in alcoholics and controls respectively. Thus, as indicated, the increased amounts of stage REM found in alcoholics were due to accelerated REM periodicity rather than increased REM period durations. The modes on the left in Figure 3 also illustrate the considerably higher proportion of REM disruptions in alcoholics than in controls, a difference which is significant beyond the 0.001 level.

Autonomic and phasic variables. Among the autonomic measures, alcoholics had higher rates per minute of nonspecific GSR responses than controls during waking and in all stages of sleep ($p<.01$). As Table 4 indicates, in alcoholics the GSR rate during stage REM (3.6/min) approached the waking rate, an unusual finding. Spontaneous GSR responses are rare during stage

TABLE 3.

Other Measures of Sleep

		Controls	Alcoholics
Brief arousals	$\overline{X}$	32.2	97.9
(total)	s	24.9	27.5
Stage changes	$\overline{X}$	51.9	68.5
(total)	s	13.8	14.0
REM disruption*	$\overline{X}$	0.3	0.6
	s	0.1	0.1
REM duration**	$\overline{X}$	15.7	12.4
(min)	s	4.7	3.4
Latency of Sleep Onset	$\overline{X}$	20.9	31.7
(min)	s	11.2	20.4

*Proportion REM offset to REM onset intervals of 12 minutes or less.

**Average duration of all REM episodes.

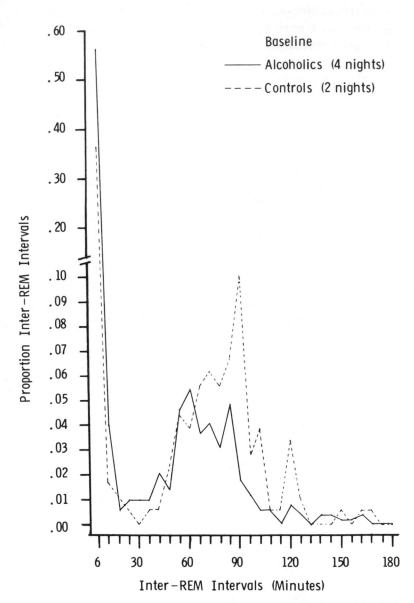

Figure 3. Proportional distribution of inter-REM intervals in 20 chronic alcoholics and age-matched controls. Note the compression of scale in upper half of ordinate.

REM in normal subjects (Johnson and Lubin 1966). The overall discharge rate for GSRs in our controls was similar to that reported by Johnson and Lubin for normal subjects, but the average rates for alcoholics were about three times higher than normal values.

Average heart rates per minute were not different for alcoholics and controls, but average respiration rates were higher for alcoholics in all stages of sleep and during waking, the differences between means being statistically significant for awake and stage 2. Rates per minute of sigma spindles in stage 2 and rapid eye movements in stage REM were not different for alcoholics and controls.

TABLE 4.

Autonomic and Phasic Variables

		GSR Rate (per min)	Respiration Rate (per min)	*Controls* Heart Rate (per min)	Spindles in Stage 2 (per min)	Eye Movement Density in REM*
Awake	$\overline{X}$	1.5	14.0	69.9		
	s	1.2	2.3	6.5		
Stage 2	$\overline{X}$	1.8	15.7	61.6	3.0	
	s	2.0	2.4	6.1	2.4	
Slow wave	$\overline{X}$	3.5	16.3	62.7		
	s	3.1	2.6	6.1		
REM	$\overline{X}$	0.7	16.6	65.7		3.9
	s	0.8	2.3	5.0		0.7
All stages	$\overline{X}$	1.9	15.6	65.0		
	s	2.2	2.6	6.8		
		GSR Rate (per min)	Respiration Rate (per min)	*Alcoholics* Heart Rate (per min)	Spindles in Stage 2 (per min)	Eye Movement Density in REM*
Awake	$\overline{X}$	5.1	17.5	69.7		
	s	2.8	3.5	5.0		
Stage 2	$\overline{X}$	5.8	19.1	66.3	3.0	
	s	3.0	4.9	5.0	2.1	
Slow wave	$\overline{X}$	9.4	18.0	64.5		
	s	2.9	3.2	6.8		
REM	$\overline{X}$	3.6	18.6	65.4		4.4
	s	2.7	4.0	4.5		1.0
All stages	$\overline{X}$	5.5	18.4	66.8		
	s	3.4	4.1	5.5		

*Number of ten-second epochs per minute containing rapid eye movements.

Effects of Two Days of Drinking on Sleep in Alcoholics

EEG stages of sleep. During the two days of drinking by the alcoholic patients, hourly BACs during the first day ranged from 130 to 180 mg/100 ml (mean = 157); for the second day, the range was 115 to 190 mg/100 ml (mean = 159). On day 1, BACs just before bedtime ranged from 110 to 165 mg/100 ml (mean = 145), and on day 2, bedtime values ranged from 110 to 190 mg/100 ml (mean = 155).

The effects of alcohol on the EEG stages of sleep were most striking in the first half of the night. For example, alcohol significantly suppressed stage REM and stage 1 and reduced waking time, while potentiating stage 4 in the first half of both alcohol nights (A-1 and A-2). Table 5 shows these effects. Stage 3 also increased during the first half of each alcohol night, the change being significant ($p<.01$) on A-1 but not quite significant on A-2 ($p<.10$). Percentage of wakefulness was further reduced in the first half of A-2 relative to A-1 but there were no other significant differences between A-1 and A-2. Alcohol effects for the second halves of A-1 and A-2 did not follow a clear-cut pattern.

Table 6, which categorizes all-night stage of sleep scores by age, shows that the relative decreases caused by alcohol in waking, stage 1, and REM were similar for both age groups, as was the increase in stage 3. These changes were statistically significant for both younger and older alcoholics on both A-1 and A-2. In the younger group, alcohol also caused a considerable and significant increase in percentage of stage 4, from about 0.6 percent on baseline nights to 7.1 percent on A-1 and 6.1 percent on A-2 ($p<.01$). However, in the older subjects, the small increase in stage 4 was not significant for either of the alcohol sessions. These differential increases in the two age groups resulted in a significant interaction between the effects of alcohol and age on percentage of stage 4. Thus, alcohol potentiated stage 4 sleep in the younger but not in the older alcoholics.

Other Measures of Sleep and Sleep Quality

The decrease found in percentage of stage REM during the first half of A-1 and A-2 was caused by a systematic increase in the latency of onset of the first REM episode, from a baseline average of 64 minutes (SD = 4) to 110 minutes (SD = 7) on A-1, and 92 minutes (SD = 6) on A-2; both changes being significant beyond the 0.001 level. As shown by the means in Table 7, alcohol also tended (NS) to reduce the frequency of REM disruptions in both halves of A-1 and A-2. Alcohol had little effect on the already shortened REM-to-REM cycle (mean baseline = 67.4 minutes, mean A-1 and A-2 = 66.1 minutes).

TABLE 5.

Alcohol and Stages of Sleep in Alcoholics

		First Half of Night				Second Half of Night			
		Baseline	Alcohol 1	Alcohol 2	Recovery	Baseline	Alcohol 1	Alcohol 2	Recovery
Awake*	$\bar{X}$	13.3	5.3	3.4	16.7	6.9	5.8	7.5	11.3
	s	8.5	5.6	4.0	16.6	6.7	8.7	9.3	19.4
Stage 1	$\bar{X}$	11.2	5.1	4.2	8.2	10.2	8.2	9.7	9.2
	s	5.6	4.4	2.9	5.3	4.4	5.7	5.2	8.5
Stage 2	$\bar{X}$	60.4	60.9	62.6	58.7	55.7	60.2	57.2	53.3
	s	9.3	17.9	13.3	10.0	5.0	9.3	6.8	9.9
Stage 3	$\bar{X}$	7.8	13.0	11.8	14.3	0.8	1.1	0.5	3.5
	s	7.6	10.4	10.5	9.8	2.2	2.8	1.6	5.6
Stage 4	$\bar{X}$	2.2	10.2	8.0	1.5	0.1	0.0	0.0	0.1
	s	4.9	13.5	10.9	3.0	0.4	0.0	0.1	0.3
REM	$\bar{X}$	18.4	10.7	13.3	17.3	33.1	30.5	32.5	33.9
	s	3.8	4.1	6.4	6.0	4.6	7.6	7.3	7.5

*Means and standard deviations for awake are based on percentage of total bedtime. All other entries are percentages of total sleep with waking excluded.

TABLE 6.

Stage of Sleep by Age in Alcoholics

		Younger Subjects** (Age 24-39)				Older Subjects (Age 40-56)		
		Baseline	Alcohol 1	Alcohol 2	Recovery	Baseline	Alcohol 1	Alcohol 2	Recovery
Awake*	X̄	9.3	4.1	4.3	10.7	11.0	7.2	6.4	16.5
	s	5.2	3.5	3.8	9.3	5.4	6.7	6.5	13.1
Stage 1	X̄	10.2	5.5	6.0	8.1	10.7	7.6	7.2	8.5
	s	3.6	2.7	3.3	4.9	4.7	5.1	2.9	7.4
Stage 2	X̄	57.8	57.4	59.1	58.3	58.3	63.3	61.5	54.4
	s	3.3	6.6	6.4	6.8	6.4	11.8	7.7	7.0
Stage 3	X̄	4.9	8.4	7.0	8.5	3.5	6.3	6.8	9.3
	s	3.3	4.9	4.7	6.8	5.3	7.7	8.7	5.1
Stage 4	X̄	0.6	7.1	6.1	0.1	1.6	3.5	2.6	1.6
	s	1.1	7.7	6.6	0.2	3.5	5.9	4.2	1.9
REM	X̄	26.4	21.5	21.8	25.0	25.9	19.2	21.8	26.2
	s	3.5	4.9	5.3	6.2	3.1	4.3	8.2	3.4

*Means and standard deviations for awake are based on percentage of total bedtime. All other entries are percentages of total sleep with waking excluded.

**Means in each column are based on N = 10.

The data in Table 7 also indicate that, with alcohol ingestion, the alcoholics had a significant decrease in the number of brief arousals, an effect that persisted throughout each alcohol session. Nevertheless, the frequency of their arousal after drinking (about 75 arousals per night) remained significantly above the average of 32 brief arousals per baseline night found in the controls (Table 3). Alcohol also decreased the latency of sleep onset on both A-1 and A-2 ($p<.001$) and the number of changes of stage was significantly reduced on A-2, but the average duration of REM episodes did not decrease significantly. There were no significant differences between means for A-1 and A-2. None of the effects just reviewed were influenced by age.

In general, the sedative effects of alcohol found in alcoholic patients were similar to those described by Rundell et al. (1972) in young normal subjects. With moderate doses of alcohol, Rundell's subjects also showed brisk onset of sleep, potentiation of slow-wave (SW) sleep, and reduced time awake. However, the magnitude and persistence of all these effects seem to have been greater in the alcoholics in our study than in Rundell's subjects. This is probably because bedtime BACs were considerably higher in the alcoholics in Rundell's study than in the normals.

Autonomic and phasic variables. As the data in Table 8 show, alcohol reduced the average frequency per minute of nonspecific electrodermal responses in the first half of A-1. These effects were statistically significant for stages 2, SW, and REM, and borderline ($p<.10$) for awake. On A-2, the

TABLE 7.

Alcohol and Other Measures of Sleep in Alcoholics

		Baseline	Alcohol 1	Alcohol 2	Recovery
Brief arousals	X̄	97.9	77.0	74.3	85.9
(total)	s	27.5	23.6	24.9	44.8
Stage changes	X̄	68.5	66.2	62.8	65.7
(total)	s	14.0	16.9	13.6	29.1
REM disruption*	X̄	0.6	0.5	0.5	0.5
	s	0.1	0.2	0.2	0.2
REM duration**	X̄	12.4	11.4	10.9	13.7
(min)	s	3.4	3.5	3.7	5.4
Latency of sleep onset	X̄	31.8	12.3	10.5	34.5
(min)	s	20.4	11.6	10.6	22.2

*Proportion REM offset to REM onset intervals of 12 minutes or less.

**Average duration of all REM episodes.

TABLE 8.

Autonomic and Phasic Variables in Alcoholics

		First Half of Night				
		GSR Rate (per min)	Respiration Rate (per min)	Heart Rate (per min)	Spindles in Stage 2 (per min)	Eye Movement Density in REM*
Baseline	$\overline{X}$	5.4	19.1	67.8	2.5	4.3
	s	3.1	3.9	5.6	2.2	1.1
Alcohol 1	$\overline{X}$	2.1	19.8	84.9	1.8	3.5
	s	3.3	4.7	8.2	2.3	1.4
Alcohol 2	$\overline{X}$	2.7	20.6	83.9	1.8	3.9
	s	3.9	3.9	4.4	1.1	1.2
Recovery	$\overline{X}$	4.2	19.0	68.3	2.6	4.6
	s	3.3	3.7	5.3	1.6	0.8

		Second Half of Night				
		GSR Rate (per min)	Respiration Rate (per min)	Heart Rate (per min)	Spindles in Stage 2 (per min)	Eye Movement Density in REM*
Baseline	$\overline{X}$	5.8	17.2	65.6	3.4	4.5
	s	4.3	4.5	5.7	2.0	0.9
Alcohol 1	$\overline{X}$	4.8	17.5	83.5	2.3	4.0
	s	6.5	4.0	8.3	1.8	1.2
Alcohol 2	$\overline{X}$	3.3	18.8	76.8	2.0	4.2
	s	3.6	3.5	6.5	1.3	1.2
Recovery	$\overline{X}$	3.5	18.8	67.1	3.4	4.5
	s	4.0	3.9	6.6	1.4	0.8

*Number of ten-second epochs per minute containing rapid eye movements.

reduced GSR responses continued as trends $(p<.10)$ except for stage SW in which the reduction maintained significance $(p<.01)$. Average heart rates which had not been different for sober alcoholic patients and matched controls were systematically increased by alcohol in alcoholics throughout each alcohol session and in all states of consciousness. Alcohol had no systematic effect on rate of respiration. The frequency per minute (density) of sigma spindles in stage 2 decreased significantly on both halves of A-1 and A-2, but the density of rapid eye movements was reduced only on A-1. None of the alcohol effects on phasic and autonomic variables were related to age.

Except for respiration, the pattern of changes found in these autonomic and phasic variables is qualitatively similar (though more systematic from session to session) to that described by Rundell et al. (1972) in young normals, in whom alcohol also increased heart rate throughout the night and tended to decrease the density of such phasic events as GSR responses, sigma spindles in stage 2, and rapid eye movements in stage REM. Whereas the present study showed no alcohol effects on respiratory rates, Rundell et al. (1972) found an increase over three nights of alcohol ingestion.

Changes in Sleep Patterns from Baseline Sessions to Final Recovery

As reported above, the sleep patterns of sober alcoholic patients differed in several ways from those of their age-matched controls. It is important to know whether these altered sleep patterns in chronic alcoholics are transient or permanent. A definitive answer depends, of course, on more extended longitudinal studies of sober alcoholics; but data from our final recovery session (R-3), obtained one week after the second alcohol recovery night (R-2), and five to six weeks after hospitalization, may provide some indication of recovery trends.

During baseline (Table 1) the alcoholic patients had higher amounts of stage REM and stage 1 than did matched controls, less stage 3, and a trend toward less stage 4, which was statistically significant in the younger (age 24 to 39) subjects. Patients did not differ significantly from controls on total time awake or percentage of stage 2. Compared to baseline, the final recovery session (R-3) in alcoholics was associated with a significant increase in stage 3 ($p<.01$), and a decrease in stage 1 ($p<.05$), with no change in percentage of stage 2 (Tables 5 and 6). These changes were significant only in the first half of the night. There was no tendency for stage REM to change either in periodicity or duration of episodes, and there was no increase in stage 4.

The poor quality of sleep in alcoholic patients manifested by frequent brief arousals, frequent disruption of REM episodes, frequent changes of stage, and a trend toward delayed sleep onset (Table 3) was not much improved on R-3. There was a tendency in the latter session (Table 7) toward normalization of some of these variables, but none of these trends was statistically significant. The frequency of REM disruption decreased significantly on R-3 in the younger patients (9 of 10 subjects), but not in the older group. Average latency of sleep onset actually increased during R-3. Cardiorespiratory and nonspecific GSR rates did not change significantly from baseline to R-3. The density of the phasic events, sigma spindles in stage 2, and rapid eye movements in stage REM, which had not differentiated sober alcoholics from controls, did not change from baseline to R-3.

Except for the differential trend in the frequency of REM disruptions, younger patients showed no greater signs of recovery than did older patients.

Discussion

Compared to normal control subjects individually matched in age, sober "middle-class" alcoholic patients in good physical health were found to have more stage REM, more descending stage 1, and less slow-wave sleep. However, the difference in stage 4 was statistically significant only for younger subjects (age 24 to 39), most of the younger controls having some stage 4, and most of the chronic alcoholics having none. Our average levels of stage 4 were lower in both younger and older normal controls than are those usually reported in the literature, probably because we used the rather stringent voltage criteria for stage 4 recommended by Rechtschaffen and Kales (1968).

The increased percentage of stage REM found in chronic alcoholics was not caused by longer REM episodes. Epochs of stage REM were shorter, on the average, in alcoholics than in controls and much more frequently disrupted. The increase in REM percentage was the result of accelerated REM periodicity and shorter latencies of REM onset. In alcoholics the average period between REM episodes (not counting fragmented single epochs) was 10 to 15 minutes shorter than in controls, while average latency from stage 2 onset to the first REM period was only 64 minutes in alcoholics compared to 102 minutes in the controls.

The quality of sleep as assessed by the "goodness of sleep" measures of Johnson, Burdick, and Smith (1970) was poor in sober alcoholics. Along with fragmentation of stage REM, they had many more brief arousals, more changes of EEG stage, and a tendency for delayed sleep onset. Surprisingly, however, they did not show significantly greater total wakefulness than did the controls.

The frequent disruption of stage REM, the numerous brief arousals, and the generally poor quality of sleep in the alcoholics might be related to chronically high levels of arousal. Our patients generated up to three times as many spontaneous GSR responses in all states of consciousness as did the controls. This phenomenon was especially noteworthy in stage REM in which GSR rates are normally very low. The alcoholics averaged about four GSRs per minute in that stage compared to rates of less than one per minute in the controls. This potentiation of nonspecific electrodermal activity was accompanied by accelerated rates of respiration in the alcoholics, about 20 percent faster on the average than in the controls. On the other hand, heart rates were not different in the two groups.

In this connection, Johnson, Burdick, and Smith (1970) found that agitation and tremor in their patients were associated with poor sleep. Patients with tremor slept less, had more waking time, more brief arousals, and less slow-wave sleep. A composite measure of goodness of sleep, similar to our measures of sleep quality, correlated -0.62 with tremor and -0.65 with ratings of agitation. Moreover, patients with high tremor ratings had more frequent REM episodes (REM interruptions). It seems likely that the agitated, tremulous patient would also show higher rates of respiration and of nonspecific GSR activity. The average of three spindles per minute found in both alcoholics and controls was exactly the value reported by Johnson, Burdick, and Smith (1970) for alcoholics, but below the approximate value of five per minute found by Feinberg, Koresko, and Hellen (1967) and Rundell et al. (1972) in young adults. The average rates of rapid eye movements in stage REM were similar in both groups to those reported for young normals (Rundell et al. 1972).

Despite relatively small samples with diverse characteristics, the literature on sleep in chronic alcoholics shows considerable agreement. For example, the data from our baseline studies replicate with gratifying specificity the findings of Johnson, Burdick, and Smith (1970). Moreover, our results reinforce the view that chronic alcohol abuse per se is the basis for the grossly disturbed sleep of the sober alcoholic.

Johnson, Burdick, and Smith (1970) and Johnson (1972) pointed out that the sleep disturbances found in chronic alcoholics are similar to those that accompany normal aging. The elderly also manifest more fragmentation of sleep, more arousals, more stage 1, shorter REM latency, and a marked loss of stage 4 (Feinberg, Koresko, and Smith 1967; Kahn and Fisher 1969). Our findings, particularly in younger alcoholics, are consistent with Johnson's notion that chronic alcoholism may be associated with premature aging of the brain.

The absence of stage 4 in the young alcoholic could also be the result of cortical damage. Quantitative analysis of several of our sleep EEG records suggested that the chronic alcoholic can generate the delta-rhythm frequencies of stage 4, but he cannot generate the voltage necessary for that classification. This finding is consistent with the observation of Johnson, Burdick, and Smith (1970) that high-voltage transients (K-complexes) are sharply reduced both in frequency of occurrence and in amplitude in the chronic alcoholic. There is reason to suppose that, although the pacemakers for various brain rhythms are located in subcortical structures, their ultimate voltage depends on the integrity of the cortex. For example, Jouvet (1961) showed that in cats an intact cerebrum was necessary for slow-wave sleep to occur, and Kogan (1969) found evidence in cats that the initiation of high-voltage sleep waves is an excitatory process that originates in deep layers of the frontal cortex. Diffuse cortical damage, particularly in frontal regions, may impair the ability of the brain to initiate high-voltage delta activity. Thus, Feinberg, Koresko, and Hellen (1967) reported a considerable deficit of stage 4 in patients with chronic brain syndromes. There is some evidence that prolonged drinking can cause permanent brain damage. Courville (1955) found deterioration in autopsied chronic alcoholics to be maximal in the dorsolateral aspects of the frontal lobes, and Haug (1968) reported that chronic alcoholics have decidedly enlarged ventricles, the increase in size being a function of duration of heavy drinking.

It is interesting and perhaps important that two days of drinking potentiated stage 4 only in the young alcoholic. Gross et al. (1973) found similar but transient increases in slow-wave sleep in alcoholics in their thirties who drank heavily for four to six days. The data indicate that in the young alcoholic, cerebral mechanisms for the generation of high-voltage delta activity can function if stimulated pharmacologically. Whether the failure to induce stage 4 in the older patients results from prolonged abuse of alcohol or normal aging or both will not be understood until older normals are given alcohol. In a pilot study conducted in our laboratory of three volunteers in their late 40s, alcohol did potentiate slow-wave sleep in two of the three subjects.

The validity of notions concerning premature aging or permanent brain damage in the chronic alcoholic depends partly on a demonstration that the disordered sleep profile does not recover with prolonged sobriety. Our data on this issue are not sufficient, but they indicate that over a period of at least five weeks of sobriety the abnormal features of sleep in alcoholics remained rather stable. Nevertheless, the increase in stage 3, and nonsignificant trends toward improved quality of sleep by the final recovery session encourage the hope that, given sufficient time, the sleep profile of the sober alcoholic may recover to age-appropriate norms.

The acute effects of alcohol are quite different from its long-range effects. Both in Rundell's (1972) young normals and in our alcoholics, ingestion of alcohol was associated with such sedative effects as reduced time to sleep onset, decreased waking time, decreased brief arousals, decreased stage 1 and stage REM, decreased spontaneous electrodermal activity, and increased slow-wave sleep. These effects were generally greater and more systematic in the chronic alcoholic than in Rundell's normals, perhaps because average bedtime BACs were about twice as high in our alcoholics as in his young adults. Our results are not entirely consistent with findings by others. Gross et al. (1973) found some transient sedative effects during the first of four to six days of heavy drinking by chronic alcoholics, but day-to-day measures were variable. Stage REM in that study was profoundly reduced throughout the entire period of heavy drinking, whereas slow-wave sleep showed a transient large increase, then declined toward the end of the drinking phase. During two days of drinking, the Johnson group's (1970) patients showed no signs of sedation. Instead, the sleep disturbance peaked during the initial period of intoxication and gradually declined over the subsequent ten days of sobriety. An explanation of the differences between our findings and theirs awaits further study. Possibly our patients were in better general health than were those of Johnson or Gross. Johnson's patients may have been in acute withdrawal at the onset of drinking. Gross's patients ingested much larger quantities of alcohol each day than did ours, and they drank for a much longer period. In any case, our data indicate that alcohol may have transient "normalizing" effects on the sleep of the chronic alcoholic, and they support the notion that the alcoholic drinks, in part, to correct his own insomnia. Prolonged drinking, however, leads to further disturbance of sleep, and cessation of heavy drinking leads to the acute withdrawal patterns elegantly described by Gross and his co-workers (Gross et al. 1972), that is, a "self-perpetuating disregulation" (Yules, Freedman, and Chandler 1966).

The sedative effects and the transient potentiation of slow-wave sleep associated with alcohol ingestion in both normal subjects and alcoholics are similar to the effects produced by the serotonin precursor, tryptophan (Wyatt et al. 1970, Griffiths et al. 1972). Tryptophan loading probably increases serotonin levels in the brain, and, as is well known, the studies of Jouvet (1969) have strongly implicated serotonin in the mechanisms of slow-wave sleep.

Perhaps alcohol potentiates serontonin production in the brain. Kuriyama, Rauscher, and Sze (1971) found that chronic alcohol administration in mice caused an increase in rate of serotonin turnover in the brain, although there was no change in steady-state level. Further, during alcohol loading the increased excretion of tryptamine in human urine, accompanied by a concordant increase in percentage of slow-wave sleep (Kissin, Gross, and Schutz 1973), could reflect an alcohol-induced increase in serotonin turnover in brain and body. Because of the similarities of the indoleamine and catecholamine systems in biosynthesis, metabolism, and response to drugs, one might expect to find similar alcohol effects for norepinephrine. Corrodi, Fuxe, and Hökfelt (1966) found similar evidence for increased activity of catecholamine neurons in the brains of alcoholized cats. Moreover, when the synthesis of norepinephrine and dopamine was blocked pharmacologically, alcohol potentiated the depletion of brain catecholamines. Thus the transient enhancement of slow-wave sleep found with alcohol may be mediated by increased brain activity of the biogenic amines.

The loss of slow-wave sleep, the acceleration of REM periodicity, the fragmentation of REM episodes, and the increase in brief arousals found in sober alcoholics are remarkably similar to the changes in sleep caused by single and repeated doses of reserpine (Coulter, Lester, and Williams 1971). Thus one wonders whether the biochemical mechanisms for the states of the chronic alcoholic and the normal subject receiving reserpine might be similar. Reserpine impairs the storage sites for the catechol- and indoleamines, releasing them for degradation, and it blocks their further uptake from inter-neuronal pools. Possibly the final result of chronic alcohol abuse is also depletion of the monoamines from brain and body. The data of Corrodi and co-workers (1966) in rats showed that, when synthesis of the catecholamines was blocked, alcohol potentiated catecholamine depletion in the brain. The increased excretion of tryptamine in human urine during alcohol ingestion and the marked decrease during withdrawal, accompanied by concordant potentiation and then inhibition of slow-wave sleep (Kissin, Gross, and Schutz 1973), could reflect an alcohol-induced increase in serotonin turn-over, followed by serotonin depletion during the withdrawal phase. Thus Kissin and his colleagues concluded that their data and the results of animal studies by others were consistent with the hypothesis that withdrawal from chronic alcohol ingestion is associated with a reserpinelike state.

Coulter, Lester, and Williams (1971) suggested that, while the suppression of slow-wave sleep by reserpine might be related to the depletion of serotonin from brain, the associated acceleration of the REM-to-REM cycle might result from increased synthesis and turnover of serotonin mediated by steady-state feedback control mechanisms (Tozer, Neff, and Brodie 1966; Neff and Tozer 1968). Jouvet (1969) outlined a mechanism by which enhanced turnover of serotonin might accelerate the REM-to-REM cycle. On the basis of his studies of the effects of monoamine oxidase inhibitors on the sleep of cats, he proposed that the action of a deaminated catabolite of serotonin might be involved in triggering REM sleep. Presumably the rate of production of such a byproduct would increase as the rate of serotonin turnover increased following reserpine administration. Thus the accelerated REM cycle found in both normals receiving reserpine and sober chronic alcoholics is also consistent with the notion that the two states are mediated by similar alterations in the biogenic amines.

Acknowledgments

We thank Judy Smith, Sharolyn Lentz, Joe Gold, Cindy Coulter, and Robert Ebey for their help in the collection and analysis of data.

References

Allen, R.P., Wagman, A., Faillace, L.A., and McIntosh, M. 1971. Electroencephalographic (EEG) sleep recovery following prolonged alcoholic intoxication in alcoholics. *J. Nerv. Ment. Dis.* 153:424.

Burch, N., and Childers, H.E. 1963. Information processing in the time domain. In W.S. Fields and W. Abbott (eds.), *Information Storage and Neural Control.* Springfield, Ill.: Charles C Thomas.

Corrodi, H., Fuxe, K., and Hökfelt, T. 1966. The effect of ethanol on the activity of central catecholamine neurons in rat brain. *J. Pharm. Pharmacol.* 18:821.

Coulter, J.D., Lester, B.K., and Williams, H.L. 1971. Reserpine and sleep. *Psychopharmacologia* 19:134.

Courville, C.B. 1955. *Effects of Alcohol on the Nervous System of Man.* Los Angeles: San Lucas Press.

Expert Committee on Mental Health: Second Report of the Alcoholism Sub-Committee 1952. *WHO Tech. Rep. Ser.* 48:1.

Feinberg, I. 1969. Effects of age on human sleep patterns. In A. Kales (ed.), *Sleep, Physiology and Pathology: A Symposium*, p. 39. Philadelphia: J.B. Lippincott.

Feinberg, I., Koresko, R.L., and Hellen, N. 1967. EEG sleep patterns as a function of normal and pathological aging in man. *J. Psychiatr. Res.* 5:107.

Greenberg, R., and Pearlman, C. 1967. Delirium tremens and dreaming. *Am. J. Psychiatry* 124:133.

Gresham, S.C., Webb, W.B., and Williams, R.L. 1963. Alcohol and caffeine: Effect on inferred visual dreaming. *Science* 140:1266.

Griffiths, W.J., Lester, B.K., Coulter, J.D., and Williams, H.L. 1972. Tryptophan and sleep in young adults. *Psychophysiology* 9:345.

Gross, M.M., Goodenough, D.R., Tobin, M., Halpert, E., Lepore, P., Perlstein, A., Sirota, M., Dibianco, J., Fuller, R., and Kishner, I. 1966. Sleep disturbances and hallucinations in the acute alcoholic psychoses. *J. Nerv. Ment. Dis.* 142:493.

Gross, M.M., and Goodenough, D.R. 1968. Sleep disturbances in the acute alcoholic psychoses. *Psychiatric Research Report 24*, p. 132. American Psychiatric Association.

Gross, M.M., Goodenough, D.R., Hastey, J.M., Rosenblatt, S.M., and Lewis, E. 1972. Sleep disturbances in alcoholic intoxication and withdrawal. In N.K. Mello and J.H. Mendelson (eds.), *Recent Advances in Studies of Alcoholism*, p. 317. Washington, D.C.: U.S. Govt. Printing Office.

Gross, M.M., Goodenough, D.R., Nagarajan, M., and Hastey, J.M. 1973. Sleep changes induced by experimental alcoholization. In M.M. Gross (ed.), *Alcohol Intoxication and Withdrawal: Experimental Studies*, vol. 35, *Advances in Experimental Medicine and Biology*, p. 291. New York: Plenum Press.

Haug, J.O. 1968. Pneumoencephalographic evidence of brain damage in chronic alcoholics. *Acta Psychiatr. Scand.* 203:135.

Hawkins, D.R. 1970. Sleep, dreaming and clinical psychiatry. In E. Hartmann (ed.), *Sleep and Dreaming: International Psychiatry Clinics*, vol. 7, p. 85. Boston: Little, Brown.

Johnson, L.C. 1972. Sleep patterns in chronic alcoholics. In N.K. Mello and J.H. Mendelson (eds.), *Recent Advances in Studies of Alcoholism*, p. 288. Washington, D.C.: U.S. Govt. Printing Office.

Johnson, L.C., and Lubin, A. 1966. Spontaneous electrodermal activity during waking and sleeping. *Psychophysiology* 3:8.

Johnson, L.C., Burdick, J.A., and Smith, J. 1970. Sleep during alcohol intake and withdrawal in the chronic alcoholic. *Arch. Gen. Psychiatry* 22:406.

Jouvet, M. 1961. Telencephalic and rhombencephalic sleep in the cat. In G.E.W. Wolstenholme and M. O'Connor (eds.), *Ciba Foundation Symposium on the Nature of Sleep*. Boston: Little, Brown.

Jouvet, M. 1969. Biogenic amines and the states of sleep. *Science* 163:32.

Kahn, E., and Fisher, C.F. 1969. The sleep characteristics of the normal aged male. *J. Nerv. Ment. Dis.* 148:477.

Kissin, B., Gross, M.M., and Schutz, I. 1973. Correlation of urinary biogenic amines with sleep stages. In M.M. Gross (ed.), *Alcohol Intoxication and Withdrawal: Experimental Studies*, vol. 35, *Advances in Experimental Medicine and Biology*, p. 281. New York: Plenum Press.

Kogan, A.B. 1969. On physiological mechanisms of sleep inhibition irradiation over the cerebral cortex. *Act. Nerv. Super.* (Praha) 11:141.

Kuriyama, K., Rauscher, G.E., and Sze, P.Y. 1971. Effect of acute and chronic administration of ethanol on the 5-hydroxytryptamine turnover and tryptophane hydroxylase activity of the mouse brain. *Brain Res.* 26:450.

Lester, B.K., Chanes, R.E., and Condit, P.T. 1969. A clinical syndrome and EEG sleep changes associated with amino acid deprivation. *Am. J. Psychiatry* 126:185.

Mello, N.K., and Mendelson, J.H. 1970. Behavioral studies of sleep patterns in alcoholics during intoxication and withdrawal. *J. Pharmacol. Exp. Ther.* 175:94.

Meltzer, H.Y., Kupfer, D.J., Wyatt, R., and Snyder, F. 1970. Sleep disturbances and serum CPK activity in acute psychosis. *Arch. Gen. Psychiatry* 22:398.

Neff, N.H., and Tozer, T.N. 1968. *In vivo* measurement of brain serotonin turnover. In S. Garrattini and P.A. Shore (eds.), E. Costa and M. Sandler (assoc. eds.), *Advances in Pharmacology, Biological Role of Indolealkylamine Derivatives*, vol. 6, p. 97. New York: Academic Press.

Rechtschaffen, A., and Kales, A. (eds.) 1968. *A Manual of Standardized Terminology, Techniques and Scoring System for Sleep Stages of Human Subjects.* Washington, D.C.: U.S. Govt. Printing Office.

Rundell, O.H., Lester, B.K., Griffiths, W.J., and Williams, H.L. 1972. Alcohol and sleep in young adults. *Psychopharmacologia* 26:201.

Snyder, F. 1969. Dynamic aspects of sleep disturbances in relation to mental illness. *Biol. Psychiatry* 1:119.

Tozer, T.N., Neff, N.H., and Brodie, B.B. 1966. Application of steady state kinetics to the synthesis and turnover time of serotonin in the brain of normal and reserpine-treated rats. *J. Pharmacol. Exp. Ther.* 153:177.

Webb, W.B., and Agnew, H.W., Jr. 1968. Measurement and characteristics of nocturnal sleep. In L.E. Abt and B.F. Reise (eds.), *Progress in Clinical Psychology*, vol. 8, p. 2. New York: Grune & Stratton.

Wyatt, R.J., Engelman, K., Kupfer, D.J., Fram, D.H., Sjoerdsma, A., and Snyder, F. 1970. Effects of L-tryptophan (a natural sedative) on human sleep. *Lancet* 2:842.

Yules, R.B., Freedman, D.X., and Chandler, K.A. 1966. The effect of ethyl alcohol on man's electroencephalographic sleep cycle. *Electroencephalogr. Clin. Neurophysiol.* 20:109.

sleep profiles of insomnia and hypnotic drug effectiveness

Anthony Kales, M.D., and
Edward Bixler, Ph.D.

Sleep Research and Treatment Facility and
Department of Psychiatry
Pennsylvania State University
Milton S. Hershey Medical Center
Hershey, Pennsylvania

In recent years there has been an increasing emphasis on using the sleep laboratory to evaluate sleep disorders (Kales and Kales 1972, Kales 1973, Kales and Kales 1974). In our Sleep Research and Treatment Facility which includes a Sleep Laboratory and Sleep Disorders Clinic, we have used a multidimensional approach in evaluating the most prevalent sleep disorder—insomnia. This approach has included epidemiological research, psychological evaluation and treatment, the evaluation of sleep patterns in insomniac subjects, the evaluation of the effects of hypnotic drugs on sleep stages and the assessment of hypnotic drug effectiveness, that is, pharmacological treatment. These varied studies have provided comprehensive profiles of the insomniac patient and of the action of hypnotic drugs (Kales and Kales 1972 and 1974).

In order to obtain a more accurate assessment of the incidence of insomnia in a major metropolitan population, we participated in the 1973 Los Angeles Metropolitan Area Survey (LAMAS) by including a number of questions relating to various aspects of disturbed sleep. LAMAS is a shared-time omnibus survey of Los Angeles County residents, repeated twice a year. It enables research investigators to obtain data from a representative sample of 1000 Los Angeles metropolitan households.

Our analysis of the information on sleep difficulty from the LAMAS survey is only preliminary at this time. The incidence for each type of sleep difficulty was as follows: (1) trouble falling asleep, 14.4 percent; (2) waking up during the night, 22.8 percent; and (3) early final awakening, 13.7 percent. This would indicate that the incidence of at least one of these types of sleep difficulties is likely to be in the range of 30 to 35 percent. Seventy-seven percent of the population estimated that they fell asleep within 30 minutes, while 23 percent estimated that it took 30 minutes or longer to fall asleep. Seventy-nine percent had two or less awakenings each night, while 21 percent awakened two or more times per night.

Our data relating to the psychological evaluation of insomniac patients have been described in detail elsewhere (Kales and Kales 1972 and 1974). Briefly, our data indicate that the majority of insomniac patients demonstrate various degrees of psychopathology either on psychological testing or psychiatric interviews, or both. The most consistent finding in these patients has been the presence of depression, with the characteristics of depression varying from one age group to another.

Sleep Profiles of Insomnia

"Home" vs. "Laboratory" Sleep Environments

While the sleep laboratory is clearly recognized as a rigorous and objective means for evaluating sleep patterns, there has been some question whether sleep in the sleep laboratory environment is representative of that in the home environment. We were interested in comparing the sleep of the patients at home with their sleep in the laboratory across the conditions of placebo-baseline, drug, and placebo-withdrawal. We were particularly interested in the question of whether sleep in the laboratory was more disturbed (even after adaptation) than sleep at home under a given condition.

To answer this question, the effectiveness of a hypnotic drug in inducing and maintaining sleep was evaluated in a study in which patients were recorded both at home with telemetry and in the sleep laboratory (Kales et al. 1973a). The protocol was as follows: nights 1-4, placebo-home; nights 5-8, placebo-laboratory; nights 9-11, drug-laboratory; nights 12-19, drug-home; nights 20-22, drug-laboratory; nights 23-33, drug-home; nights 34-36, drug-laboratory; nights 37-40, placebo-laboratory; nights 41-48, placebo-home; nights 49-51, placebo-laboratory. Two of the patients were recorded at various times during their home periods by an FM/AM telemetry system designed by the Space Biology Laboratory, Brain Research Institute, University of California-Los Angeles Center for Health Sciences (Hanley et al. 1969).

In terms of sleep induction and maintenance, findings were similar in both the laboratory and at home, that is, a marked decrease in total wake time with drug administration as compared to baseline values. There was a suggestion that the two patients slept slightly better in terms of total sleep time in the laboratory as compared to at home. There also was a trend toward a slight decrease in rapid eye movement (REM) sleep on home nights as compared to laboratory nights.

These data suggest that the sleep laboratory does not bias the data toward a greater degree of sleep disturbance. This may, of course, vary from patient to patient or subject to subject depending on his psychological status and personal reaction toward the laboratory environment (Kales et al. 1973a).

Sleep Laboratory Findings in Insomnia

In an earlier study, Monroe (1967) compared the sleep patterns of "good" and "poor" sleepers. He found that the poor sleepers spent less time in REM sleep and more time in stage 2 than the good sleepers. However, subsequent studies of subjects with more severe insomnia have shown that stage 4 sleep is decreased while the percentage of REM sleep is similar to controls.

In our laboratory (Kales 1969b, Kales and Kales 1972, Kales 1972), we compared the sleep patterns of insomniac subjects (ages 21 to 33) with age-matched controls on nights 3 and 4 of four consecutive nights in the sleep laboratory. There were significant differences in sleep latency and total wake time, with these parameters being higher in the insomniacs. There were no statistically significant differences in REM percentage or in percentage of stage 4 sleep. Although the insomniac patients had less stage 4 sleep than the controls, an occasional insomniac patient had a normal amount of stage 4 sleep, thus making this difference nonsignificant. The percentage of stage 3 was quite similar for both groups. Over the four consecutive nights, the insomniac subjects showed considerable variability from night to night in sleep latency, percentage of sleep time, and percentage of stage REM.

Subjective Estimates vs. Sleep Laboratory Findings

One important clinical application of sleep laboratory research involves the determination of the relationship between the subjective complaint and the objective electroencephalographic (EEG) finding. How well does a patient's complaint of insomnia correlate with an actual sleep difficulty in the laboratory? In the sleep laboratory, what is the relationship between the subjective estimates and the objective EEG values? Can the subjective estimates be used to accurately predict the objective data, and, if so, does this predictability hold across different conditions, that is, placebo-baseline, drug administration, and placebo-withdrawal?

Using a criterion of sleep difficulty as being a sleep latency of longer than 30 minutes, we demonstrated a positive correlation between the clinical complaint and the presence of an actual sleep difficulty (Bixler et al. 1973). These data support the work of Monroe (1967) who found, in comparing good and poor sleepers, a positive relationship between a clinical complaint of sleep difficulty and the presence of objective sleep disturbance in the laboratory.

In comparing the subjective and objective data from our sleep laboratory studies (Bixler et al. 1973) we found that our patients tended to overestimate sleep latency and underestimate total sleep time and number of awakenings. There was a significant difference between the subjective and objective values for sleep latency, total wake time, and number of awakenings across all nights and conditions. This meant that the patients were not accurate in terms of estimating the absolute amount of their sleep difficulty.

Although there was a significant difference between the subjective and objective values for the three variables, the subjective and objective data were significantly related; that is, changes across various conditions were in the same direction. Using various tests to determine the predictability of the objective from the subjective, we found that predictability was significantly better than chance but that the degree of predictability was still quite low.

These data indicate that physicians may rely in great part on the patient's complaint of disturbed sleep as being valid, although the patient may be inaccurate in estimating the absolute amount of difficulty. The data also indicate that while subjective estimates move in the same direction as the objective values, they are poor predictors of the absolute objective values. This, in turn, has implications for drug evaluation studies.

Physiological Correlates of Insomnia

Monroe's study (1967) also compared various physiological parameters of the good and poor sleepers. There was an increased heart rate, peripheral vasoconstriction, and higher rectal temperature during sleep for the poor sleepers compared to the good sleepers. This suggests that poor sleepers have a higher level of physiological arousal during sleep and that the sleep of insomniacs is different not only in quantity but also in quality from that of normal individuals.

Aserinsky (1965) has reported considerable variability in the respiratory rate of normal subjects during REM sleep. In association with the actual bursts of eye movement, there is a marked decrease in the rate and amplitude of respiration.

Sleep apnea has been reported to be a universal occurrence in normal infants between one and three months of age. This finding is of critical importance since sleep apnea has been implicated in sudden infant death syndrome (SIDS) (Steinschneider 1972). Sleep apnea in infants occurs most frequently during REM sleep.

The sleep apnea noted in hypersomnia, narcolepsy, and insomnia occurred out of both REM and nonREM sleep and was not related to any specific sleep stage. The sleep apnea associated with insomnia is a recent finding. Guilleminault and associates (1973) suggest that as many as 10 percent of all insomniacs may have associated sleep apnea. However, in 50 insomniac patients studied in our laboratory, none were found to have sleep apnea. This suggests that the incidence of sleep apnea in insomnia is much lower and may be restricted to patients with specific central and/or cardiopulmonary deficits.

Sleep Profiles of Hypnotic Drugs

Effects of Short-Term Hypnotic Drug Use on Sleep Stages

Initially, in our laboratory, we used a standard eight-night protocol (Table 1) to determine whether hypnotic drugs altered sleep patterns (Kales 1969a). The first placebo night allows for adaptation to the laboratory, while the second and third placebo nights are used for baseline measurements. On the next three nights the active drug is administered at "lights out" and the initial and short-term cumulative effects of the drug on sleep patterns can be measured. On the last two nights placebo is again administered and withdrawal effects, if any, are observed.

A number of our short-term studies based on this eight-night protocol have shown that many drugs produce significant alterations in REM sleep. The following drugs, in the doses listed, produced a decrease in REM sleep and were followed by a rebound of REM sleep (increase above baseline levels) on withdrawal: glutethimide (Doriden), 500 mg; secobarbital sodium

TABLE 1. Eight-Night Drug Evaluation Protocol

Nights	Substance	Administration
1-3	placebo	baseline in laboratory
4-6	active drug	taken in laboratory
7-8	placebo	withdrawal in laboratory

(Seconal), 100 mg; pentobarbital sodium (Nembutal), 100 mg; methyprylon (Noludar), 300 mg; methaqualone (Quaalude), 300 mg; and diphenhydramine (Benadryl), 50 mg. On the other hand, the following drugs produced either no decrease or minimal changes in REM sleep in the doses given, nor were they (with one exception) followed by REM rebound on withdrawal: chloral hydrate (Noctec), 500 and 1000 mg; chlordiazepoxide (Librium), 50 mg; diazepam (Valium), 10 mg; and promethazine (Phenergan), 25 mg. However, following the withdrawal of promethazine there was a marked increase in REM sleep on withdrawal.

Because we scored all stages of sleep (often not previously done), our studies also demonstrated that in addition to producing changes in REM sleep, some drugs produce decreases in stage 4 sleep. These included three hypnotics: flurazepam, 30 mg; glutethimide, 500 mg; and pentobarbital, 100 mg; and two tranquilizers: chlordiazepoxide, 50 mg, and diazepam, 10 mg. The most marked decreases in stage 4 sleep occurred after the administration of the benzodiazepine drugs, flurazepam and diazepam. The decrease in stage 4 sleep occurred on the first night of pentobarbital administration, while the decrease in stage 4 sleep with the other four drugs did not occur until the second or third consecutive drug nights. This demonstrates just one of the advantages of a protocol that has several consecutive drug nights rather than a single one (Kales and Kales 1970).

While much information has been amassed from modern sleep-research laboratory studies, we do not know the specific significance of the presence or absence of a given sleep stage (Kales and Kales 1970, Kales et al. 1970b). For example, it was previously thought that REM deprivation led to gross psychological changes, but the current consensus is that these changes do not occur. Thus, at this time it would not be correct to state that REM sleep, stage 4 sleep, etc. are "necessary."

The only clinical correlate we noted with any sleep-stage alteration relates to changes in dreaming which frequently accompany the marked increase in REM sleep (REM rebound) following the withdrawal of certain drugs (Kales et al. 1970b). These changes in dreaming, originally described by Oswald and Priest (1965), may include increased dreaming, vivid or unpleasant dreams, and on occasion even nightmares, particularly if the drug is used in multiple doses over long periods and the withdrawal is abrupt.

Effects of Chronic Hypnotic Use on Sleep Stages

In other related studies we evaluated the effects and effectiveness of hypnotic drugs used chronically (Kales and Kales 1972, Kales et al. 1974). Ten patients, eight women and two men, who were regularly taking hypnotic drugs for insomnia, were evaluated in the sleep laboratory while they continued to use their medication in the accustomed manner. With the exception of one patient who had been taking a hypnotic for only four months, all of the patients had taken hypnotics for one to ten years. Of the ten patients, two were taking single doses of glutethimide, 500 mg nightly, while the remaining patients were taking multiple doses of a hypnotic each night. Three of these remaining patients were taking pentobarbital, one was taking glutethimide, two were taking a combination of secobarbital-amobarbital, one glutethimide and pentobarbital, and one chloral hydrate.

Patients who were chronically taking two or three times the single clinical dose of pentobarbital, glutethimide, or the amobarbital-secobarbital combination demonstrated a continued REM suppression. In addition, in one patient this effect of continued REM suppression was observed with the chronic use of only a single therapeutic dose. Statistical analysis supported the finding of REM alteration by demonstrating a significant difference between insomniac patients chronically taking drugs and those taking no medication (Figure 1).

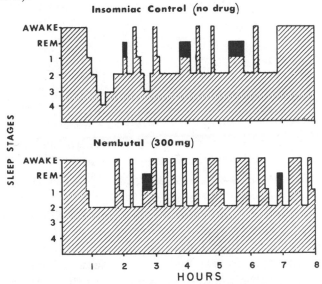

Figure 1. Sleep patterns of patient chronically taking 300 mg of Nembutal compared to composite of insomniac subjects not taking medication. In spite of the multiple drug dose, sleep latency is just as prolonged and there are many more awakenings (12) than in the nondrug insomniac controls (6). In addition, REM sleep (darkened areas) is decreased and stages 3 and 4 are absent in the chronic drug patient. (From Kales et al. 1974.)

It has generally been assumed that with continued use of REM-suppressant hypnotics, the percentage of REM sleep would gradually return to baseline levels. In a previously reported study of two patients who were chronically taking massive hypnotic doses (1000 mg of pentobarbital and 1200 mg of an amobarbital-secobarbital combination), we demonstrated marked and persistent REM suppression. This study demonstrates that with the chronic use of several doses of various hypnotic drugs, a moderate to marked REM sleep suppression can be maintained. Whether persistent REM suppression can also occur with the chronic use of single therapeutic doses of certain REM-suppressant hypnotics needs to be evaluated in further studies.

Evaluation of Hypnotic Drug Effectiveness

A particular focus of our studies has been the evaluation of the degree and length of the effectiveness of these drugs in inducing and maintaining sleep in insomniac patients (Kales et al. 1970a, Kales and Kales 1972). The experimental protocol for these studies is described in Table 2.

TABLE 2. 22-Night Drug Evaluation Protocol

Nights	Substance	Administration
1-4	placebo	baseline in laboratory
5-7	active drug	taken in laboratory
8-15	active drug	taken in home
16-18	active drug	taken in laboratory
19-22	placebo	withdrawal in laboratory

The first placebo night allows for adaptation to the laboratory environment; on nights 2 to 4 baseline measurements are obtained. On nights 5 to 7 initial and short-term drug effectiveness in inducing and maintaining sleep is measured. Nights 17 to 18 mark the end of the two-week period of drug administration, and these laboratory nights allow for determining whether the drug is still effective or whether tolerance has developed.

We have evaluated individually the following drugs and dosages with this 22-night protocol: chloral hydrate (Noctec), 1000 mg; ethclorvynol (Placidyl), 500 mg; glutethimide (Doriden), 500 mg; methaqualone (Sopor), 150 and 300 mg; methaqualone HCl (Parest), 400 mg; and secobarbital (Seconal), 100 mg.

We found that all of the drugs were initially moderately to markedly effective in inducing or maintaining sleep, or both. We found, however, that at the end of the two-week period of drug administration, a loss of effectiveness for sleep induction or maintenance, or both, had developed with all of these drugs (Kales et al. 1970, Kales and Kales 1972).

Effectiveness of Hypnotic Drugs Used Chronically

The most striking finding in the study of chronic hypnotic drug users was the poor sleep experienced by these insomniac patients in spite of their continued hypnotic use (Figure 1). The results showed that all of these patients had as great or greater difficulty either in falling asleep, staying asleep, or both, when compared to age-matched insomniac control subjects who were not taking drugs. Seven of the ten patients taking medication had values for total wake time that were either similar to or greater than those of the insomniac controls. At least one of the three key parameters for measuring hypnotic drug effectiveness—sleep latency, wake time after sleep onset, or total wake time—was elevated in every patient over the insomniac controls (Kales and Kales 1972, Kales et al. 1974).

We consider the continued effectiveness and safety of a hypnotic drug to be the primary factor in recommending its use. There have been very few studies, however, in which the effectiveness of a hypnotic drug has been evaluated beyond several consecutive nights to one week of drug administration, let alone for periods of months. The major implication of our sleep laboratory studies evaluating hypnotic drug effectiveness relates to the need for clearly establishing the effectiveness of a hypnotic drug for specific periods of time.

Drug-Withdrawal Insomnia

We have described a condition to which we refer as drug-withdrawal insomnia, which results from both psychological factors and physiological changes involved in drug withdrawal (Kales et al. 1974). When a patient abruptly withdraws from the regular and prolonged use of multiple doses of a hypnotic, he frequently first experiences marked insomnia, that is, difficulty in falling asleep. The insomnia is the result of apprehension over his ability to get along without the drug and an abstinence syndrome that includes jitteriness and nervousness. In addition, once the patient falls asleep, his sleep is frequently fragmented and disrupted.

Sleep research has helped to explain how altered sleep and dream patterns disturb sleep and contribute additionally to the drug-withdrawal insomnia. If the hypnotic which is abruptly withdrawn is a REM suppressant, there is a marked increase or rebound in REM sleep associated with an increased intensity and frequency of dreaming (Oswald and Priest 1965, Kales et al. 1970). At times even nightmares occur. It should be emphasized that altered sleep patterns and drug-withdrawal insomnia may occur not only when a drug is intentionally withdrawn, but also on an actual drug night when the patient sleeps past the duration of pharmacologic action of the drug (Kales et al. 1970a, 1970b, and 1974).

Summary

These studies suggest the following: Insomnia is indeed quite common and there is a need for improved methods of psychological evaluation and treatment of the disorder. The sleep laboratory is not only an objective environment for investigative studies, but the sleep obtained in this environment is a reliable index of sleep at home. Clinical complaints of insomnia have been substantiated in sleep laboratory studies. Subjective estimates are to a certain extent predictive of the presence of sleep difficulty but not of its severity. Most hypnotic drugs quickly lose their effectiveness for inducing or maintaining sleep, or both. When used chronically, they not only are ineffective, but they produce marked sleep-stage alterations that may additionally contribute to the sleep difficulty by resulting in drug-withdrawal insomnia. Finally, these studies underscore the critical need for extended evaluations of hypnotic drug effectiveness in the sleep laboratory.

Acknowledgment

Work supported in part by NASA Grant, NGR 39-009-204, NASA Contract, NAS 9-10835, NIMH Grant 1 PO7 RR00576-03, and the Foundation for Psychobiological Research.

References

Aserinsky, E. 1965. Periodic respiratory pattern occurring in conjunction with eye movement during sleep. *Science* 150:763.

Bixler, E.O., Kales, A., Leo, L.A., and Slye, E.S. 1973. A comparison of subjective estimates and objective sleep laboratory findings in insomniac patients. *Sleep Research* 2:143.

Guilleminault, C., Eldridge, E.L., and Dement, W.C. 1973. Insomnia with sleep apnea: a new syndrome. *Science* 181:856.

Hanley, J., Zweizig, J.R., Kado, R.T., Adey, W.R., and Rovner, L.D. 1969. Combined telephone and radiotelemetry of the EEG. *Electroencephalogr. Clin. Neurophysiol.* 26:323.

Kales, A. 1969a. Drug dependency, investigations of stimulants and depressants. UCLA Interdepartmental Conference. *Ann. Intern. Med.* 70:591.

Kales, A. 1969b. Psychophysiological studies of insomnia. *Ann. Intern. Med.* 71:625.

Kales, A. 1972. The evaluation and treatment of sleep disorders: pharmacological and psychological studies. In M. Chase (ed.), *The Sleeping Brain*, p. 447. Los Angeles: UCLA Brain Information Service/Brain Research Institute.

Kales, A. 1973. Treating sleep disorders. *American Family Physician* 8:158.

Kales, A., Bixler, E.O., and Scharf, M.B. 1973a. A comparison of home telemetry and sleep laboratory recordings with insomniac subjects. *Sleep Research* 2:178.

Kales, A., Bixler, E.O., Tan, T.L., Scharf, M.B., and Kales, J.D. 1974. Chronic hypnotic use: ineffectiveness, drug withdrawal insomnia and hypnotic drug dependence. *JAMA* 227:513.

Kales, A., and Kales, J.D. 1970. Sleep laboratory evaluation of psychoactive drugs. *Pharmacology for Physicians.* 4:1.

Kales, A., and Kales, J.D. 1972. Recent advances in the diagnosis and treatment of sleep disorders. In G. Usdin (ed.), *The Relevance of Sleep Research to Clinical Practice*, p. 61. New York: Brunner/Mazel.

Kales, A., and Kales, J.D. 1974. Sleep disorders: recent findings in the diagnosis and treatment of disturbed sleep. *New Engl. J. Med.* 290:487.

Kales, A., Kales, J.D., Leo, L.A., and Bixler, E.O. 1973b. Evaluation of the effectiveness of hypnotic drugs under conditions of prolonged use. *Sleep Research* 2:157.

Kales, A., Kales, J.D., Scharf, M.B., and Tan, T.L. 1970a. Hypnotics and altered sleep-dream patterns II. All-night EEG studies of chloral hydrate, flurazepam and methaqualone. *Arch. Gen. Psychiatry* 23:219.

Kales, A., Preston, T.A., Tan, T.L., and Allen, C. 1970b. Hypnotics and altered sleep-dream cycle I. All-night EEG studies of glutethimide, methyprylon, and pentobarbital. *Arch. Gen. Psychiatry* 23:211.

Monroe, L.J. 1967. Psychological and physiological differences between good and poor sleepers. *J. Abnorm. Psychol.* 72:255.

Oswald, I., and Priest, R.G. 1965. Five weeks to escape the sleeping pill habit. *Brit. Med. J.* 2:1093.

Steinschneider, A. 1972. Prolonged apnea and the sudden infant death syndrome: clinical and laboratory observations. *Pediatrics* 50:646.

effect of sleep-wake cycle shifts on sleep and neuroendocrine function

Elliot D. Weitzman, M.D.

Montefiore Hospital and Medical Center
and The Albert Einstein College of Medicine, Bronx, New York

Interest in the effect of phase-shifting of the sleep-waking rhythm in man has been accelerated because of the recent demonstration of important relationships between sleep, sleep stages, and hypothalamic-pituitary neuro-endocrine function (Weitzman and Hellman 1974). The past history of studies concerned with the effect of altering the sleep-waking pattern has emphasized biochemical and physiological changes occurring when the individual was subject to either a 180-degree inversion, partial phase shift, or change in the length of the "day" (Mills 1966, Halberg 1969, Elliott et al. 1972). The use of such experimental manipulations of defined circadian rhythmic processes has led to several general principles regarding differing modes of response patterns to such cyclic shifts. It is clear that a number of circadian rhythmic processes are quite resistant to shift, requiring several weeks for the establishment of an inverted rhythm. The body temperature cycle, urinary potassium rhythm, and the 24-hour adrenocorticotropic hormone (ACTH)-cortisol secretory pattern are examples of such resistant rhythms (Sharp 1960; Sharp, Slorach, and Vipond 1961; Weitzman et al. 1968; Aschoff 1969; Elliott et al. 1972). Other measured functions have been shown to be rapidly inverted or shifted. These functions include urinary phosphates, water excretion, and the 24-hour pattern of plasma growth hormone (Sassin, Parker, and Johnson 1969), prolactin (Sassin et al. 1973), and luteinizing hormones in pubertal children (Boyar et al. 1972a). The concept of desynchronization of rhythmic physiologic function as a consequence of

93

phase shift has been an attractive one to describe the disorganization that takes place during the adaptive transition period to such cyclic phase shifts (Aschoff 1969).

Most studies have also concluded that it is not possible for a number of biological rhythms to establish a new period length which is *much* greater or *much* less than 24 hours (Halberg 1969). Indeed those processes which are most resistant to a phase shift are also quite resistant to a widely divergent non-24-hour rhythm.

It was not until recently that sleep itself, with sleep stage measurement, was incorporated into the experimental protocols of human rhythmic disturbances (Weitzman et al. 1968 and 1970a). The elaboration and quantitative definition of the characteristic sleep patterns during the past fifteen years have emphasized the multidimensional and intrinsic short-term rhythmic quality of sleep itself (Chase 1972). During the past five years, therefore, polygraphic measurements of sleep and the correlative relationships between sleep stages and physiologic parameters have been incorporated as an important part of the experimental paradigms in regard to the effect of phase shifts in man.

During the past five years our research program has been studying the effect of manipulation of the 24-hour sleep-wake cycle on sleep stages, body temperature, and several neuroendocrine secretory systems.

Sleep Stage Patterns

Effect of 180-Degree Inversion and Establishment of a Three-Hour Sleep-Wake Schedule

A group of normal young adult subjects was subjected to an acute 180-degree inversion of their sleep-waking cycle in a laboratory environment (Weitzman et al. 1968 and 1970a). The subjects slept for one week at night (10 p.m. to 6 a.m.) followed by two weeks of day sleep (10 a.m. to 6 p.m.) (Figure 1).

There was a persistent tendency for spontaneous waking to occur in the latter third of sleep during the inverted sleep period. This was associated with a shift of rapid eye movement (REM) sleep to an earlier time. Further evidence of disturbed REM sleep was shown by the increased frequency of interrupted REM and interruptions of REM sleep epochs. However, the basic 90-minute REM cycle persisted during the day sleep period.

In contradistinction to the disturbances of REM sleep, stages 3 and 4 appeared to shift immediately with the cycle shift. These stages of sleep continued to be present during the first two hours of the sleep period after the 180-degree shift, as in several previous studies, which suggests that the

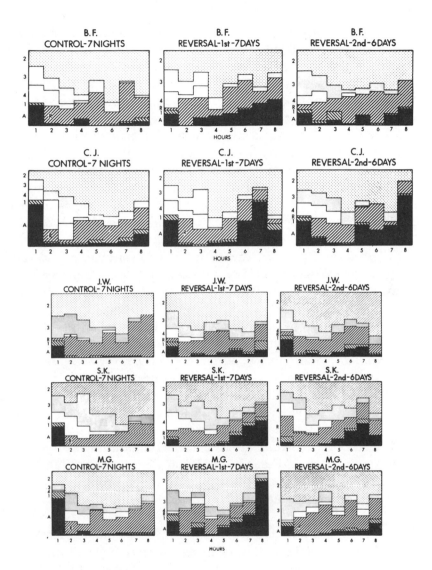

Figure 1. Average sleep stage and waking time proportions for five subjects of 8-hour sleep time available during the control period (10 p.m.-6 a.m.) and the reversal period (10 a.m.-6 p.m.). The numbers and letters on the ordinate represent percentage of polygraphically scored sleep and waking stages; R = REM sleep, A = Awake, stages 1, 2, 3, and 4 sleep.

duration and quality of the waking period may be a factor in determining the timing and amount of stage 3 to 4 sleep. In our study a waking period of 16 hours was always followed upon going to sleep by a similar period of stage 3 to 4 sleep whether the subject went to sleep at 10 p.m. or 10 a.m.

In a second study, lasting a total of nine weeks for each subject, a group of five young adults was subjected to a schedule consisting of three weeks' sleep in the laboratory at night (11 p.m. to 7 a.m.), followed by three weeks of sleep during the day (11 a.m. to 7 p.m.), and then followed by a reinversion of three weeks at night (11 p.m. to 7 a.m.); all sleep periods were monitored by continuous polygraphic recording (Weitzman et al. 1970a). In this study the findings essentially confirmed our previous results that early spontaneous awakening occurred at the end of the daytime sleep periods, with a reduction of REM sleep as a percentage of total sleep time, and a shift of REM time to a time earlier in the day sleep period. These changes were less prominent in the third week of the day sleep period, indicating that some degree of adaptation had taken place. When reinversion occurred, a rebound took place with an increase in total sleep and stage REM. By the second week of the return to night sleep, the nocturnal sleep stage pattern had essentially returned to that found in the control baseline period. Thus an asymmetry was produced by the two reversals. The effects persisted longer in the inverted than in the reinverted three-week period, and no sleep or REM rebound occurred even at the end of three weeks in the inverted period, whereas it was found immediately on reinversion. This latter finding is of some interest since it suggests that even though the percentages of sleep stages had returned toward normal at the end of the reversal phase, they had not made up the "debt" incurred during this period.

As part of our study of the effect of sleep-wake cycle shift on sleep and neuroendocrine patterns, we carried out a study of the effects of a prolonged 3-hour sleep-wake cycle on a group of seven subjects (Weitzman et al. in press). At the end of a baseline week of normal nocturnal sleep with polygraphic monitoring, each of the subjects began a 3-hour sleep-wake schedule which was adhered to for ten 24-hour periods. The subjects were allowed eight 1-hour sleep times (lights out) for each 24-hour period (9 to 10 a.m., 12 p.m. to 1 p.m., 3 to 4 p.m., 6 to 7 p.m., 12 a.m. to 1 a.m., 3 to 4 a.m., 6 to 7 a.m.). Each subject was instructed that he had 8 equally spaced hours of the day available for sleep and that lights would remain out during this time whether he slept or not. The subjects slept in a comfortable bed, in a sound-attenuated room in almost total darkness. At the end of each of the above dark hours, the lights were turned on, and the subjects were awakened if they were asleep. A major change in the utilization of the time allotted for sleep occurred during the ten-day 3-hour sleep-wake period. In spite of the availability of 8 hours of time for sleep (lights out), the subjects slept only an average of 56 percent, compared with 90 percent of the baseline period of 8 hours (Figure 2). REM sleep time was most affected; this was reduced to an average of 30 minutes (11 percent of total sleep time) for the first two days and stabilized at 60 minutes (22 percent of total sleep time) for the last five days of the 3-hour sleep-wake period. In spite of a significant amount of sleep deprivation, a striking persistence of a circadian pattern of total sleep time was evident throughout the ten-day, 3-hour sleep-wake condition. The distribution and amount of REM sleep time was most affected, with stages 3 to 4 sleep least affected.

Body Temperature Rhythm

The body temperature rhythm has been shown to be a highly reliable and stable indicator of the phase-state relationship of human circadian functions (Kleitman 1963). Our results are fully in conformity with past observations that a period of one to several weeks is necessary before a 180-degree inversion of the body temperature will take place (Weitzman et al. 1968

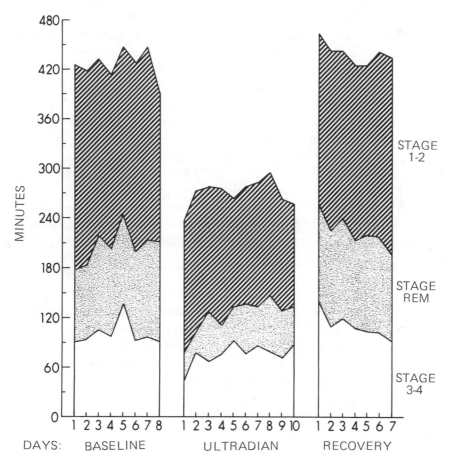

Figure 2. Average sleep-stage amounts in minutes during the baseline, ultradian, and recovery days for seven young adult subjects.

and 1970b). During both the two-week and three-week periods of inversion for the two studies of 180-degree inversion, the range of daily temperature difference decreased. Full inversion of the 24-hour temperature curve did not take place by two weeks of sleep-wake inversion. However, an apparent reversal of the curve took place for the third week of the longer study. The pattern of reversal is of some interest since it was *not* found to be a process of progressive shift of the acrophase (phase at peak of 24-hour curve). Rather the normal monophasic 24-hour temperature curve was changed to a disphasic one, in which the two 12-hour clock time periods showed a differential shift of the mean temperature value; that is, during the daytime sleep period the temperature progressively fell, and during the waking night period the temperature progressively rose.

Of considerable interest is the rate at which the body temperature curve was reestablished following the reinversion of the sleep-waking cycle in the nine-week study (Figure 3). This took place very rapidly—actually within the first few days. This indicates that in spite of an apparent inversion of the 24-hour temperature curve after three weeks of daytime sleep, the central nervous system "memory" of the past, well-established temporal pattern was still present, and, given the opportunity, immediately reestablished itself. This later finding indicates that the evidence of a reversed curve is not necessarily a good indication that the mechanisms producing the pattern are fully shifted in their temporal function.

ACTH Cortisol Pattern

Recent studies by our group, which have been confirmed by others, indicate that episodic secretion of ACTH and cortisol is present throughout the entire 24-hour period, and that the "circadian" or 24-hour pattern results from the temporal pattern (clustering) of the episodes (Hellman et al. 1970, Weitzman et al. 1971). These findings have suggested to us that the temporal sequence of episode initiation appears to be under CNS control as a "programmed" sequence, and that with a stable, repetitive daily life pattern the association of the ACTH-adrenal secretory events with the sleep-waking cycle is part of a general program of biological rhythms.

We have carried out several studies investigating the effect of altering the sleep-waking cycle on the 24-hour pattern of cortisol secretion. In the same studies outlined above, a group of normal subjects was subjected to a two-week 180-degree inverted sleep-wake cycle following one week of baseline measurements, and in the second study normal subjects were subjected to a three-week 180-degree sleep-wake cycle inversion, preceded by a three-week baseline and followed by a three-week reinversion recovery period (Weitzman et al. 1968, 1970a, and 1970b). Both studies demonstrated a

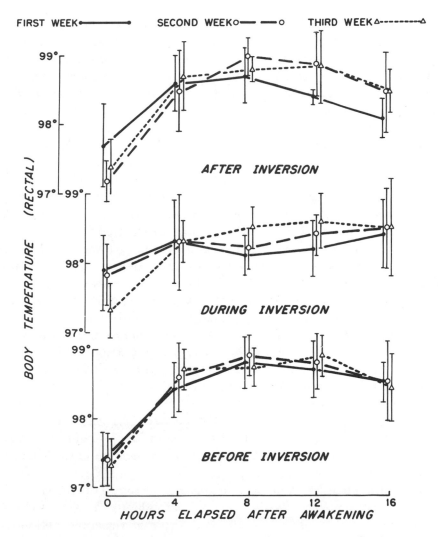

Figure 3. Mean and standard deviation values of body temperature (rectal) of five subjects before, during, and after 180-degree inversion of their sleep-waking cycle. Each value represents the average of rectal temperatures for each of three sequential weeks during the three experimental periods (total of nine weeks) and is presented in terms of hours elapsed after awakening. Time of awakening was 7 a.m. for the "before" and "after" condition and 7 p.m. for the "during inversion" condition.

delay of one to three weeks before evidence of inversion of the circadian cortisol rhythm could be seen. Following sleep-waking reversal, the characteristic pattern of a series of peak elevations of plasma cortisol, occurring during the latter part of the sleep period, was disrupted. Some subjects demonstrated a major decrease in steroid values on several reversed day sleep periods, whereas others demonstrated peak elevations very early in the day-time sleep period. A signficant delay in the reestablishment of the circadian 17-hydroxycorticosteroids (17-OHCS) occurred, and a dissociation between sleep-stage patterns and plasma cortisol levels was present after sleep reversal. Although considerable variability in the 24-hour rhythm of urinary 17-OHCS took place during the three-week inverted portion of the experiment, a rapid reinversion (return to baseline pattern) occurred within the first week.

We also studied the 24-hour plasma cortisol pattern in the prolonged three-hour sleep-wake cycle study outlined above (Weitzman et al. in press). Analysis of the pattern of cortisol secretory activity for both a baseline 24-hour period and the eighth 24-hour period of the 3-hour sleep-wake cycle revealed no significant differences in average 24-hour cortisol output, num-ber of secretory episodes, and total secretory time. However, in the 3-hour experimental condition the secretory episodes appeared to be entrained to the 3-hour sleep-wake cycle. In this 3-hour cycle cortisol output and secre-tory time were maximal for the first hour after awakening, less for the second hour of awakening, and minimal for the third hour, that is, the hour of the next available sleep period. Despite the establishment of this 3-hour pattern, a clear circadian rhythm was also present, with maximal secretory activity occurring between 4 a.m. and 4 p.m., which coincided with that of the baseline rhythm and with the time of maximal sleep. However, the usual maximal secretory phase seen in baseline, between 4 a.m. and 8 a.m., was not prominent on the experimental 24-hour curves. These findings demon-strate the resistance present when altering both the 24-hour (circadian) as well as the short-term episodic secretory pattern by manipulation of sleep-wake cycles.

The 24-hour organization of the episodic secretion of ACTH-cortisol is correlated with circadian events, including light-dark changes as well as the sleep-waking cycle. In order to evaluate the role of visual perception of the 24-hour light-dark cycle in the control of these neuroendocrine temporal events, we recently studied a group of seven blind subjects, all with total absence of light perception (Weitzman et al. 1972). Five were totally blind from birth, one had both eyes removed during the first year of life, and one lost all vision progressively between ages 9 and 11. Utilizing our indwelling catheter technique, we found that cortisol was secreted episodically in all blind subjects, in patterns similar to those we previously reported in normal subjects. Five subjects had a definite circadian pattern of the cortisol epi-sodic secretory events with a lower concentration in the evening and a higher concentration during the early morning sleep period and subsequent waking period (Figure 4). Two of the subjects had an atypical cortisol pattern and did not clearly demonstrate a 24-hour rhythm. However, there was no rela-

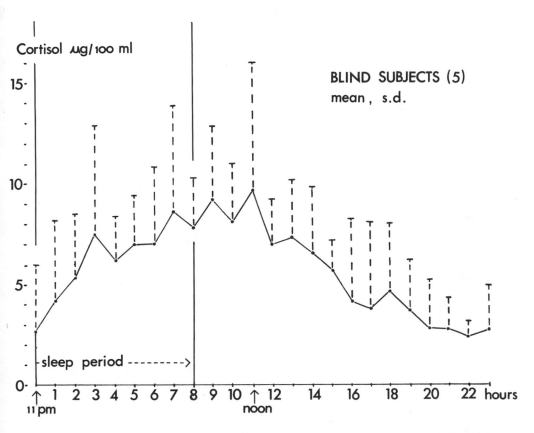

Figure 4. Mean and standard deviation (SD) of plasma cortisol concentrations for five blind adults during a 24-hour period. Each hourly value is the average of three samples taken every 20 minutes for each subject.

tion between the 24-hour pattern, and whether the subjects had congenital or adventitious blindness.

Growth Hormone and Prolactin Hormone Pattern

It has been repeatedly confirmed that growth hormone (GH) is secreted during the first two hours of sleep under normal sleep-waking conditions (Takahashi, Kipnis, and Daughaday 1968; Honda et al. 1969; Parker et al. 1969). If sleep onset is shifted a few hours or prevented until 12 hours later, the release of GH has been shown to be related to time of sleep onset, and no release of GH takes place at the expected time if the subject does not sleep at night (Sassin, Parker, and Johnson 1969).

Comparison of sleep-stage patterns with the time of GH released suggested a relation to the electroencephalographic pattern associated with stages 3 to 4 sleep. In a recent study in our laboratory, plasma was sampled at 4-minute intervals during and for about 90 minutes after the transition period from waking to sleep (Pawel, Sassin, and Weitzman 1972). The polygraphic sleep-stage scoring was carried out for both 10- and 30-second epochs during this time, and correlation was made regarding sleep-stage pattern and the rise in GH concentration. The results demonstrated that the transitional events between waking and definitive sleep (stage 1 and brief periods of stage 2 sleep) were not sufficient to elicit this release. Subsequent to this transitional period, release of GH coincided with the development of definitive sleep characterized by slow synchronous electrocortical activity. It should be emphasized that the presence of slow-wave (stages 3 to 4) sleep is not always associated with GH release since it has been shown that, especially during the latter portion of the night, stages 3 to 4 have been recorded without accompanying human growth hormone release. However, the consistent correlative temporal pattern found in the above study, as well as in other reports, suggests that an underlying mechanism precipitates both the onset of slow-wave sleep and release of GH.

We also studied the plasma GH concentration patterns during sleep in our studies of totally blind subjects (Figure 5) (Weitzman et al. 1972). Six of the seven blind subjects had a sleep-related release of GH; five had peak concentrations at sleep onset greater than 7 ng/ml and the sixth had a small rise to a peak of 1.6 ng/ml. The two subjects with low or absent sleep-related release of GH had the most abnormal sleep patterns. These results differ from a recent study by Krieger and Glick (1971) who reported the absence of GH release during sleep in a group of blind subjects. Their sleep patterns were apparently quite abnormal and may explain in part our different results. The importance of relating the GH response to polygraphically defined sleep-stage pattern is strongly emphasized.

In a study carried out by our laboratory group with A. Frantz of Columbia College of Physicians and Surgeons, we demonstrated that a clear increment in plasma prolactin concentration took place 60 to 90 minutes after sleep onset (Sassin et al. 1972). This initial nocturnal peak was followed by a series of larger secretory episodes resulting in progressively higher plasma concentrations during the remaining hours of sleep, with peak concentrations occurring at about 5 to 7 a.m. toward the end of the sleep period. A rapid fall in concentration occurred during the hour following awakening, with low values reached between 10 a.m. and noon. The pattern of release during the waking and sleeping times was clearly episodic but never fell to undetectable values. We were unable to readily detect a clear relation between the prolactin peaks during sleep and a specific sleep stage. One subject, however, had a delay in sleep onset of about two hours and had

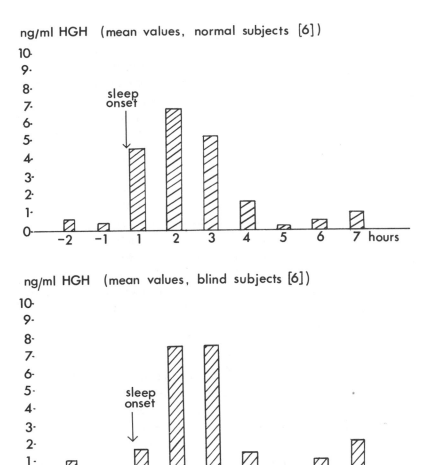

Figure 5. Mean Growth hormone concentrations for six normal and six blind subjects just before and during a nocturnal sleep period. The hourly values are the average of three samples taken every 20 minutes for each subject. Sleep onset was defined by the time of the first appearance of stage 2 sleep.

a similar delay in the initial nocturnal sleep elevation and fall at the end of sleep. Although the initial rise in prolactin after sleep onset usually began at the same time as the GH rise, the prolactin peak occurred an average of 40 minutes after the GH peak. In addition, with the exception of this sleep-onset secretion episode, no consistent relation between the GH and prolactin episodes could be identified for the remaining 24-hour period. Indeed, the episodic pattern of prolactin release cannot be directly correlated in temporal sequence with the other hormonal systems.

We measured 24-hour plasma prolactin levels in a group of normal young adults who underwent partial or complete inversion of their sleep-waking cycles (Sassin et al. 1973). Prolactin release shifted immediately and completely with shifts of sleep onset of 3, 6, and 12 hours. Thus the nocturnal rise is dependent on the occurrence of sleep and is not based on an inherent rhythm related to time of day. After shift of sleep onset, prolactin and GH are not secreted in increased amounts at the time of day in which increased secretion occurred during baseline sleep, indicating that the 24-hour pattern cannot be described as a circadian or inherent rhythm, as is the case for the ACTH-cortisol system.

Gonadotrophic Hormone (Luteinizing Hormone) Secretory 24-Hour Patterns

Several years ago, our research group undertook a study of the temporal pattern of luteinizing hormone (LH) secretion in man, using the technique of frequent plasma sampling over a 24-hour period in association with the polygraphic definition of sleep states during the nocturnal sleep period. We have studied a group of normal young adult men, pubertal boys and girls, prepubertal children, and normal women during different segments of the menstrual cycle.

In the group of normal men we found that all subjects showed discrete LH secretory episodes which were characterized by rapid rises and slower declines in concentration (Boyar et al. 1972b). The initiation and cessation of these secretory episodes occurred within narrow, well-defined LH concentration ranges. Using the 20-minute sampling technique, about 12 secretory episodes occurred for a 24-hour period with one third present during the sleep period. In this group of adult men, we were unable to demonstrate a 24-hour rhythm, nor was there evidence of a clustering of episodes as a function of the time of day. The interval between episodes was quite irregular, and no clear relationship could be recognized between initiation of an episode and a specific sleep stage. Rubin et al. have recently reported that LH values during sleep in men were 14 percent greater during REM periods when compared to other sleep stages combined (Rubin et al. 1972).

A different 24-hour pattern was found in pubertal boys and girls (Boyar et al. 1972a). In both early and late puberty a major increment in LH concentration occurred during the sleep period. The episodes of secretion were clearly augmented during the entire sleep period. In the late pubertal group higher amplitude daytime waking LH secretory episodes began to occur, resulting in a mean LH concentration approaching the adult range. However, the mean sleep LH values were still higher than waking values in the late pubertal group. These unequivocal differences between sleep and waking portions of the 24 hours showed no sex differences. In pubertal boys it was demonstrated that delayed sleep onset to 5:30 a.m. resulted in a similar delay in the augmentation of LH secretion, strongly suggesting that this release is related directly to sleep, like that found with the sleep-related GH and prolactin release pattern (Figure 6).

For the prepubertal children (ages 6 to 11) no difference was found between LH concentration during the sleeping and waking state, and the values were all in a low range of concentration. The exciting developments linking the anatomy and physiology of the CNS biogenic amines in the control of both sleep and reproductive physiology emphasize the need for cross-disciplinary programs in these areas of research interest.

Studies of the 24-hour pattern of LH secretion in adult women are complicated by the changes occurring in gonadotrophic hormones in relation to the monthly menstrual cycle (Yen et al. 1972). The day-to-day pattern of plasma LH concentration has been well documented. Following menstruation the concentration of LH in the plasma progressively rises until the midcycle ovulatory period when the "LH surge" occurs and when peak plasma concentrations are two or more times greater than during other phases of the menstrual cycle. During the luteal phase, LH declines several days after the LH surge, and then low values are maintained through menses.

In order to study the 24-hour sleep-waking LH pattern in menstruating women, we therefore have carried out such studies during selected portions of the monthly cycle (Kapen et al. 1973a and 1973b). During the early follicular phase of the menstrual cycle (first five days), the pattern of LH secretion was characterized by a sequence of 10 to 15 secretory episodes during the 24-hour period. The average interval between secretory episodes was about 120 minutes, and no consistent differences between the inter-episode interval were found between the night and day periods. No major increment in LH occurred during sleep like that found in the pubertal children. There was, however, a significant decrease in the plasma LH concentration during the first 3 hours after sleep onset in all five subjects studied. When the onset of the first stage 2 sleep of the night was used as a reference, an approximately 33-percent decrease in mean plasma LH was present for the third hour after the onset of stage 2. There was thus a clear decrease in LH concentration in the first half of the sleep period of the night, with a subsequent rise in the latter half. Comparison with an age-matched, normal male group revealed that no such pattern could be recognized for the males.

In a recent study a group of five women, who demonstrated the decrease in LH during the third hour of sleep, underwent an acute 180-degree inversion of their sleep-waking cycle during the early follicular phase of the menstrual cycle with concomitant measurement of the 24-hour plasma LH pattern (Kapen 1974). It was found that a similar decrease in LH concentration took place during the second to third hour after sleep onset as occurred during the night's sleep period (Figure 7). Since the shift was an acute one, the results suggest that the LH decrease at night during sleep is not an "inherent," or circadian, rhythm, but again one dependent on sleep. In one woman studied in the 3-hour sleep-wake study, there appeared to be a relationship with daytime nonREM sleep periods and a drop in LH concentration (Figure 8) (Weitzman et al. in press).

During the periovulatory phase of the menstrual cycle, measurement of the nocturnal (8- to 10-hour) pattern of LH secretion revealed again recurrent episodic secretory events during both the sleeping and waking periods (Kapen et al. 1973a). During the time of the LH surge, as defined by plasma LH concentrations greater than 40 mIU/ml, the secretory episodes were superimposed on a progressive elevation of the baseline concentration. In several subjects the presumptive onset of the LH surge could be recognized by an abrupt, large increase in the plasma LH concentration. These occurred in close proximity to the end of the sleep period. On the succeeding night increments in LH values to greater than 40 mIU/ml continued. These findings again emphasize the importance of short-term temporal events in the organization of hormone secretion and the importance of frequent sampling in defining these patterns.

References

Aschoff, J. 1969. Desynchronization and resynchronization of human circadian rhythms. *Aerosp. Med.* 40:844.

Boyar, R., Finkelstein, J., Roffwarg, H., Kapen, S., Weitzman, E.D., and Hellman, L. 1972a. Synchronization of augmented LH secretion with sleep during puberty. *N. Engl. J. Med.* 287:582.

Boyar, R., Perlow, M., Hellman, L., Kapen, S., and Weitzman, E.D. 1972b. Twenty-four hour pattern of luteinizing hormone secretion in normal man with sleep stage recording. *J. Clin. Endocrinol. Metab.* 35:73.

Chase, M.H. (ed.). 1972. *The Sleeping Brain.* Los Angeles: Brain Research Institute, University of California at Los Angeles.

Elliott, A.J., Mills, J.N., Minors, D.S., and Waterhouse, J.M. 1972. The effect of real and simulated time zone shifts upon the circadian rhythms of body temperature, plasma 11-hydroxycorticosteroids, and renal excretion in human subjects. *J. Physiol.* 221:227.

Halberg, F. 1969. Chronobiology. *Ann. Rev. Physiol.* 31:675.

Hellman, L., Nakada, F., Curti, J., Weitzman, E.D., Kream, J., Roffwarg, H., Ellman, S., Fukushima, D.K., and Gallagher, T.F. 1970. Cortisol is secreted episodically by normal man. *J. Clin. Endocrinol. Metab.* 30:411.

Honda, Y., Takahashi, K., Takahashi, S., Azumi, K., Irie, M., Sakuma, M., Tsushima, T., and Shizume, K. 1969. Growth hormone secretion during nocturnal sleep in normal subjects. *J. Clin. Endocrinol. Metab.* 29:20.

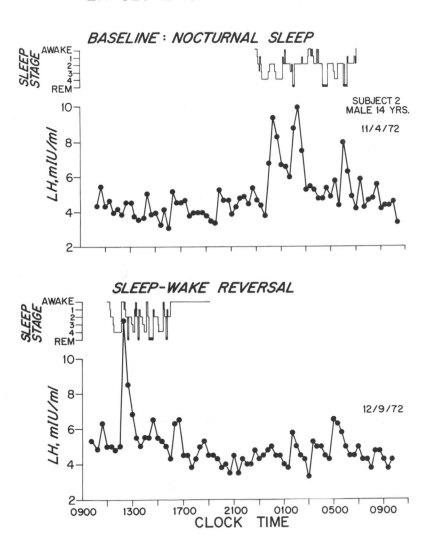

Figure 6. Plasma luteinizing hormone (LH) concentrations and sleep-stage pattern during two 24-hour periods in a 14-year-old healthy pubertal boy. Samples were obtained every 20 minutes with an indwelling venous catheter. **Top graph:** *subject slept from 11 p.m. to 7 a.m.;* **bottom graph:** *subject slept from 11 a.m. to 4 p.m.*

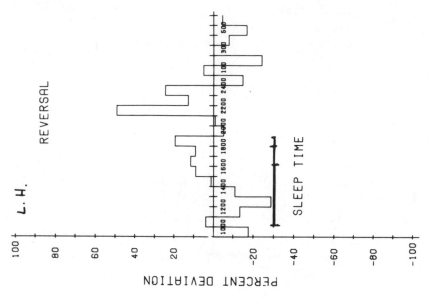

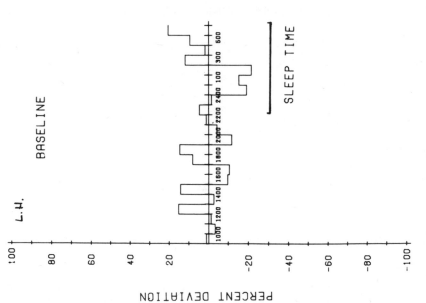

Figure 7. Average hourly percentage deviation from the mean 24-hour luteinizing hormone (LH) concentration for five women sleeping at night (10 p.m.-6 a.m.) and during the day (10 a.m.-6 p.m.). Each hourly value represents the average of three plasma samples taken every 20 minutes.

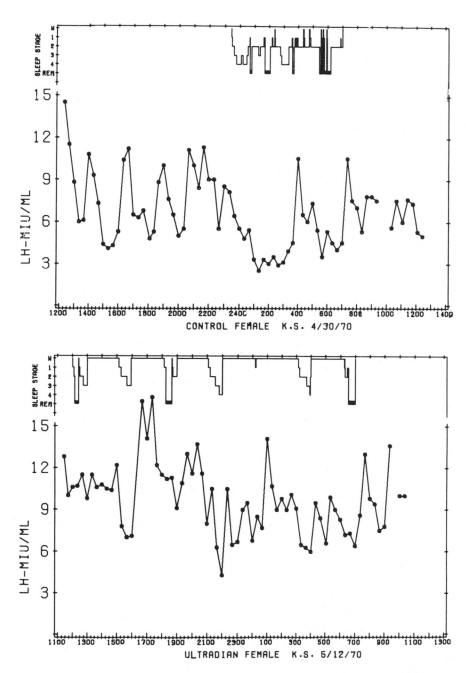

Figure 8. Plasma luteinizing hormone (LH) concentrations and sleep-stage patterns during two 24-hour periods in a 24-year-old healthy woman. Samples were obtained every 20 minutes with an indwelling venous catheter. **Top graph**: *subject slept from 11 p.m. to 7 a.m.;* **bottom graph**: *subject slept during six separate hourly periods. (See text for description of three-hour ultradian study.)*

Kapen, S., Boyar, R., Perlow, M., Hellman, L., and Weitzman, E.D. 1973a. Episodic release of luteinizing hormone at mid-menstrual cycle in normal adult women. *J. Clin. Endocrinol. Metab.* 36:724.

Kapen, S., Boyar, R., Perlow, M., Hellman, L., and Weitzman, E.D. 1973b. Luteinizing hormone: Changes in secretory patterns during sleep in adult women. *Life Sci.* 13:693.

Kapen, S., Boyar, R., Hellman, L., and Weitzman, E.D. 1974. Unpublished data.

Kleitman, N. 1963. *Sleep and Wakefulness.* Chicago: University of Chicago Press.

Krieger, D.T., and Glick, S. 1971. Absent sleep peak of GH release in blind subjects: Correlation with sleep EEG stages. *J. Clin. Endocrinol. Metab.* 33:847.

Mills, J.N. 1966. Human circadian rhythms. *Physiol. Rev.* 46:128.

Parker, D.C., Sassin, J.F., Gotlin, R.W., Mace, J.W., and Rossman, L.G. 1969. Human growth hormone release during sleep: Electroencephalographic correlation. *J. Clin. Endocrinol. Metab.* 29:871.

Pawel, M.A., Sassin, J., and Weitzman, E.D. 1972. The temporal relation between HGH release and sleep stage changes at nocturnal sleep onset in man. *Life Sci.* 11:587.

Rubin, R., Kales, A., Adler, R., Fagan, T., and Odell, W. 1972. Gonadotropin secretion during sleep in normal adult men. *Science* 175:196.

Sassin, J.F., Frantz, A.G., Weitzman, E.D., and Kapen, S. 1972. Human prolactin: 24-hour pattern with increased release during sleep. *Science* 177:1205.

Sassin, J.F., Frantz, A., Kapen, S., and Weitzman, E.D. 1973. The nocturnal rise of human prolactin is dependent on sleep. *J. Clin. Endocrinol. Metab.* 37:436.

Sassin, J., Parker, D.C., and Johnson, L. 1969. Human growth hormone release: Relation to slow wave sleep and sleep waking cycles. *Science* 165:513.

Sharp, G.W.G. 1960. Reversal of diurnal rhythms of water and electrolyte excretion in man. *J. Endocrinol.* 21:97.

Sharp, G.W.G., Slorach, S.A., and Vipond, H.J. 1961. Diurnal rhythms of keto- and ketogenic steroid excretion and the adaptation to changes of the activity-sleep routine. *J. Endocrinol.* 22:377.

Takahashi, Y., Kipnis, D.M., and Daughaday, W.H. 1968. Growth hormone secretion during sleep. *J. Clin. Invest.* 47:2079.

Weitzman, E.D., Fukushima, D., Nogeire, C., Hellman, L., Sassin, J., Perlow, M., and Gallagher, T.F. 1974. Studies on ultradian rhythmicity in human sleep and associated neuro-endocrine rhythms. In L.E. Scheving, F. Halberg, and J.E. Pauly (eds.), *Chronobiology:* Proceedings of the International Society for the Study of Biological Rhythms, Little Rock, Arkansas. Tokyo: Igaku Shoin.

Weitzman, E.D., Fukushima, D., Nogeire, C., Roffwarg, H., Gallagher, T.F., and Hellman, L. 1971. The twenty-four hour pattern of the episodic secretion of cortisol in normal subjects. *J. Clin. Endocrinol. Metab.* 33:14.

Weitzman, E.D., Goldmacher, D., Kripke, D., McGregor, P., Kream, J., and Hellman, L. 1968. Reversal of sleep-waking cycle: Effect on sleep stage pattern and certain neuro-endocrine rhythms. *Trans. Am. Neurol. Assoc.* 93:153.

Weitzman, E.D., and Hellman, L. 1974. Temporal organization of the 24 hour pattern of the hypothalamic-pituitary axis. In M. Ferin (ed.), *Biorhythms and Human Reproduction.* New York: John Wiley.

Weitzman, E.D., Kripke, D., Goldmacher, D., McGregor, P., and Nogeire, C. 1970a. Acute reversal of the sleep-waking cycle in man: Effect on sleep stage patterns. *Arch. Neurol.* 22:485.

Weitzman, E.D., Kripke, D.S., Kream, J., McGregor, P., and Hellman, L. 1970b. The effect of a prolonged non-geographic 180° sleep-wake shift on body temperature, plasma growth hormone and cortisol and urinary 17-OHCS. *Psychophysiology* 7:307.

Weitzman, E.D., Nogeire, C., Perlow, M., Fukushima, D., Sassin, J., McGregor, P., Gallagher, T.F., and Hellman, L. Effects of a prolonged 3 hour sleep-wake cycle on sleep stages, plasma cortisol, growth hormone and body temperature in man. *J. Clin. Endocrinol. Metab.* (in press).

Weitzman, E.D., Perlow, M., Sassin, J.F., Fukushima, D., Burack, B., and Hellman, L. 1972. Persistence of the twenty-four hour pattern of episodic cortisol secretion and growth hormone release in blind subjects. *Trans. Am. Neurol. Assoc.* 97:197.

Yen, S.S.C., Tsai, C.C., Naftolin, F., VandenBerg, G., and Ajabor, L. 1972. Pulsatile patterns of gonadotropin release in subjects with and without ovarian function. *J. Clin. Endocrinol. Metab.* 34:671.

electrophysiological home-recorded sleep study in insomnia

James D. Frost, Jr., M.D. and
Milton R. DeLucchi, Ph.D.

Neurophysiology Service
The Methodist Hospital, and
Department of Physiology
Baylor College of Medicine
Houston, Texas

Since the discovery in 1953 by Aserinsky and Kleitman of what is now recognized as the REM (rapid eye movement) stage of sleep, and the subsequent precise definition of the human sleep-stage profile by Dement and Kleitman (1957), there has been a tremendous upsurge in the volume of sleep research. Physiological monitoring, including measurement of the electroencephalogram (EEG), electrooculogram (EOG), and electromyogram (EMG), has provided a reliable, objective tool for studying the inherently subjective phenomena of sleep. An important practical application of sleep-laboratory research has been the ability to accurately assess the clinical efficacy of various hypnotic drugs. Thus, much information now exists on the effects of hypnotic drugs with respect to both quantitative factors (for example, sleep latency, total sleep time, etc.) and qualitative factors (for example, alterations in sleep-stage characteristics, number of arousals, etc.).

Most investigators of hypnotic drugs have followed a relatively standardized basic protocol. A number of potential subjects are initially selected from the general population on the basis of their subjective complaints of insomnia, that is, prolonged sleep-onset latency, prolonged arousals throughout the night, or early awakenings. Subjects are further evaluated medically and psychologically, and they participate in baseline sessions in which physiological monitoring is used to obtain objective data. Finally, drug effectiveness is evaluated in subjects showing objective evidence of insomnia by continued all-night monitoring sessions. Drug efficacy is assessed by comparison of the objective results obtained during the baseline and drug-administration periods.

Such objective sleep-laboratory studies have yielded invaluable information and have contributed significantly to our understanding of the mechanisms of hypnotic drug action. In terms of understanding insomnia, however, from the point of view of the individual patient, the protocol is in some ways restrictive. In our experience, for example, it is not unusual for individuals complaining of severe insomnia prior to the study to sleep quite well in the laboratory setting. This phenomenon is often recognized by the subject, who reports far better sleep in the hospital than at home. In fact, while noninsomniacs often complain when made to sleep in the laboratory, such complaints are almost nonexistent among the group who consider themselves insomniacs.

In these instances insomnia seems to depend on certain factors in the subject's typical environment, factors that are not present in the laboratory. While these aspects are apparent and have been recognized by other workers, the technology associated with the objective assessment of sleep (that is, EEG, EOG, and EMG monitoring) has, until recently, confined such studies to the laboratory. The study described here was undertaken with the hope of achieving two goals: (1) the practical evaluation of a new system that would permit insomniac subjects to monitor their sleep at home while following their usual sleep-waking schedules and (2) the objective evaluation of the efficacy of an established hypnotic agent (flurazepam hydrochloride) when used in an unsupervised setting, as if it has been prescribed by the patient's physician.

Methods

Frost et al. (these proceedings) described the sleep experiments of the NASA Skylab program. In each long-term flight, one crew member's sleep status was continuously monitored during selected eight-hour rest periods. The flight hardware (an elastic cap containing prefilled sponge electrodes, a preamplifier unit, and a control-panel assembly/magnetic-tape recorder) was designed so that the astronaut could monitor his own sleep. Electroencephalographic, electrooculographic, and head-motion activity were detected, analyzed onboard by an automatic sleep analyzer, and recorded for postflight analysis. A sleep-recording system modeled after the Skylab hardware was utilized in this home-enviroment study of insomnia. The apparatus was easy to operate, and it permitted considerable freedom from the usual recording constraints. Sleep monitoring in familiar home surroundings was done with the expectation of obtaining a more realistic picture of the insomniac's nocturnal habits than might be expected in the laboratory situation. The object was to disturb the subjects' normal routines as little as possible; they were asked to follow their customary life patterns during the study. Each individual decided when to go to bed and when to arise. They had no fixed schedules regarding what to do on any particular night of the study, except that they were required to take the test medication at bedtime each night.

Subject Selection

All participants accepted into this study met certain criteria regarding general health, subjective estimate of sleep difficulty, use of medication (which could influence study results), and objective measures of sleep quality and quantity. Individuals who had been treated with phenothiazine or reserpine in the past, as well as persons with major medical or psychiatric disorders, were not accepted. In the selection interview, the acceptable subject had to estimate that he averaged less than six hours' sleep per night, or that he had a sleep latency of more than 45 minutes. No medication, including oral contraceptives, was permitted for 14 days prior to the first recording night. Each subject underwent four nights of baseline recording. The first recorded night was to allow familiarization with procedure and equipment and was not included in the baseline results. Continuation in the home study of sleep required that during two of the three baseline nights recorded sleep parameters objectively indicated 6.5 hours or less of sleep, or a sleep latency in excess of 45 minutes.

One female and four male volunteers, ranging in age from 20 to 22 years, were selected as insomniacs on the basis of the interviews and the objective sleep findings during the baseline nights.

Equipment

The complete home sleep-monitoring system consisted of three components: recording cap, preamplifier/accelerometer unit, and control panel/magnetic-tape recorder.

The recording cap (Figure 1) was constructed from an elastic material and was designed to fit closely to provide sufficient tension for good scalp-electrode contact. The cap was available in three sizes, small, medium, and large, to accommodate various head sizes. Proper electrode location was assured when the cap was snugly but comfortably secured by the padded chin strap.

Prefilled, electrolyte-saturated, conical, silicone-rubber electrodes were attached to the inside of the cap for recording EEG and EOG signals. Wires led from the electrodes to a miniature electrical connector at the cap vertex. Similar electrodes in the chin strap recorded the EMG.

The preamplifier/accelerometer unit provided initial amplification of the EEG, EOG, and EMG signals, in addition to supplying head-motion information. This unit fastened to the connector at the cap vertex to assure minimal interference with the subjects' comfort. Amplified signals passed through a 7-ft cable to the control-panel assembly (Figure 2), which provided final amplification of the signals, subject-operated controls, and electrode-check circuitry.

The control panel, usually placed adjacent to the bed and thus easily visible to the subject while preparing for recording, contained a series of indicator lamps, each representing one sponge-electrode sensor. After cutting off the tips of the electrodes to expose the electrolyte and after donning the cap, the subject simply moved the panel selector switch from the "off" to the "check" position, activating automatic electrode-check circuitry. A small test current ($0-10\mu$ A) passed through the ground electrode to each recording electrode and was sensed to indicate interelectrode resistance. When a given electrode was in proper contact with the scalp, its average resistance was 50,000 Ω or less, and this condition was indicated by illumination of a lamp on the control panel corresponding to that electrode. Improper contact resulted in no illumination of the particular electrode represented, and this problem could usually be resolved by slightly rocking the sensor to reposition the sponge through the hair and against the scalp.

Subject Training

A few days before the first recording night, the subject visited the laboratory and was fitted with a properly sized sleep cap. Each subject was taught to connect the preamplifier to the cap, to connect the preamplifier cable to the control panel, to prepare the electrodes, to don the cap correctly, and to perform the electrode-check procedure. The subject was then instructed on the proper care of the cap between recording sessions and the technique for refilling the sponge electrodes with fresh electrolyte prior to each sleep period. Following the detailed demonstration, the subject practiced the procedures until he was confident of performing them at home.

On the first day of sleep recording, the subject returned to the laboratory and once more practiced the sleep-recording procedure before taking the equipment home. Although somewhat less than one hour was required to train a subject, this training was critical to successful home sleep monitoring.

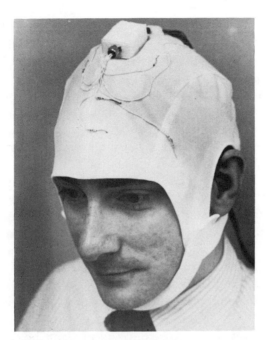

Figure 1. Subject wearing properly positioned recording cap. The preamplifier/accelerometer unit (top of cap) performs initial amplification of signals from the recording electrodes and also supplies head-motion information.

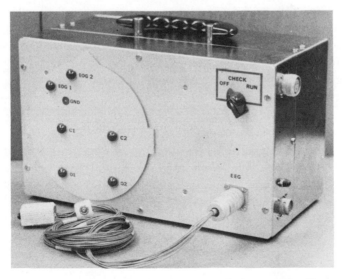

Figure 2. Control-panel assembly used in the home sleep study. **Upper right:** *modeselector switch.* **Lower right:** *connector for preamplifier/accelerometer cable (cable and preamp unit connected).* **Left:** *electrode-check configuration, containing lamps corresponding to each electrode in the cap.*

Protocol

All participants followed the same medication schedule throughout the study. Each night the subjects took the capsule supplied for that night (one capsule was issued each day) and prepared for recording, following the practiced procedure. The subjects were not informed about what kind of medications they were receiving and were told only that several drugs were being evaluated. The first four nights, subjects received placebos, the next seven, flurazepam hydrochloride (Dalmane, 30 mg), and the last three nights they again received placebos.

EEG, EOG, EMG, and head-motion signals were monitored continuously throughout the sleep period. The EEG was obtained using a paired-central to paired-occipital derivation, C_1C_2 to O_1O_2 (International Federation 1958). The EOG was recorded between one electrode positioned laterally to the outer canthus and another located centrally above the eye. The EMG was recorded from two submental electrodes in the chin strap, positioned 3 cm apart. The dual-axis accelerometer associated with the preamplifier recorded lateral and vertical head motion, which assisted in artifact detection.

If the subject decided to arise during the night, he merely disconnected the cable from the recorder and, without removing the cap, got out of bed. The recorder continued to run, thus producing a time reference for the period that the subject was out of bed. Returning to bed, the subject simply reconnected the cable to the recording unit and repeated the electrode-check procedure to ascertain that all electrodes remained properly seated against the scalp; when satisfied that all was in proper order, he again switched to the record mode.

Each morning the recording unit was returned to the laboratory, where the tape was removed for analysis. The unit was recharged during the day, and new tape was installed. The subject returned in the evening to pick up the recording unit and to obtain medication for that night.

Participants kept a daily log of their time to bed and time of arising and also noted their subjective impressions of sleep. Tape-recorded data were played back onto a conventional polygraphic recorder, and all sleep records were scored visually. Results were evaluated using the standardized criteria for scoring of sleep stages as established by the Association for the Psychophysiological Study of Sleep (Rechtschaffen and Kales 1968).

Results

The results of the study are summarized in Table 1, which indicates the average values of selected sleep parameters for each of the subjects. The baseline values were obtained by averaging the last three nights of the first four sessions during which placebo was administered. The drug results are the average of the seven nights when the subject received flurazepam hydrochloride (30 mg), and the withdrawal period is the average of the last three nights of the study, during which the subject again received a placebo.

Objective findings during the three baseline nights indicated that all subjects were insomniac according to the criteria selected for this study in that they either had a sleep latency exceeding 45 minutes or they obtained 6.5 or less hours' sleep during two of the three baseline nights.

Thus, all the subjects were correct in the evaluation that their sleep was inappropriate. However, similar to findings reported by Kales and Bixler (these proceedings), they could not assess in what way their sleep was improper.

During baseline, medication, and recovery nights, these aspects of sleep were determined: sleep latency, total bed time, total sleep time, total sleep percentage, number of awakenings, stage percentage, and REM latency.

Sleep Latency

During baseline monitoring, it was found that average sleep latency among subjects ranged from 23 to 51 minutes. This contrasted with their estimation of their sleep latency, which ranged from 30 minutes to as long as 2 hours. Table 2 compares the subjective estimates with the results found during baseline monitoring nights. It is evident that the subjective estimations of sleep latency were very inaccurate; all overestimated the time required to fall asleep. Table 1 compares the results of baseline monitoring with those obtained during medication and withdrawal. The average reduction in sleep latency was 9 minutes. This reduction continued into the post-drug period, during which time the average reduction in sleep latency was 11.5 minutes (compared to baseline).

In one subject (CD), the sleep latency increased during drug nights (9.5 minutes average increase) and returned to baseline upon withdrawal of medication.

Total Bed Time

During baseline nights, the four subjects' overall average time in bed was only 6 hours and 37 minutes. In all cases, during drug administration, the total time they spent in bed increased (Table 1), with the overall average becoming 7 hours and 20 minutes, a 43-minute increase. The increase varied from as little as 2 minutes to 1 hour and 54 minutes in the average of individual subjects. Upon drug withdrawal, they again decreased the time

TABLE 1. Objective Results

	Subject SS			Subject RM			Subject ED			Subject CD		
	Base-line	Drug	With-drawal	Base-line	Drug	With-drawal	Base-line	Drug	With-drawal	Base-line	Drug	With-drawal
Sleep latency (min)	22.7	16.2	19.7	51.2	27.9	27.9	35.6	21.4	15.0	28.6	38.1	29.4
Total bed time (hr)	6.8	6.9	6.0	7.6	7.8	7.7	6.2	8.1	6.5	5.8	6.5	5.7
Total sleep time (hr)	6.5	6.6	5.7	6.6	7.4	6.8	5.6	8.0	6.2	5.4	5.8	5.3
Total sleep %	94.7	95.7	94.2	86.6	94.1	89.4	89.3	95.4	95.8	91.9	88.9	92.7
No. of awakenings	3.7	3.6	2.3	12.0	7.1	13.7	4.3	5.8	4.7	2.3	3.6	2.0
Stage 1 %	4.5	3.7	5.1	3.9	3.5	5.5	4.6	4.6	7.4	5.3	3.2	2.0
Stage 2 %	69.4	71.3	71.4	65.8	76.7	71.7	51.9	66.3	65.4	60.3	69.9	65.4
Stage 3 %	8.2	6.7	7.2	7.1	2.0	3.9	13.4	9.7	11.2	18.0	8.7	11.8
Stage 4 %	0.4	0.2	0.1	1.1	0.0	0.0	2.7	0.7	0.1	1.0	0.2	0.1
Stage REM %	17.5	18.1	16.2	22.1	17.8	19.0	27.4	18.9	16.2	15.3	18.1	20.7
REM latency (min)	104.1	117.0	146.9	111.4	162.7	159.3	101.6	121.0	128.3	96.4	137.6	129.9

TABLE 2. Sleep Latency

Subject	Subjective Estimate	Baseline Monitoring (3-night average)
ED	?	36 minutes
CD	1-2 hours	29 minutes
RM	1½-2 hours	51 minutes
SS	1½-? hours	23 minutes

TABLE 3. Total Sleep

Subject	Subjective Estimate	Baseline Monitoring (3-night average)
ED	4 hours	5 hours, 36 minutes
CD	5½-6 hours	5 hours, 22 minutes
RM	1½-2 hours	6 hours, 36 minutes
SS	5½-6 hours	6 hours, 29 minutes

they spent in bed. In two cases, they reduced their bed time to less than it was on baseline nights.

Total Sleep Time

Table 3 provides a comparison of total sleep time observed during baseline nights and the subject's own estimate of this parameter. One subject (CD) overestimated his total sleep, while the others underestimated theirs.

In all subjects, the total length of sleep increased upon taking medication (overall average increase, 55 minutes) and decreased upon withdrawal of the drug (Table 1).

Total Sleep Percentage

In all subjects, the absolute sleep time increased upon taking medication. However, the percentage of total bed time spent asleep (Table 1) varied greatly (1 percent, 6.1 percent, 7.5 percent increase, and 3 percent decrease), reflecting the coincident changes in total bed time.

Number of Awakenings

No significant changes in this parameter were noted among the subjects of this study (Table 1).

Sleep-Stage Characteristics

In three subjects, the percentage of stage 1 sleep decreased slightly upon drug administration, while it was unchanged in one subject (ED). In all subjects, the percentage of stage 2 sleep increased upon drug administration. In all four subjects it continued well above the baseline during the recovery nights.

The baseline percentage of stages 3 and 4 sleep combined was low in all four insomniac subjects (range, 8.2 to 19 percent), almost all of this being stage 3. Upon drug administration it dropped further (range, 2.0 to 10.4 percent of total sleep time), with stage 4 being essentially eliminated (average, 0.3 percent). Following drug withdrawal, the percentage of stages 3 and 4 continued to remain well below the baseline.

The percentage of stage REM decreased while on medication for two subjects (RM, ED); it was essentially unchanged in one subject (SS) and increased in another (CD). Upon withdrawal it decreased for two subjects (SS, ED), remained below baseline for three subjects (SS, RM, ED), and continued to increase for one subject (CD).

The number of REM periods was variable, with no consistent pattern.

REM Latency

In all subjects, the REM latency was increased during the drug nights. There was an average increase of REM latency of 31.2 minutes. Upon drug withdrawal the REM latency in all subjects continued to be greater than during the baseline nights (average, 35.2 minutes). In two subjects (ED, SS), the latency further increased over the drug nights.

Discussion and Conclusions

The observed effects of flurazepam hydrochloride on the sleep of these insomniacs were consistent with previously reported studies (Jick et al. 1966; Jick 1969; Kales et al. 1969a, 1969b, 1970a, 1970b; Kales and Scharf 1973; Dement et al. 1973). All subjects experienced an increase in the percentage of stage 2 sleep. In all subjects the percentage of stages 3 and 4 was reduced. This occurred even though their sleep was atypical, in that little stage 3 or stage 4 was observed during the baseline sleep nights. The REM latency was increased above baseline for all subjects, while the effect upon REM time and the number of REMs was inconsistent.

Excessive sleep latency and insufficient total sleep were the primary complaints of those who volunteered for this home study. The test medication clearly modified these sleep shortcomings, as illustrated in Figures 3 and

4, which comprise the plots of sleep stage versus time for two subjects during baseline, medication, and postmedication nights.

This home-recorded sleep study revealed an important aspect of an insomniac's sleep difficulty which would not have been disclosed in a laboratory study in which fixed bedtimes are typical. When the subjects were permitted to follow their customary sleep habits, they spent far less than 8 hours in bed. They usually went to bed very late, even though they had to arise in the morning to meet their daily commitments, and complained of feeling tired upon getting up. In home surroundings the insomniac may lack sleep discipline; that is, he finds it easy to avoid going to bed and tends to do things other than lie in bed until sleep comes.

It has been our experience that subjects frequently state that they sleep better in the laboratory than they do at home. They express surprise and

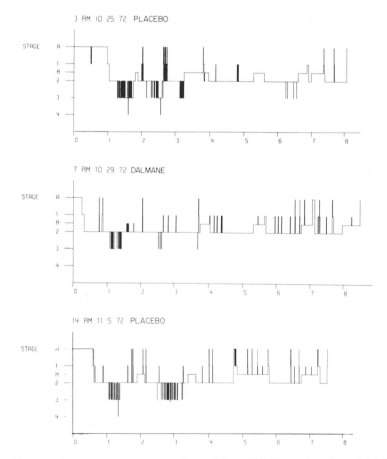

Figure 3. Plots of sleep stage versus time for subject RM. **Upper** tracing: *night 3, placebo administration.* **Center** tracing: *night 7, Dalmane administration.* **Lower** tracing: *night 14, placebo administration.*

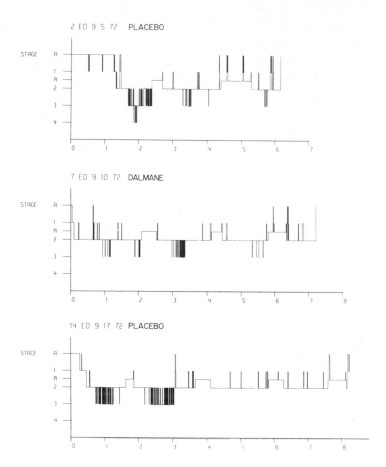

Figure 4. Plots of sleep stage versus time for subject ED. **Upper** tracing: *night 2, placebo administration.* **Center** tracing: *night 7, Dalmane administration.* **Lower** tracing: *night 14, placebo administration.*

indicate that they really thought they would have difficulty sleeping with electrodes attached to their scalp and lead wires going to the EEG head-board. On two occasions, subjects telephoned us a few days following the conclusion of sleep monitoring in our laboratory to tell us that since they were home they were once again having sleep difficulties. It is not un-common to have insomniac subjects say that they have a greater sense of security in the laboratory than at home. Apparently they are not aware of the feeling of insecurity before their monitoring sessions in the laboratory; at that time they realize that their sleep is considerably better than at home, and they try to account for the change.

Sleep monitoring in the home environment by the sleep subject himself is a practical technique. It must, of course, be used selectively, when consideration of the home environment and the individual's sleep habits is required in assessing his sleep problem. Home sleep recording has inherent special requirements and potential shortcomings. The subject must master the recording procedures and must follow instructions carefully. Since a technician is not present through the night, a technical problem with the monitoring apparatus may not be discovered until morning. During our study we lost few data because of such problems; in all, we had two data-loss periods (totaling less than 3 hours) in 66 recording nights.

Appropriate equipment and proper protocol design consequently provide a useful method for examining sleep in various environments which may affect the objective measure of sleep.

References

Aserinsky, E., and Kleitman, N. 1953. Regularly occurring periods of eye motility and concomitant phenomena during sleep. *Science* 118:273.

Dement, W., and Kleitman, N. 1957. The relation of eye movements during sleep to dream activity: an objective method for the study of dreaming. *J. Exp. Psychol.* 53:339.

Dement, W.C., Zarcone, V.P., Hoddes, E., Smythe, H., and Carskadon, M. 1973. Sleep laboratory and clinical studies with flurazepam. In S. Garattini, E. Mussini, and L.O. Randall (eds.), *The Benzodiazepines*, p. 599. New York: Raven Press.

Jick, H. 1969. Clinical evaluation of hypnotics. In A. Kales (ed.), *Sleep: Physiology and Pathology*, p. 289. Philadelphia: J.B. Lippincott.

Jick, H., Slone, D., Dinan, B. and Muench, H. 1966. Evaluation of drug efficiency by a preference technic. *N. Engl. J. Med.* 275:1399.

Kales, A., Allen, C., Scharf, M.B., and Kales, J.D. 1970a. Hypnotic drugs and their effectiveness. All-night EEG studies of insomniac subjects. *Arch. Gen. Psychiatry* 23:226.

Kales, A., Kales, J.D., Scharf, M.B., and Tan, T.-L. 1970b. Hypnotics and altered sleep-dream patterns. II. All-night EEG studies of chloral hydrate, flurazepam, and methaqualone. *Arch. Gen. Psychiatry* 23:219.

Kales, A., Ling Tan, T., Scharf, M., Kales, J., and Malmstrom, E. 1969a. Effects of long and short term administration of flurazepam (Dalmane) in subjects with insomnia. *Psychophysiology* 6:260.

Kales, A., Malmstrom, E.J., Scharf, M.B., and Rubin, R.T. 1969b. Psychophysiological and biochemical changes following use and withdrawal of hypnotics. In A. Kales (ed.), *Sleep: Physiology and Pathology*, p. 331. Philadelphia: J.B. Lippincott.

Kales, A., and Scharf, M.B. 1973. Sleep laboratory and clinical studies of the effects of benzodiazepines on sleep: flurazepam, diazepam, chlordiazepoxide, and RO 5-4200. In S. Garattini, E. Mussini, and L.O. Randall (eds.), *The Benzodiazepines*, p. 577. New York: Raven Press.

Rechtschaffen, A., and Kales, A. (eds.). 1968. *A Manual of Standardized Terminology, Techniques and Scoring System for Sleep Stages of Human Subjects*. Washington, D.C.: Public Health Service, U.S. Govt. Printing Office.

The ten twenty electrode system of the International Federation 1958. *Electroencephalogr. Clin. Neurophysiol.* 10:371.

parameter selection and optimization in brain wave research

Bernard Saltzberg, Ph.D.

Department of Psychiatry and Neurology
Tulane University School of Medicine
New Orleans, Louisiana

The increasingly important role of mathematical methods and computer analysis in brain wave research has created an urgent need to effectively communicate mathematical and computational concepts to neurophysiologists and other medical investigators engaged in behavioral and clinical research. I hope this paper will partly serve that need. The material presented is not intended as a mathematically rigorous treatment of parameter abstraction, but rather as a neurophysiologically motivated introduction to the mathematical notions underlying the selection and measurement of certain parameters. The ultimate objective is the correlation of these parameters with neurophysiological factors as a basis for studying the electrical activity of the brain and behavior.

As a consequence of the many properties of brain electrical activity that can be quantified, a problem of central concern in electroencephalographic research is the selection and effective measurement of those properties of the EEG which are most likely to correlate with behavior, clinical states, or physiological factors. In the context of this paper, any quantifiable property of electrophysiological signal activity is defined as a parameter. To emphasize the broad meaning of the words "parameter selection" in the title, the values of power spectral density (PSD) at a set of discrete frequencies constitute a set of parameters, and the parameter selection problem may simply be one of choosing particular subsets of frequencies which experience suggests are clinically useful. For example, in some experimental designs, one might sum the PSD values over frequencies in the range of 8 to 12 Hz and monitor the energy in that band to provide a single tracking parameter to be correlated with the state of the subject. In other investigations, it may be desirable to study all the lines in the complex spectrum, or it may be desirable to reduce the parameter space by summing the PSD over different subsets of lines in the spectrum as a means of monitoring the division of signal energy among the familiar delta, theta, alpha, and beta frequency bands. In still other experimental designs, spectral-moment parameters or period-analytic parameters are useful for monitoring long-term changes in state, while time-lag parameters or parameters which describe transient events in the EEG might be more appropriate in evoked potential studies. In summary, the choice of relevant parameters in the analysis of brain electrical activity is determined by (1) the experimental design and the hypotheses to be tested, (2) historical experience with such data, and (3) the ease and accuracy with which the parameter can be computed given the limitations of measurement and the presence of noise. At another level, not addressed in this paper, a set of candidate parameters can be evaluated by multivariate statistical procedures to determine which of these parameters possess the greatest discriminating power. This paper, however, is addressed to the problems involved in the measurement and computation of selected parameters.

Unfortunately, there are no universal methods for selecting parameters, and there are no general methods for optimizing their determination. However, a few examples can go a long way in illustrating the essential nature of this problem and the types of constraints that limit accuracy and dictate trade-offs in the optimization process. The optimization problem refers to the best methods for obtaining a parameter where "best" is defined with respect to some criterion or set of criteria. In such optimization problems, it is essential to understand the constraints on the data and the kinds of trade-offs that result when several criteria are involved and/or when the experiment limits the data base. For example, in spectral analysis, if one wishes to determine accurately *when* a particular frequency is present and also determine accurately *how much* of that frequency is present in the data, then trade-offs must be considered as a result of the conflict in these requirements. The problems associated with the optimization of spectral parameters are treated in great detail in the standard literature on this subject and will not be discussed here. This paper will attempt to discuss a number of specific EEG parameters and evoked potential parameters which are useful in a broad range of experimental designs requiring the analysis of brain electrical activity. Sections 2, 3, and 4 are primarily concerned with parameters that arise in the context of evoked potential studies. Sections 4, 5, and 6 are primarily concerned with parameters which reveal statistical properties of single-channel and multiple-channel EEG recordings.

1. Optimization of Latency Determination

A parameter of interest in EEG evoked potential (EP) studies is the latency of certain events such as peaks in the response. Frequently it is desired to test a hypothesis concerned with causally relating a change in latency to an altered physiological or behavioral state of the subject. In order to test such a hypothesis it is essential that the inherent variability in latency due to background random activity (noise) be determined. This knowledge is essential in experimental designs where one wishes to test the significance of a shift in average evoked potential (AEP) latency due to an altered experimental state or the significance of the latency differences among subjects. This section deals with an analysis of the factors governing latency variability due to noise and the determination of the type of filtering that will decrease the variability (that is, increase precision).

The analysis goes along the following lines: Assume a noise-free version of the EP is available and designate this as

$$y(t_i) = \text{value of the noise-free EP at time } t_i \qquad (1)$$

Also let

$$S(t_i) = \text{value of the EP at time } t_i \text{ in the presence of additive noise,} \qquad (2)$$
so that (2) may be written

$$S(t_i) = y(t_i) + n(t_i) \qquad (3)$$

where

$$n(t_i) = \text{noise value at time } t_i \qquad (4)$$

The error in lag (or latency) can be determined by shifting $y(t)$ by some amount τ until a best fit (in the least squares sense) is obtained between y and S. This is accomplished by choosing τ so that the following sum of squared differences, Q, is minimized:

$$Q = \sum_{i=1}^{k} [S(t_i) - y(t_i + \tau)]^2 \qquad (5)$$

By substituting $S(t_i) = y(t_i) + n(t_i)$ into *(5)* and noting that for small τ we may approximate $y(t_i + \tau)$ as a linear function of τ, viz.:

$$y(t_i+\tau) = y(t_i) + \frac{\partial y(t_i)}{\partial t_i} \tau \tag{6}$$

then *(5)* becomes

$$Q = \sum_{i=1}^{k} [n(t_i) - \frac{\partial y(t_i)}{\partial t_i} \tau]^2 \tag{7}$$

The value of τ which minimizes *(7)* is determined by setting $\dfrac{\partial Q}{\partial \tau} = O$, which yields:

$$\tau = \frac{\displaystyle\sum_{i=1}^{k} n(t_i) \frac{\partial y}{\partial t_i}}{\displaystyle\sum_{i=1}^{k} (\frac{\partial y}{\partial t_i})^2} \tag{8}$$

The mean or expected value of τ is zero since the expected value of the noise is assumed to be zero, and if it is further assumed that the noise samples are uncorrelated, then the ensemble variance (expected value of τ^2) can be simplified, viz.:

$$\sigma_\tau^2 = \frac{\displaystyle\sum_{i=1}^{k} n^2(t_i)}{\displaystyle\sum_{i=1}^{k} (\frac{\partial y}{\partial t_i})^2} \tag{9}$$

This expression says that places on the AEP where the derivative is large make the smallest contribution to the error in latency, which is intuitively quite reasonable. An alternate form of *(9)* is desirable in considering methods of modifying the EP input data (that is, determining an optimum filter) to reduce the latency error. Noting that

$$\sum_{i=1}^{k} n^2(t_i) = \int_\Omega P_n(\omega)\, d\omega \tag{10}$$

and

$$\sum_{i=1}^{k} \left(\frac{\partial y}{\partial t_i}\right)^2 = \int_{\Omega} \omega^2 P_s(\omega)\, d\omega \tag{11}$$

where

$P_n(\omega)$ = power spectral density of the noise

and

$P_s(\omega)$ = power spectral density of the signal

$\omega^2 P_s(\omega)$ = power spectral density of the derivative of the signal

and substituting *(10)* and *(11)* into *(9)* gives

$$\sigma_T^2 = \frac{\int_{\Omega} P_n(\omega)\, d\omega}{\int_{\Omega} \omega^2 P_s(\omega)\, d\omega} \tag{12}$$

We now introduce a filter which modifies the PSD by a factor $H(\omega)$ and the resulting postfiltered variance is

$$\sigma_T^2 = \frac{\int_{\Omega} P_n(\omega) H(\omega)\, d\omega}{\int_{\Omega} \omega^2 P_s(\omega) H(\omega)\, d\omega} \tag{13}$$

The $H(\omega)$ which minimizes the variance corresponds to a "notch" filter at a frequency, ω_o, where the function $P_n(\omega)/\omega^2 P_s(\omega)$ has an absolute minimum. Thus ω_o is a root of the equation:

$$\frac{d}{d\omega} \left[\frac{P_n(\omega)}{\omega^2 P_s(\omega)} \right] = 0 \tag{14}$$

Therefore, an approximation to the variance after optimum filtering is given by

$$\sigma_T{}^2 = \frac{P_n(\omega_0)}{\omega_0{}^2 P_s(\omega_0)} \tag{15}$$

The standard deviation, σ_T, is

$$\sigma_T = \frac{1}{\omega_0}\sqrt{\frac{P_n(\omega_0)}{P_s(\omega_0)}} \tag{16}$$

For illustration, consider a single EP with a minimum noise-to-signal ratio of two in the vicinity of 5 Hz which is reduced by a factor of eight by averaging 64 replications. In this situation, the error in latency due to noise is

$$\sigma_T = \frac{\sqrt{2}}{2\pi \times 5 \times 8}\ \text{sec} = 5.6\ \text{msec} \tag{17}$$

Therefore, to be biologically or clinically significant, a shift in latency would need to be large compared to 5.6 msec. It should be noted that without optimization, the standard error in latency would be determined by the average noise-to-signal ratio over all frequencies. In many applications, the EP is imbedded in large average noise backgrounds compared to the optimally filtered EP, and therefore a much larger number of replications would be necessary to reduce the latency error in the case of averaging without filtering. Increasing the number of replications, however, increases the time to complete the experiment and sometimes this presents problems because it may be difficult to maintain the constancy of a given experimental state over long periods of stimulation.

The following examples illustrate how one may determine the center frequency of the optimum filter analytically, given the functional form of the noise PSD and the signal PSD.

Example 1:

Given

$$P_n = \text{constant} > 0$$
$$P_s \propto \omega \, (\omega_1 - \omega)$$
$$\left. \right\} \quad 0 < \omega < \omega_1$$

$$P_n = P_s = 0 \qquad \text{outside } (0, \, \omega_1)$$

In accordance with *(14)*, the center frequency is a root of:

$$\frac{d}{d\omega} \left[\frac{1}{\omega^3 \, (\omega_1 - \omega)} \right] = 0$$

which gives,

$$\omega_o = 3/4 \, \omega_1$$

Example 2:

Given

$$P_s \propto e^{-\omega/\omega_s}$$
$$P_n = \text{constant} > 0$$
$$\left. \right\} \quad 0 < \omega < \omega_1$$

$$P_s = P_n = 0 \qquad \text{outside } (0, \, \omega_1)$$

The center frequency is a root of:

$$\frac{d}{d\omega} \left[\frac{1}{\omega^2 e^{-\omega/\omega_s}} \right] = 0$$

which gives

$$\omega_o = 2\omega_s$$

Example 3:

Given

$$P_n \propto \omega^a$$

$$P_s \propto \omega^b (\omega_1 - \omega)$$

$$\left.\begin{matrix}\\ \\ \end{matrix}\right\} \quad 0 < \omega < \omega_1$$

$$P_n = P_s = 0 \qquad\qquad \text{outside } (0, \omega_1)$$

The center frequency is a root of:

$$\frac{d}{d\omega}\left[\frac{\omega^a}{\omega^{b+2}(\omega_1 - \omega)}\right] = 0$$

which gives

$$\omega_0 = \frac{b-a+2}{b-a+3} \cdot \omega_1$$

The following example illustrates how one may proceed from experimental data. The case illustrated is taken from an EEG evoked potential study, and the specific steps in the filter design are outlined using the experimental data from this study. First, compute the PSD of the EEG background as shown in Figure 1a. Then obtain the derivative of the AEP and compute its PSD. (The unfiltered AEP represents our best estimate of the noise-free EP.) Examining Figures 1a and 1b, select a small portion of the spectrum where the ratio of intensities is smallest. This occurs at about 3 Hz in this example. We then select a filter which consists of one cycle of a 3-Hz sine wave which is convolved with the EP to obtain a response which is optimized for minimum latency error. Figure 2a shows a single EP before filtering to optimize latency determination, and Figure 2b shows the same response after filtering to optimize the measurement of latency.

2. Parameters That Arise in the Analysis of Overlapping Evoked Potentials

This section will describe two methods for studying overlapping evoked reponses. In the first method, the parameters will be derived from a regression model, and in the second method, the parameters will be derived by a deconvolution approach involving a procedure known as cepstral smoothing.

In studies directed to questions concerning the nervous system's ability to resolve closely spaced stimuli, experiments are frequently conducted that give rise to overlapping evoked responses. The two approaches described are easily generalized to any number of overlapping identical responses, but for simplicity the methods will be described for the case of two responses.

The first method assumes that the response to a single stimulus is known and that the response to a stimulus pair is the superposition of the known response to a single stimulus, plus a time-delayed and attenuated version of this known response. In AEP experiments, if the successive stimuli are presented with sufficient separation in time so that the response to a stimulus is over before its successor is applied, then this is called a single-stimulus AEP. In the paired-stimulus AEP, the response to the first stimulus of the pair is still going on at the time the next stimulus is applied. In the second method (the cepstral smoothing approach) the single-stimulus response need not be known. All that is necessary is that the shape of the initial response and the time-delayed response be identical.

Method 1:

For investigations in which the single-stimulus response is assumed known, useful parameters can sometimes be simply obtained from a regression analysis model.

The experiment usually involves a pattern of stimulation consisting of periodic short bursts of closely spaced stimulus events such as a pair of sharp

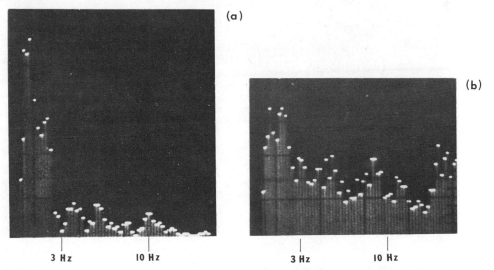

Figure 1. (a) Power spectral density (PSD) of EEG background. (b) PSD of signal derivative.

clicks (say, 50 msec apart) presented every two seconds. In these investigations the separation between the paired stimuli is varied until the pattern of paired stimulation produces an AEP that is indistinguishable from the AEP due to single stimulation, holding the interstimulus interval constant; two seconds in the example mentioned. The analysis usually includes comparison of the shape of the single-stimulus AEP against the paired-stimulus AEP by several methods. When the separation between the paired-stimulus events is large, direct visual comparison of the AEP traces is usually adequate. In fact, when the response contains well-defined sharp peaks, fairly good quantitative estimates can be made of the latency and amplitude attenuation of the second response relative to the first. However, when the separation between the paired-stimulus events is very small (or for large separations, when more precision is desired in estimating latency and amplitude attenuation), more rigorous procedures are required for comparing and assessing the AEPs obtained. This is necessary because a response to the second stimulus is fre-

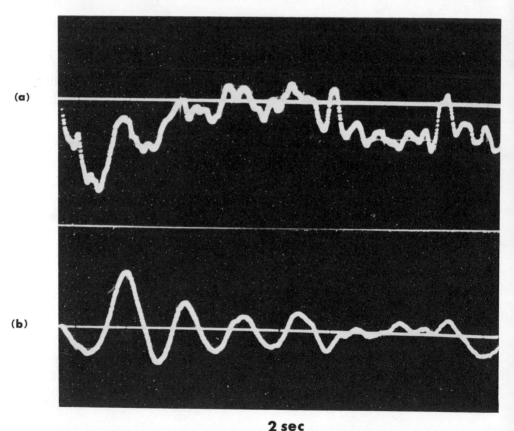

2 sec

Figure 2. (a) Evoked response without filter. (b) Same evoked response using latency enhancement filter.

quently masked by the ongoing response to the first stimulus event.

The following regression model has been used to serve this purpose. A least squares fit of the AEP due to paired stimulation is calculated using a regression model consisting of the single-stimulus AEP combined with an attenuated and delayed single-stimulus AEP. Three useful parameters are obtained in this type of analysis, namely, (1) a delay parameter to compare with the actual stimulus separation, (2) an amplitude parameter to determine the relative reduction in response to the second of the paired stimuli as compared to the response to the first stimulus, and (3) the residual or mean square error of fit which gives a quantitative basis for assessing the accuracy and suitability of the regression model. Expressed in mathematical terms, this method of paired stimulation analysis consists of the following:

Let $S(t)$ = the AEP due to single stimulation

$S_p(t)$ = the AEP due to paired stimulation

Then the regression model estimates $S_p(t)$ as follows:

$$S_p'(t) = S(t) + aS(t-\tau)$$

where $S_p'(t)$ is the least squares best fit to $S_p(t)$ and $S(t-\tau)$ is the delayed version of the AEP due to single stimulation. Note: $S(t-\tau) = 0$ for $t < \tau$.

The regression parameters τ and a have been chosen to minimize the residual, or mean, square error of fit, $\overline{\epsilon^2}$:

Thus, $\overline{\epsilon^2} = 1/T \int_o^T [S_p'(t) - S_p(t)]^2 \, dt,$

where T = the epoch over which the evoked potential is being analyzed.

The parameters τ and a give information about latency and relative amplitude, respectively. The latency is expected to be approximately equal to the separation between the paired-stimulus events and a significant positive deviation from this nominal latency might imply an inhibitory effect due to the first stimulus. The relative amplitude, a, may be associated with the relative number of neural elements that participate in the second response. If the residual, ϵ^2, is small compared to the average power in $S_p(t)$, $\{1/T \int_o^T S_p^2(t) \, dt\}$, then the regression model selected is supported by the AEP data and the parameters τ and a can be estimated with reasonable accuracy. On the other hand, if the residual is large compared to the average power in $S_p(t)$, then the parameters cannot be estimated accurately and the regression model selected is not suitable for representing the paired-stimulus AEP. In this circumstance, the response to paired stimulation cannot be modeled as a linear superposition of single responses; this implies that a complex nonlinear mechanism may be involved or that the system responds to the paired pattern as if it were a new type of single stimulus of longer duration. However, the residual error term can be used to meaningfully quantify the deviation from the regression model and thus serve as a useful descriptor of individual differences in neural response. This error parameter describes the departure from linearity as measured by the percentage of variance not accounted for by the linear model.

Method 2:

When $S(t)$ is unknown, an approach based on deconvolution and cepstral analysis procedures is capable of resolving overlapping responses. In order to separate targets or account for multiple reflections that produce overlapping echoes, such procedures have proved useful in radar and sonar applications. The cepstral analysis approach is illustrated by noting that $S_p(t) = S(t) + aS(t-\tau)$ can be written in the alternate form,

$$S_p(t) = S(t) * [\delta(t) + a\delta(t-\tau)] \tag{1}$$

where $*$ denotes convolution

and $\delta(t)$ is the Dirac delta function.

The Fourier transform of *(1)* is the product of the Fourier transforms of the convolved functions, giving

$$\bar{S}_p(\omega) = \bar{S}(\omega)[1 + ae^{-i\omega\tau}] \tag{2}$$

where the bar denotes Fourier transform, and 1 and $e^{-i\omega\tau}$ are the Fourier transforms of $\delta(t)$ and $\delta(t-\tau)$, respectively. Now take the logarithm of *(2)* giving

$$\log \bar{S}_p(\omega) = \log \bar{S}(\omega) + \log(1 + ae^{-i\omega\tau}) \tag{3}$$

and note that the first term is the logarithm of the spectrum of the unknown response function while the second term is due to the echo property and is independent of the shape of S(t). Also, the second term is a periodic function of ω with period $2\pi/\tau$. The periodicity may be seen by writing the series expansion:

$$\log(1 + ae^{-i\omega\tau}) = \sum_{n=1}^{\infty} (-1)^{n+1} \frac{a^n}{n} e^{-in\omega\tau} \tag{4}$$

A procedure for attempting to remove the echo term in *(3)* is called cepstral smoothing. It consists of taking the inverse Fourier transform of *(3)* so that:

$$F^{-1} [\log \bar{S}_p(\omega)] = F^{-1} [\log \bar{S}(\omega)]$$
$$+F^{-1} [\log(1 + ae^{-i\omega\tau})] \tag{5}$$

Equation *(5)* is called the complex cepstrum of $\bar{S}_p(t)$. Using *(4)*, the second term in *(5)* can be written

$$F^{-1} [\log(1 + ae^{i\omega\tau})] = F^{-1} [\sum_{n=1}^{\infty} (-1)^{n+1} \frac{a^n}{n} e^{in\omega\tau}]$$
$$= \sum_{n=1}^{\infty} (-1)^{n+1} \frac{a^n}{n} \delta(x - n\tau) \tag{6}$$

From *(6)*, it can be seen that the contribution to the cepstrum of the echo term is a series of impulses τ units apart with intensities a^n/n. Intuitively, it can be seen from *(6)* that the effect of the echo terms can be largely removed by smoothing through the peaks in the cepstrum produced by the delta functions. This process is called cepstral smoothing, and it represents a method of deconvolving the convolution of two functions by recognizing that in echo phenomena the inverse of the log spectrum of the echo function produces peaks separated by integer multiples of the echo delay. Therefore, this procedure may be useful in applications in which echo delay is a relevant parameter and in which the basic wave shape of a complex signal composed of the time-delayed addition of unknown but identical waveforms is of interest.

In order to reconstruct the basic waveform, several additional steps are required after cepstral smoothing. First, the smoothed cepstrum is Fourier transformed, and then the exponential of this transform is computed. Finally, the inverse transform of this result yields an estimate of the basic waveform.

The above discussion of deconvolution via cepstral smoothing approaches is intended only to suggest a possible direction of analysis in certain studies of brain electrical activity. Details such as the special consideration required in computing the phase function of the complex log spectrum have been omitted, as have discussions of the effects of noise, and many other theoretical questions which need study in this problem area.

The bibliography at the end of this chapter is recommended to the reader wishing a more rigorous and detailed theoretical view of this approach, as well as a broader understanding of its applications and limitations.

3. Clustering of Evoked Potentials

The use of averaging procedures to detect the presence of evoked potentials which are small compared to the noise background is based on the assumption that each evoked potential pattern is time-locked to the stimulus event. This section presents an approach to the problem for cases in which this assumption does not necessarily hold, that is, for cases where response variability may be a confounding factor. In order to obtain a square root of N (where N is the number of responses) improvement in the signal-to-noise ratio, it is necessary that only identical responses be included in the average. The clustering procedure described here establishes the groupings of an ensemble of evoked potentials in accordance with a variance criterion. This procedure establishes the optimum groupings of members of an ensemble of evoked potentials that are similar to one another. The need for such a procedure in evoked potential applications arises from the fact that the response of a system to identical stimuli is not identical unless the initial state of the system at each of the stimulation times is identical. In EEG evoked potential research, the experimenter ordinarily does not have control of the initial conditions of the biological system involved, and therefore response variability is inevitable. On the assumption that a small number of basically different responses result from alterations in initial conditions during the course of the experiment, the clustering procedure will arrange the ensemble of evoked potentials into a number of groups, with each group containing responses of similar shape. The average evoked potentials can then be obtained for each group and the square root of N (where N is the number in each group) signal-to-noise enhancement will be approached. A further advantage of this separation of responses into groups is that the characteristics of the response are not smeared, as would be the case when dissimilar shapes are averaged together.

A description of the computational procedures involved in performing the clustering analysis will convey the essential ideas in terms of the intended application to evoked potentials, and therefore the following discussion will be limited to a description of these procedures.

Vector notation is useful in describing the procedures, and therefore the sample point values of each evoked potential will be considered the components of a k-dimensional vector, where k is the number of components in each vector and N represents the number of vectors. We will therefore be studying the optimum grouping of N k-dimensional vectors. The possible number of groupings ranges from one to N; the case of a one-group optimum represents the condition in which all the evoked potentials are sufficiently similar in shape, so that it is appropriate to average all of them in the evoked potential analysis. At the other extreme of N groups being optimum, all of the evoked potentials are so dissimilar that each response should be considered a group of its own. Among all the possible groupings from one to N, the clustering procedure establishes the number of groups that is most likely based on the closest Euclidian distance between point pairs in a k-dimensional vector space. The computational task is significantly reduced if one starts the clustering procedure by assuming N groups and proceeding to N-1 groups, N-2 groups, etc. It is clear that if we assume N groups in which each vector is its own mean vector, then the variance of each group is zero. If we now move to N-1 groups, then only the two closest of the N vectors need to be joined, and the clustering algorithm selects those two such that the sums of the squares of the differences of their component values are smallest among all the possible pairings of vectors. The possible pairings of vectors are the combinations of N things taken two at a time, $\frac{N(N-1)}{2}$. The two vectors most similar by this criterion are eliminated from the clustering set and replaced by their mean vector. The procedure is now repeated on the N-1 vectors in this new set. This involves a combination of N-1 things taken two at a time and the two vectors most similar are again joined. The procedure is then reapplied to the N-2 vectors that remain in the set and is repeated until only one group remains. The change in variance is computed at each step and that grouping is considered optimum which, if further reduced, would produce a significant increase in variance (where significance may be established with an F test). For example, if the evoked potentials clustered naturally into three groupings, then the procedure would result in a large increase in variance when the number of groupings were reduced from three to two. This large increase in variance would suggest that any further reduction in the number of groupings would force distinctly different evoked potentials to be combined into the same group. When one proceeds as described, the machine time required is proportional to k (the number of components in the vector, that is, the number of sample points), and to N^3 (the cube of the number of vectors, that is, the number of evoked potentials).

It should be emphasized that if one were to approach this problem by assuming three groups and then perform the distance calculations on all the possible ways by forming three groups from N vectors, the number of computations would be very large, compared to the procedure described whereby one proceeds systematically from N groups to one group. A further advantage is that, by examining the incremental variances as the program proceeds from N groups to one group, it is not only possible to select the number of groups that make the most sense in terms of the variance criterion, but also to determine to what extent one can assume that a different number of groups is present.

Figures 3 and 4 illustrate the results of applying this clustering procedure to a set of 20 evoked potentials where the initial portion of each evoked potential is characterized by a 10-dimensional vector, that is, 10 sample points. The (a) curve in Figure 3 shows the AEP that results when all 20 responses are averaged together. The (b) and (c) curves in Figure 3 are the two AEPs that result when the ensemble of 20 responses is clustered into two groups. The numbers alongside each of these AEPs indicate the particular EP replications that belong to each group. There are 9 in group (b) and 11 in group (c). The three curves in Figure 4 are the three AEPs that result from clustering the 20 responses into three groups. It should be noted that the (c) group of Figure 3 remained intact, while the nine responses in the (b) group separated into a group of five responses plus a group of four responses. This example illustrates how clustering procedures can provide the investigator with insights into the nature of the evoked response under conditions of response variability, as well as possible insights to aid in the formulation of hypotheses on the nature of the initial conditions that may be responsible for this variability.

4. Parameters that Reveal EEG Nonlinearities (Polycoherence)

Polycoherence analysis can be applied to the problem of determining whether a particular random-appearing EEG record is composed of a sum of independent (uncoupled) frequency components or whether it is composed of dependent or coupled components. With this approach one can investigate whether a completely random signal source (that is, a signal composed of independent spectral components) has been modified by a nonlinear transmission medium. It should be pointed out first that a signal composed of independent spectral components will retain this spectral independence when modified by a linear medium. Therefore the question at issue in electroencephalography is whether a random-appearing, scalp-recorded signal is the result of a linear operation only on a random but otherwise unspecified signal source, or whether it is the result of nonlinear operations as well.

For example, one of the questions addressed in a study (Barnett et al.

1971) is whether, under certain conditions, the beta activity in the EEG is due to the alpha activity, or whether the alpha and beta activities are independent of one another. An alternate way of phrasing this question should help to clarify why nonlinearities are implied by dependence of alpha on beta. For specificity, if the 10-Hz component is called the a component and

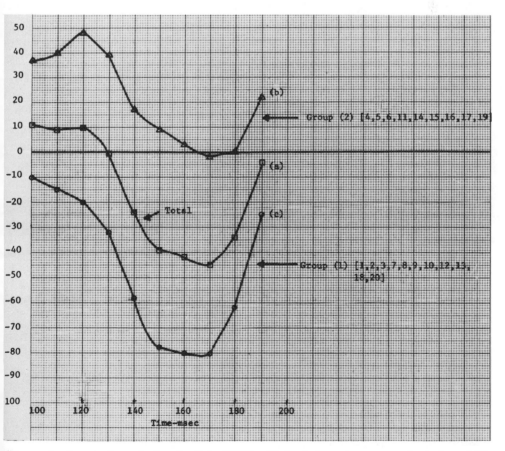

Figure 3. Averaged evoked potentials (AEP) obtained from two-group clustering of 20 evoked potentials (EP).

20 Hz the β component, then the alternate question might be: Was the 20-Hz component created by squaring the 10-Hz component contained in the source signal, or was the source signal composed of independent 10-Hz and 20-Hz components? To determine which of these conditions exist, some simple properties of sinusoids need to be used. The first property is that the

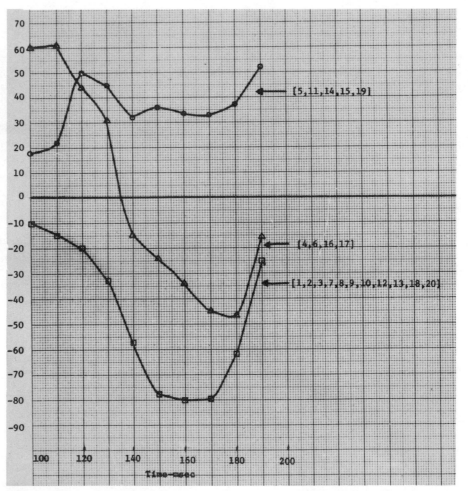

Figure 4. Averaged evoked potentials obtained from three-group clustering of 20 evoked potentials.

square of a sinusoid results in another sinusoid at twice the frequency. The second obvious but important property is that the sinusoid created by squaring has a fixed phase relative to the original sinusoid. Therefore, if independent random generators were responsible for the 10-Hz and the 20-Hz components in the EEG, then the relative phase of these componenets would not remain fixed but would vary randomly from analysis epoch to analysis epoch. It is this random variation of the relative phase of certain frequency components in the output of a linear system with a random input signal, as opposed to the fixed relative phase of these frequency components in the output when system nonlinearities exist, that provides the basis for distinguishing between these states (linear vs. nonlinear) by the use of polyspectral analysis techniques. The polyspectrum with appropriate normalization is called the polycoherence function. The second order spectrum is called the bispectrum, and when normalized it is called the bicoherence function. The generalization to higher order coherence functions is straightforward. Since bicoherence illustrates the principles involved in the applications of this approach to the identification of nonlinearities, the following heuristic discussion will be limited to bicoherence analysis of the EEG.

To gain some intuitive understanding of how the properties of the bicoherence function reveal nonlinearities, consider a number of epochs (say, N) of a single EEG channel. Compute the complex Fourier series of each epoch and select the complex Fourier coefficients at each of three frequencies, ω_1, ω_2, and $\omega_3 = \omega_1 + \omega_2$.

For the kth epoch, denote the complex amplitude at each of these frequencies as follows:

$$A_k(\omega_1) = a_k(\omega_1) + ib_k(\omega_1) = r_k(\omega_1)\, e^{i\theta\, k(\omega_1)} \tag{1}$$

$$A_k(\omega_2) = a_k(\omega_2) + ib_k(\omega_2) = r_k(\omega_2)\, e^{i\theta\, k(\omega_2)} \tag{2}$$

$$A_k(\omega_3) = a_k(\omega_3) + ib_k(\omega_3) = r_k(\omega_3)\, e^{i\theta\, k(\omega_3)} \tag{3}$$

where

$$\left| A_k \right| = \sqrt{a_k^2 + b_k^2} = r_k \tag{4}$$

Using *(1)*, *(2)* and *(3)*, the bicoherence function is defined as follows:

$$
\text{Bicoh } (\omega_1,\omega_2) = \frac{\sum\limits_{k=1}^{N} A_k(\omega_1)A_k(\omega_2)A_k^*(\omega_3)}{\sum\limits_{k=1}^{N} \left|A_k(\omega_1)\right| \left|A_k(\omega_2\right| \left|A_k(\omega_3)\right|} \tag{5}
$$

where * denotes the complex conjugate and $\omega_3 = \omega_1+\omega_2$.

In polar form *(5)* becomes

$$
\text{Bicoh } (\omega_1,\omega_2) = \frac{\sum\limits_{k=1}^{N} r_k(\omega_1)r_k(\omega_2)r_k(\omega_3)\, e^{i[\theta_k(\omega_1)+\theta_k(\omega_2)-\theta_k(\omega_3)]}}{\sum\limits_{k=1}^{N} r_k(\omega_1)r_k(\omega_2)r_k(\omega_3)} \tag{6}
$$

If in each epoch (i.e., for all k),

$$
\theta_k(\omega_1)+\theta_k(\omega_2)-\theta_k(\omega_1+\omega_2) = \phi \tag{7}
$$

is a constant independent of k, then the exponential term in *(6)* can be factored out of the numerator summation, and the sum of triple products of the r_k in the numerator is then identical to the denominator, giving:

$$
\text{Bicoh } (\omega_1,\omega_2) = e^{i\phi} \tag{8}
$$

$$
\left| \text{Bicoh } (\omega_1,\omega_2) \right| = 1 \tag{9}
$$

The result *(9)* implies that the phase of the Fourier componenet at frequency $(\omega_1+\omega_2)$ is locked to the sum of the phases of the components at frequency ω_1 and ω_2. On the other hand, in a truly random signal, the relative phases of all components are independent so that,

$$
\theta_k(\omega_1)+\theta_k(\omega_2)-\theta_k(\omega_1+\omega_2) = \phi_k \tag{10}
$$

varies randomly from epoch to epoch. The expected value of *(6)* under this condition is zero as opposed to the completely phase-locked condition under which it takes on its maximum absolute value of unity. Thus, the absolute value of bicoherence can take on values from zero to one, depending upon the relative amounts of coupled (phase-locked) versus uncoupled energy at the frequencies examined. Although the expected value of bicoherence is zero for a truly random signal, one must take into account that deviations from this expected value depend upon factors such as ensemble size (that is, the number of epochs chosen), the length of each epoch, and stationarity of the signal. Therefore, in estimating the significance of a particular departure from zero bicoherence, the value must be compared to the expected error of estimating bicoherence before attributing the observed departure to a non-linear mechanism in the generation of EEG.

The preceding discussion has indicated that a significant departure from zero bicoherence implies phase-locked, rather than independent, Fourier components. To complete the argument, it is necessary to show that phase-locked components imply system nonlinearities. To do this without resorting to involved mathematical methods, let $Y(t)$ denote the brain electrical activity at the scalp due to a signal source $X(t)$ that is assumed random. Let us further assume that a nonlinear mechanism exists, such that $X^2(t)$ as well as $X(t)$ contribute to the composition of $Y(t)$. Now denote the two Fourier components at frequencies ω_1 and ω_2 in the source signal $X(t)$ as λ_{1k} and λ_{2k} (where k again denotes a particular analysis epoch), and examine the consequences of squaring the sum of these terms. To emphasize phase relations, a Fourier component may be written in the following form:

$$\lambda_{1k} = c_{1k} \cos(\omega_1 t + \theta_{1k}) \tag{11}$$

$$\lambda_{2k} = c_{2k} \cos(\omega_2 t + \theta_{2k}) \tag{12}$$

$$(\lambda_{1k} + \lambda_{2k})^2 = \lambda_k^2 + 2\lambda_{1k}\lambda_{2k} + \lambda_{2k}^2 \tag{13}$$

The $2\lambda_{1k}\lambda_{2k}$ product term in (13) can be rewritten using the trigonometric identity for the product of cosines as follows:

$$2\lambda_{1k}\lambda_{2k} = c_{1k}c_{2k}[\cos\left\{(\omega_1+\omega_2)t+(\theta_{1k}+\theta_{2k})\right\}$$
$$+ \cos\left\{(\omega_1-\omega_2)t+(\theta_{1k}-\theta_{2k})\right\}] \tag{14}$$

Note that the first term on the right-hand side of (14) is at the frequency $(\omega_1+\omega_2)$, and designate it as $\lambda_{(1+2)k}$, so that

$$\lambda_{(1+2)k} = c_{1k}c_{2k} \cos\left\{(\omega_1+\omega_2)t+\theta_{1k}+\theta_{2k}\right\} \tag{15}$$

By comparing *(15)* with *(11)* and *(12)*, we note that the phase of the Fourier component at $(\omega_1+\omega_2)$ is the sum of the phases of the components at ω_1 and ω_2. Referring to *(6)*, the definition of bicoherence, we note that it is an operation on the data that subtracts the phase at frequency $(\omega_1+\omega_2)$ from the sum of the phases at ω_1 and ω_2. In the example above, where the component at $(\omega_1+\omega_2)$ resulted from a squaring operation on the signal source X(t), the phase term of the bicoherence function would therefore be identical for all epochs (in this example, zero for all k = 1 to N). This constancy of the phase term in the bicoherence function results in a significant nonzero value of bicoherence at the frequencies chosen, as opposed to the linear condition where the phase term would vary randomly with k, and consequently result in an expected value of zero bicoherence at these frequencies. Rather than averaging over a number of successive epochs of the EEG to calculate bicoherence as in the foregoing discussion, one may use a single epoch and average over a number of frequency components in the vicinity of ω_1, ω_2, and $\omega_1+\omega_2$ to calculate bicoherence. The variance of the estimates of bicoherence is again a function of many factors, including the length of the epoch and the size and shape of the spectral window used, as in the general case for lower order spectral estimators.

5. Tracking Parameters (Period Analysis and Spectral Moments)

In applications in which the information to be abstracted from long-term EEG recordings appears in the form of generalized changes in the complex structure of the signal, one seeks parameters that effectively monitor or track these changes. Because very long records are involved (for example, eight hours of multiple-channel sleep EEG recordings for sleep-staging studies), it is essential that these parameters be capable of substantially compressing the data at reasonable computational cost, as well as being suitable for tracking general changes in complex EEG structure. This section, therefore, will describe methods for monitoring slow changes in the complex structure of a time series, with the objective of developing efficient methods for computing EEG statistical parameters that correlate with physiological change in state (such as in drug effect studies and in sleep staging).

The tracking parameters described in this section are derived from the EEG's autospectrum, its autocorrelation function, and from the average zero-crossing rates of the EEG and its time derivatives. The parameters represent even-ordered moments of the power spectral density (PSD), and it is shown that for complex signals such as the EEG, the parameters of period analysis (major, intermediate, and minor period parameters) are equivalent statistical measures of the EEG. The computational operations to derive these parameters, as well as the mathematical properties and relationships among these parameters, are summarized. The specific parameters to be discussed are:

(a) Moments of the autospectrum; that is, power spectral density (PSD)
(b) Average zero-crossing rate of the signal and its derivatives (period analysis)
(c) Even-ordered derivatives of the correlation function at zero lag, and
(d) Average power of derivatives of the signal.

Since tracking procedures are designed for application to the monitoring of long runs of data, it is important that efficient computational procedures be developed for deriving the tracking parameters. In this section it is shown that certain parameters can be computed efficiently with indirect methods. The equivalence of certain spectral parameters to other parameters, whose derivations are computationally simple and fast, are mathematically analyzed and experimentally verified in the context of an investigation of EEG parameter tracking.

Power Spectral Density, Autocorrelation Function,
and their Relation to Period Analysis Parameters

The following equation which relates the average rate of zero crossings to the power spectral density holds for a normally distributed zero mean process. (Experimental data are presented in subsequent sections to demonstrate that the EEG spectrum and zero-crossing properties approximate this equality accurately.)

$$\left(\frac{N_k}{2}\right)^2 = \frac{\int_o^\infty f^{2k+2} P(f)\, df}{\int_o^\infty f^{2k} P(f)\, df} \qquad (1)$$

where

N_k = average rate of zero crossings of the kth derivative of the signal process $S(t)$

$P(f)$ = power spectral density of the signal process $S(t)$

In period analysis we are concerned with N_k for $K = 0, 1, 2$ only, and therefore the data of interest correspond to points of baseline crossings, points of maxima and minima, and to points of inflection of the signal $S(t)$.

Thus

N_O = the average rate at which S(t) passes through its zero mean value

N_1 = the average rate at which $\dfrac{dS(t)}{dt}$ passes through its zero mean value

N_2 = the average rate at which $\dfrac{d^2S(t)}{dt^2}$ passes through its zero mean value

Since we wish to demonstrate the validity of *(1)* for electroencephalography, it is necessary to compute the spectral moments defined by the right-hand side of *(1)*. This implies a lengthy computation to estimate the components of the Fourier spectra, followed by integration to compute the moments of these spectra. However, moments of the power spectral density can be derived from simple operations on the autocorrelation function to avoid this tedious and, for the volume of data generated in many EEG applications, prohibitive computation.

The finite epoch autocorrelation function and power spectral density are defined as follows:

$$\phi(\tau) = \frac{1}{T} \int_{-T/2}^{T/2} S(t)\, S(t+\tau)\, dt \tag{2}$$

$$P(f) = \frac{1}{T} \left| \int_{-T/2}^{T/2} S(t)\, e^{-i2\pi f}\, dt \right|^2 \tag{3}$$

In the limit as T→∞, the above equations are related through the integral transform pair:

$$P(f) = \int_{-\infty}^{+\infty} \phi(\tau)\, e^{-i2\pi f\tau}\, d\tau$$

$$= 2 \int_{0}^{\infty} \phi(\tau)\, \cos 2\pi f\tau\, d\tau \tag{4}$$

$$\phi(\tau) = \int_{-\infty}^{+\infty} P(f)\, e^{i2\pi f\tau}\, df$$

$$= 2\int_{0}^{\infty} P(f)\, \cos 2\pi f\tau\, df \tag{5}$$

Equation (5) is independent of any conditions on the amplitude probability distribution of S(t) so long as P(f) exists, and therefore it may be used in general as a basis for generating moments of P(f), as shown in equations (6) and (7).

Since only even moments do not vanish, consider the even-ordered derivates of $\phi(\tau)$,

$$\frac{d^{2n}\phi(\tau)}{d\tau^{2n}} = 2\int_{0}^{\infty} (-1)^n\, (2\pi f)^{2n}\, P(f)\, \cos 2\pi f\tau\, df \tag{6}$$

setting $\tau = 0$ and rearranging terms

$$\int_{0}^{\infty} f^{2n}\, P(f)\, df = \frac{(-1)^n}{2(2\pi)^{2n}}\; \frac{d^{2n}\phi(0)}{d\tau^{2n}} \tag{7}$$

Thus the moments of the power spectral density are proportional to the zero lag derivatives of the autocorrelation function. Equation (7) represents a major computational efficiency because, instead of computing the components of P(f) and then integrating $f^{2n}P(f)$ to derive moments, all one needs to do is compute the values of $\phi(\tau)$ at $2n + 1$ increments of lag $\{\phi(0), \phi(\Delta\tau), \ldots \phi(2n\Delta\tau)\}$, and perform simple finite differencing operations on these values to obtain the desired spectral moment. A further computational efficiency is gained by observing that odd-ordered derivatives are known a priori to be zero. Thus, in computing the second moment of P(f), we need calculate only two correlation values rather than three, namely:

From equation *(7)*

$$\int_0^\infty f^2\, P(f)\, df = -\frac{1}{8\pi^2} \frac{d^2\phi(0)}{d\tau^2} \qquad (8)$$

denote

$$\frac{d\psi}{d\tau} \equiv \phi' \text{ and } \frac{d^2\phi}{d\tau^2} \equiv \phi''$$

From the mean value theorem for differentiation we have

$$\phi'\left(\frac{\Delta\tau}{2}\right) \simeq \frac{\phi(\Delta\tau) - \phi(0)}{\Delta\tau} \qquad (9)$$

Using *(9)* to compute $\phi''(0)$ we have

$$\phi''(0) = \frac{\phi'\left(\frac{\Delta\tau}{2}\right) - \phi'(0)}{\Delta\tau/2} \qquad (10)$$

but $\phi'(0) = 0$ and $\phi'\left(\frac{\Delta\tau}{2}\right)$ is given by *(9)*, so *(10)* reduces to

$$\phi''(0) = 2\,\frac{\phi(\Delta\tau) - \phi(0)}{(\Delta\tau)^2} \qquad (11)$$

Substituting *(11)* into *(8)* we have

$$\int_0^\infty f^2\, P(f)df = \frac{1}{(2\pi)^2} \frac{\phi(0) - \phi(\Delta\tau)}{(\Delta\tau)^2} \qquad (12)$$

but from *(1)* under the previously stated conditions on S(t)

$$\left(\frac{N_o}{2}\right)^2 = \frac{\displaystyle\int_o^\infty f^2\, P(f)\, df}{\displaystyle\int_o^\infty P(f)\, df} \tag{13}$$

or using *(12)*

$$\frac{N_o}{2} = \frac{1}{2\pi\Delta\tau}\left(1 - \frac{\phi(\Delta\tau)}{\phi(0)}\right)^{1/2} \tag{14}$$

In the EEG data analysis that follows, we shall demonstrate that the second moment of the normalized power spectral density is accurately approximated by N_o, the average zero-cross rate of S(t). The parameter N_o is called "major period count," and it provides an important measure for signal tracking because its computational simplicity makes large-scale EEG analysis of spectral moments quite practical. It has been shown in *(12)* that the second moment may be approximated from two values of the autocorrelation function and that this result is independent of the constraints imposed on *(13)*, which relates zero crossings to the second moment. Therefore, a demonstration of the validity of zero-crossing approaches to spectral moment calculations is obtained by comparing the values obtained from both methods of computation. This comparison is shown in the context of an EEG drug study in Figures 5, 6, and 7.

A further demonstration of the utility and validity of the zero-crossing approach is obtained by comparing the autocorrelation function of typical EEGs with their polarity correlation functions. This comparison is shown in Figures 8 and 9. Since the polarity correlation function is computed from the sign function of S(t) [defined in *(15)*], it depends only on the location of zero crossings, and thus agreement of standard correlation function computations and polarity correlation function computations of EEGs establishes the validity of zero-crossing data for representing general properties of the power spectral density beyond the second moment.

$$\text{sgn}\,[S(t)] = 1 \qquad \text{when } S(t) \geq 0$$
$$\tag{15}$$
$$= -1 \qquad \text{when } S(t) < 0$$

If we denote the autocorrelation function of sgn [S(t)] as ϕ_c, then

$$\phi_c(\tau) = \frac{1}{T} \int_0^T \text{sgn}\,[S(t)]\,\text{sgn}\,[S(t+\tau)]\,dt \qquad (16)$$

Equation (16) is sometimes referred to as the autocorrelation of the infinitely clipped (that is, infinitely amplified and then clipped) EEG. The polarity autocorrelation function, denoted by ϕ_p, is a better estimate of the autocorrelation function, and it is given by a simple transformation on ϕ_c, as shown below.

$$\phi_p(\tau) = \sin\left[\frac{\pi}{2}\,\phi_c(\tau)\right] \qquad (17)$$

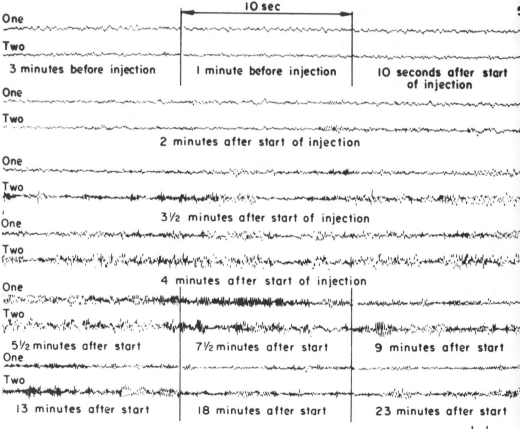

Figure 5. Typical EEG recording before, during, and after seven-minute injection of 500 mg of sodium amytal.

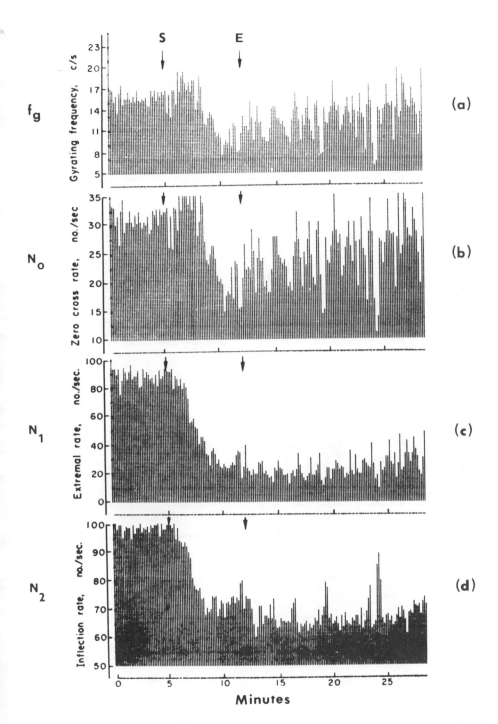

Figure 6. Monitoring of drug study, lead one, using four tracking parameters: f_g, N_O, N_1, *and* N_2. *S—start of injection. E—end of injection.*

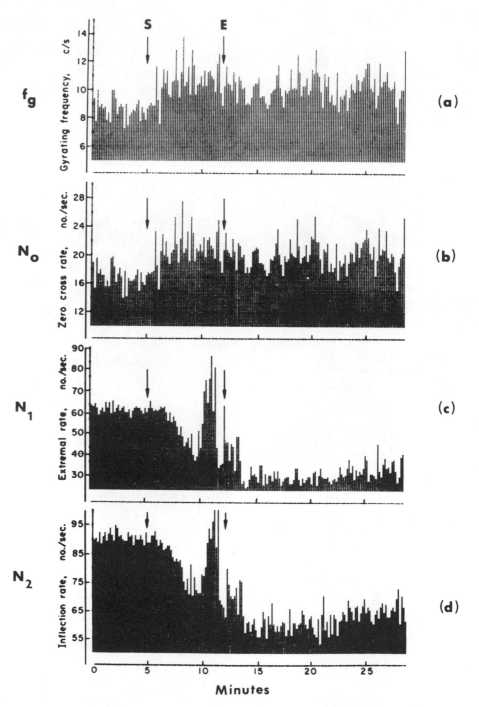

Figure 7. Monitoring of drug study, lead two, using four tracking parameters: f_g, N_o, N_1, and N_2. S—start of injection. E—end of injection.

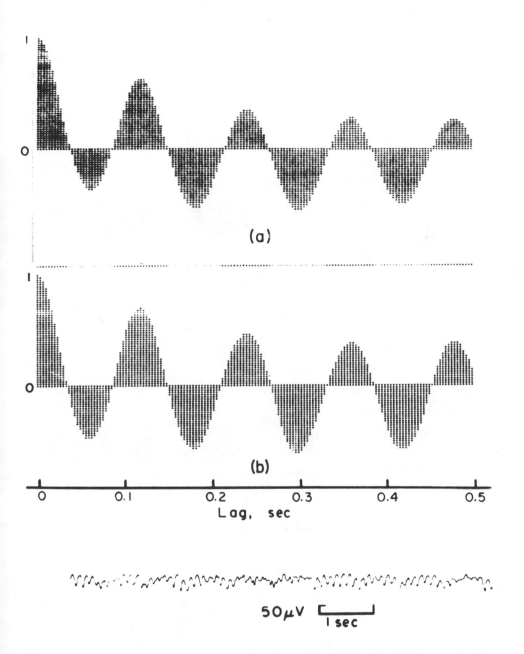

Figure 8. Comparison of autocorrelation function of the EEG with SGN approximation based on EEG zero crossings only. (a) Autocorrelation function. (b) SGN approximation of (a).

The computer-analyzed EEG signals presented below establish the accuracy and effectiveness of these approximations. The evaluation was based on a variety of EEG signals collected in an experimental study of the effect of certain drugs on the electrical activity of the nervous system.

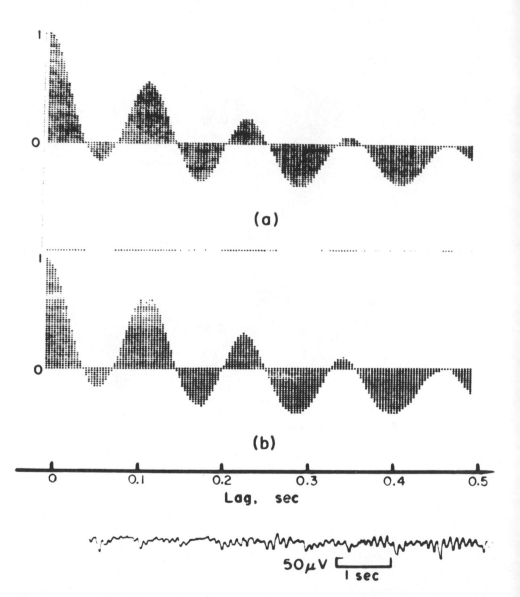

Figure 9. *Comparison of Autocorrelation function of the EEG with SGN approximation based on EEG zero crossings only. (a) Autocorrelation function. (b) SGN approximation of (a).*

Results

This section describes the experimental results obtained in the application of zero crossing and spectral moment methods to the evaluation of EEG drug effects.

Two channels of EEG were monitored in an experimental design[1] in which sodium amytal was administered to the subject to ascertain whether significant EEG alterations were reflected in spectral moments and zero-crossing tracking parameters. For convenience we will refer to the square root of the second moment of the PSD as the "gyrating frequency." This terminology seems appropriate since this quantity has the dimensions of frequency and since the equation representing it has the same form as that for the radius of gyration in mechanics. In addition to showing the efficacy of these tracking parameters, this experiment demonstrates with a long data sample that the gyrating frequency of each analysis epoch (360 ten-second epochs representing one hour of EEG were analyzed) is consistently equal to half the measured average zero-crossing rate for the corresponding epoch.

Verification of the equality,

$$f_g = \frac{N_o}{2}$$

where

$$f_g = \frac{\int_o^\infty f^2\, P(f)\, df}{\int_o^\infty P(f)\, df}$$

and

$$N_o = \text{average zero-crossing rate}$$

establishes the validity of using zero-crossing rate in EEG to monitor spectral moments.

---

[1] A specific experimental design was selected that would provide a clear test of the applicability to electroencephalography of the analytical methods being investigated. Although the design is specific to a particular drug, it seems reasonable to expect that these methods will be equally effective in most experimental designs involving the assessment of long-term changes in the complex structure of the EEG.

Figure 5 is representative of the raw EEG data subjected to analysis in this part of the study. EEG records typical of before, during, and after the injection of the drug are shown in this figure. Figures 6(a) and 7(a) are independent 30-minute monitoring runs using f_g as the tracking parameter. Figures 6(b) and 7(b) are 30-minute monitoring runs of the same EEG data as Figures 6(a) and 7(a), respectively, using N_o as the tracking parameter. Comparison of Figures 6(a) with 6(b) and 7(a) with 7(b) clearly demonstrates the essential equivalence of these tracking parameters for monitoring EEG. From these data, as well as from the striking similarity of these parameters over long runs of typical EEG recordings, it may be concluded that the constraints on EEG signal statistics justify the application of simplified zero-crossing count procedures to estimate the integrals required to compute spectral moments.

Figures 6(c) and 7(c) are EEG monitoring runs using N_1 as the tracking parameter. It also follows from the previous analysis that N_1 is essentially equivalent to the gyrating frequency of the first derivative of the EEG. Figures 6(d) and 7(d) are monitoring runs using N_2 as the tracking parameter. Similarly, N_2 is essentially equivalent to the gyrating frequency of the second derivative of the EEG.

It can be noted in Figures 6 and 7 that the profiles of f_g and N_o are practically identical, and more importantly it can be noted that dramatic changes in the profile of the tracking parameters N_1 and N_2 accompany the drug injection. The significant reduction in the values of these tracking parameters following drug injection, as opposed to the less significant changes in f_g and N_o, indicates that drug effects are monitored more effectively by zero crossings of the first and second derivatives of the EEG. The implications of the greater sensitivity of N_1 and N_2 to these drug-induced EEG changes are that only a small change in the ratio of high-frequency power to low-frequency power takes place in response to the injection. This sensitivity is true of N_1 and N_2 but not of N_o, because the higher moments (4th and 6th, respectively) magnify the effect of small shifts in the spectral distribution. As expected, the parameters derived from the lower ordered moment, N_o, did not exhibit as much sensitivity to the small shifts in spectral distribution that accompanies the administration of sodium amytal.

6. A Measure of Multiple-Channel Similarity (Concordance)

Computer techniques have mainly been directed to obtaining descriptors of single-channel EEG activity or macroscopic and microscopic measures of similarity between two channels. The purpose of this section is to describe briefly a simple method for obtaining a statistical parameter that reflects multiple-channel similarity. Although this parameter (known as Kendell's coefficient of concordance) is ordinarily applied to the problem of measuring the agreement among judges in ranking the members of a group, it is presented here as an intuitively reasonable and attractive way of studying the overall similarity of specific properties of many simultaneously recorded EEG channels.

To illustrate the concordance concept in the context of electroencephalography, suppose N channels of EEG are each divided into K epochs over the duration of the recording. Suppose further that in each epoch for every channel we compute a property of the signal (say, for example, the major period count) and then rank this property from one to K for each channel (labeling the lowest count one and the highest count K, for example). Arrange the rankings into a table of N rows (corresponding to the number of EEG channels) and K columns corresponding to the number of epochs. The rank scores across each row will run from one to K, with each score retaining its epoch position in the EEG, as illustrated in Figure 10. Now for each epoch, sum over channels and regard each sum as a summary score for that epoch. If there were perfect agreement in each epoch over all N channels, then the summary scores of the epochs would range from N to KN, with intervening values of 2N, 3N, . . . (K-1)N, though not in that order necessarily. Under this condition of perfect agreement, the variance of the summary scores is N^2 times the variance of the integers from 1 to K, which is the maximum possible variance of the summary scores. This maximum possible variance is given by

$$\sigma^2_{max} = \frac{N^2(K^2-1)}{12} \tag{1}$$

In practice, perfect agreement will rarely occur. A measure of the extent of agreement or similarity among channels is given by the ratio of the actual variance of the summary scores to the maximum possible variance. This ratio is called the coefficient of concordance, R, and is defined as

$$R = \frac{S^2}{\sigma^2_{max}} \tag{2}$$

where

$$S^2 = \frac{1}{K} \sum_{j=1}^{K} \left[T_j^2 - \left(\frac{1}{K} \sum_{j=1}^{K} T_j \right)^2 \right]$$

and T_j is the sum over all N channels of the jth epoch rank score. It is good practice to use more than seven epochs because for $K > 7$, the significance of R can be tested using

$$\chi^2_R = N(K-1)R \tag{3}$$

which follows quite closely the chi-squared distribution with K-1 degrees of freedom. A significant R (coefficient of concordance) may be interpreted as indicative of a better-than-chance agreement among the channels, that is, the particular EEG parameter being monitored (for example, the major period count) possesses rank-order similarity across all channels. On the other hand,

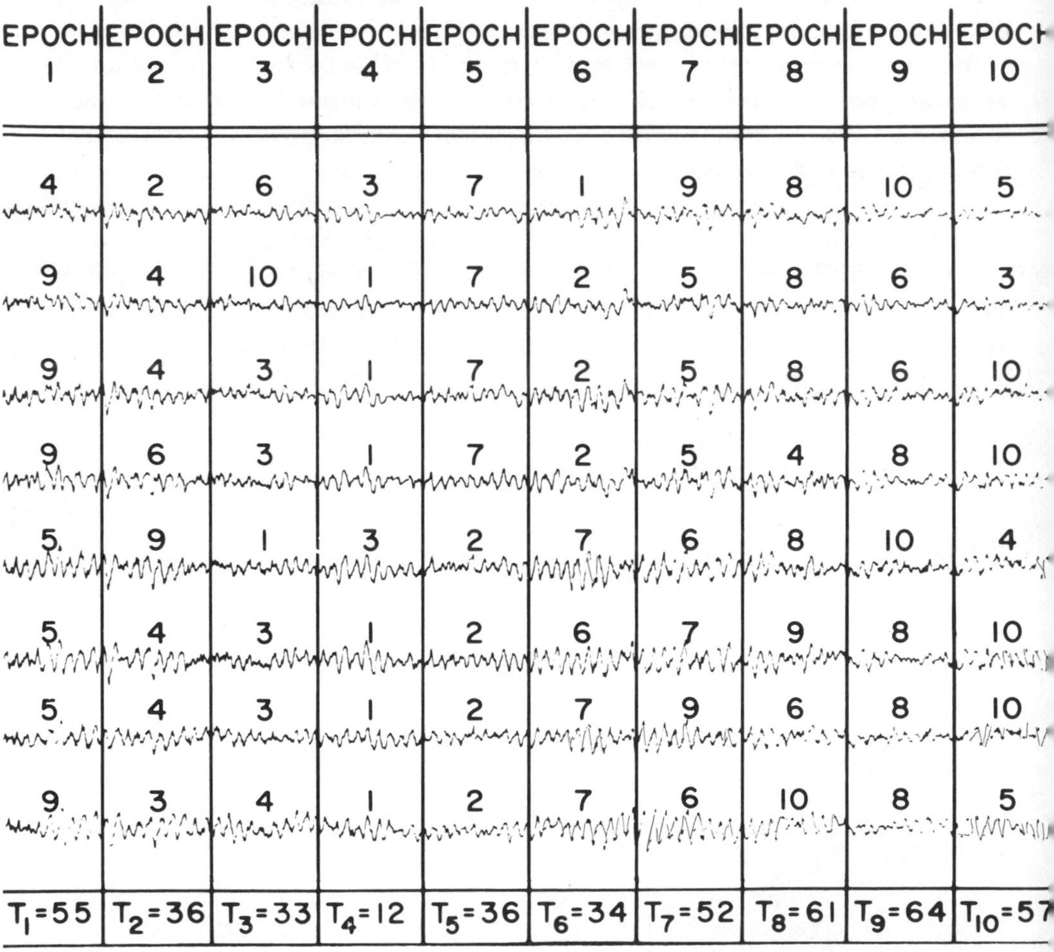

EPOCH 1	EPOCH 2	EPOCH 3	EPOCH 4	EPOCH 5	EPOCH 6	EPOCH 7	EPOCH 8	EPOCH 9	EPOCH 10
4	2	6	3	7	1	9	8	10	5
9	4	10	1	7	2	5	8	6	3
9	4	3	1	7	2	5	8	6	10
9	6	3	1	7	2	5	4	8	10
5	9	1	3	2	7	6	8	10	4
5	4	3	1	2	6	7	9	8	10
5	4	3	1	2	7	9	6	8	10
9	3	4	1	2	7	6	10	8	5
$T_1 = 55$	$T_2 = 36$	$T_3 = 33$	$T_4 = 12$	$T_5 = 36$	$T_6 = 34$	$T_7 = 52$	$T_8 = 61$	$T_9 = 64$	$T_{10} = 57$

Figure 10. Illustration of concordance calculations applied to eight channels of EEG for ten epochs.

an insignificant R may be interpreted as indicative of channel independence insofar as the particular monitoring parameter used in the test is concerned.

Acknowledgments

The methodology and the illustrative samples presented in this manuscript are drawn from research projects supported by the National Institute of Neurological Diseases and Stroke under Grants NS04705 and NS09332, and by the National Institute of Child Health and Human Development under Contract PH 43-68-1412.

Suggested Reading

Barnett, T.P., Johnson, L.C., Naitoh, P., Hicks, N., and Nute, C. 1971. Bispectrum analysis of electroencephalogram signals during waking and sleeping. *Science* 172:401.

Blackman, R.B., and Tukey, J.W. 1958. *The Measurement of Power Spectra.* New York: Dover.

Bogert, B., Healy, M., and Tukey, J. 1963. The frequency analysis of time series for echoes. In M. Rosenblatt Ed.), *Proceedings of Symposium on Time Series Analysis,* p. 209. New York: Wiley.

Callaway, E., and Halliday, R.A. 1973. Evoked potential variability: effects of age, amplitude and methods of measurement. *Electroencephalogr. Clin. Neurophysiol.* 34:125.

Hinich, M. 1962. A model for a self-adapting filter. *Information Control* 5:185.

Hinich, M. 1965. Large-sample estimation of an unknown discrete waveform which is randomly repeating in gaussian noise. *Ann. Math. Statist.* 36(2):489.

Hinich, M. 1967. Detection of an unknown waveform randomly recurring in gaussian noise. *Information Control* 10(4):394.

Noll, A.M. 1967. Cepstrum pitch determination. *J. Acoust. Soc. Am.* 41:293.

Oppenheim, A.V. 1965. Superposition in a class of non-linear systems. Research Laboratory of Electronics, Massachusetts Institute of Technology, Cambridge, Mass. *Technical Report* 432.

Oppenheim, A.V. 1965. Optimum homomorphic filters. Research Laboratory of Electronics, Massachusetts Institute of Technology, Cambridge, Mass. *Quarterly Progress Reports* 77:248.

Oppenheim, A.V. 1966. Non-linear filtering of convolved signals. Research Laboratory of Electronics, Massachusetts Institute of Technology, Cambridge, Mass. *Quarterly Progress Reports* 80:168.

Oppenheim, A.V., Schafer, R.W., and Stockham, Jr., T.G. 1968. Non-linear filtering of multiplied and convolved signals. *Proc. IEEE* 56:1264.

Robinson, E.A. 1957. Predictive decomposition of seismic traces. *Geophysics* 22:767.

Robinson, E.A. 1959. *An Introduction to Infinitely Many Variates.* New York: Hafner.

Ruchkin, D.S. 1965. An analysis of average response computations based upon aperiodic stimuli. *IEEE Trans. Biomed. Eng., BME*-12:87.

Saltzberg, B. 1971. Digital filters in neurological research. *Proceedings Symposium on Digital Filtering*. London: Imperial College of Science and Technology.

Saltzberg, B. 1973. Analysis of developmental electrophysiology. Tulane University School of Medicine, New Orleans, La. *Annual Progress Report* NINDS Grant 09332.

Saltzberg, B., and Burch, N.R. 1971. Period analytic estimates of moments of the power spectrum: a simplified EEG time domain procedure. *Electroencephalogr. Clin. Neurophysiol.* 30:568.

Saltzberg, B., Lustick, L.S., and Heath, R.G. 1971. Detection of focal depth spiking in the scalp EEG of monkeys. *Electroencephalogr. Clin. Neurophysiol.* 31:327.

Schafer, R.W. 1967. Echo removal by generalized linear filtering. *NEREM Record* p. 118.

Senmoto, S., and Childers, D.G. 1972. Adaptive decomposition of a composite signal of identical unknown wavelets in noise. *IEEE Transactions on Systems, Man, and Cybernetics*, SMC-2, 1:59.

Siegel, S. 1956. *Nonparametric Statistics*. New York: McGraw-Hill.

sequential methods for parametric discriminant analysis of the eeg during sleep [1]

L.E. Larsen, M.D., MAJ, MC[2]

Walter Reed Army Institute of Research
Washington, D.C.

In previous pattern recognition studies of the human EEG during sleep (Larsen and Walter 1969 and 1970), a method described as a "two-stage machine" was applied in order to improve classification success rates in a training/testing design (Larsen et al. 1971) with spectral based description of the electroencephalogram (EEG). The same notions were applied to chimpanzee EEG sleep data by Larsen et al. (1972 and 1973) with similar results. The method was based on the idea of a layered decision process aimed first at discriminating two aggregates of groups followed by a later discrimination for the groups within each aggregate taken separately. The aggregates of groups were determined on the basis of cross-group clustering in a discriminant space[3] of two dimensions. This paper reports further studies on a possible theoretical basis for the efficacy of the two-stage machine as well as a means to determine aggregate structure and when the technique may be

---

[1]Some results from this paper were reported at the 17th Annual U.S. Army Conference on the Design of Experiments held at the Walter Reed Army Institute of Research, September 1971.

[2]Present address: Department of Physiology, Baylor College of Medicine, Houston, Texas.

[3]The two-dimensional discriminant space is the space defined by the first to eigen vectors of $W^{-1}A$ where W is the pooled within-groups matrix of cross products of deviations and A is the among or between group matrix of cross products of deviations.

profitably employed.

The aggregation or clusters upon which the method operates are based on second-order statistics of the groups in measurement space rather than notions of distance. Whether the clusters happen to correspond to the fuzzy sets determined by a formal cluster analysis or to clusters in discriminant space is not the major concern. This is not to say these clusters have no relevance to the problem of sleep taxonomy by the EEG. Rather, the clusters we seek serve a useful purpose for extending the utility of parametric discriminant analysis in EEG pattern-recognition studies of sleep.

Data Sources

The basic problem is to classify EEG epochs into categories based on the Dement-Kleitman sleep-staging system. The EEG data that served as the basis of this study were previously described by Larsen and Walter (1970). Our original source is Johnson et al. (1969). Briefly, the data were collected from thirteen young men. The EEG samples consisted of two epochs, each one minute long, derived from a mastoid-to-P3 derivation. The epochs were agreed upon by three judges as representing each of five stages: waking, stages 1, 2, 3, 4, and stage REM. The epochs were subjected to spectral analysis at a resolution of 0.2 Hz. These narrow-band spectra were grouped into five bands: delta, 0.1 to 3.9 Hz; theta, 3.9 to 7.9 Hz; alpha, 7.9 to 12.9 Hz; sigma or $beta_1$, 12.9 to 14.9 Hz; and $beta_2$, 14.9 to 20.1 Hz. This five-variate description of the thirteen subjects is the measurement space in which the pattern recognition took place. Pattern recognition algorithms were all of the supervised and parametric class. Discriminant functions were calculated from the first of the two epochs per class per subject. The second epoch was held out for use as a testing set from which unbiased error rates were estimated. Table 1 shows the improvement in error rates obtained by use of sequential methods (see Larsen and Walter 1970 for details).

Preliminary Remarks

It should be noted that when all the assumptions underlying linear discriminant analysis are met, there cannot be any advantage to segmenting a multiple group discrimination problem. The relevant assumption underlying classical linear discriminant analysis is that the m groups being discriminated are samples from m Gaussian populations with equal variance/covariance (dispersion) matrices. Any differences are limited to unequal mean vectors. (The mean vector is an ordered one-dimensional array composed of within-group means for each variate on which the measurement space is constructed. The dispersion matrix is a symmetrical two-dimensional array of

TABLE 1.
Error Rate Improvement with Sequential Methods

		Linear		Quadratic	
		1 Stage	2 Stage	1 Stage	2 Stage
	(W	45%	64%	64%	91%
D	(1	45%	64%	51%	64%
	(REM	75%	75%	66%	66%
	(2	77%	85%	85%	85%
S	(3	77%	85%	85%	85%
	(4	69%	69%	69%	85%
	Overall	65%	74%	70%	79%

numbers containing the variances for each variate in the main diagonal and all possible pairwise covariances in the off-diagonal elements.) The dispersion matrix and mean vector occupy importance because these two parameters completely define a multivariate normal distribution. This statement is analogous to the fact that the distribution of a single Gaussian variate is determined by the population mean and variance. The assumption of equal within-groups covariance matrices allows for optimal discrimination (that is, minimal losses when costs of misclassification are equal) with linear boundaries. When this assumption is violated, the optimal boundary is no longer linear; rather, the optimal boundary (in general) is quadratic. The linear boundary obtained by BMD 07M (Dixon 1968) in such a setting is, therefore, not the optimal boundary nor is it, in general, even the best possible linear boundary. This results from the fact that the program pools across the individual groups to estimate the so-called common covariance matrix (ccm). To the extent that the assumption of equal dispersion matrices is true in the population sense, such a pooling (or "averaging" of within-group dispersions) allows a better estimate of the population dispersion matrix than any one of the individual within-groups dispersion matrices taken alone. When this assumption is violated, the resulting ccm does a variable amount of violence to the separate population values. The extent of misrepresentation depends upon how much the separate population dispersions differ.

One way to find the best linear boundary, or at least a better boundary than the one determined by simple pooling, is to weigh the estimated within-groups dispersion matrices prior to pooling (Anderson and Bahadur 1962). While this approach has generality, the determination of weights necessary to find the best linear boundary (in a multiple group discrimination with unequal within-group dispersions) is not always a simple exercise.

In certain settings another approach proposed by Rao (1966) is possible. The required conditions are that the differences in dispersion are arranged in the test space such that dispersions are homogeneous within either of two subsets, but heterogeneous between subsets. In this case the optimal boundary between subsets is quadratic, but the optimal boundary within subsets is linear; thus, two "common" covariance matrices result, each one common only to the groups within the subset. We believe this framework is the one that underlies the efficacy of the two-stage machine.[4]

Rao's formulation (1966) is a tractable specialization of the more likely situation that the subsets have greater *similarity* of dispersion within subsets than across subsets. This presents additional measurement problems, since testing equality of dispersion is simpler than indexing similarity because of the variety of ways different within-group dispersions may still be (colloquially) similar. At this point it may be useful to note that one cannot reasonably use the failure of tests for homogeneity of dispersion to judge similarity of nonequality dispersions. Such a procedure would only indicate the strength with which we reject the hypothesis of equality. It is not reasonably extendable to the assertion that strength of rejection may be used to group similar dispersions by strength of rejection of equality to one or a set of "standard" dispersion matrices. Such a statement is analogous to the fact that the significance of Wilks' lambda cannot be used to quantitatively judge group separation. Rather, a statistic such as Mahalonbois' distance is required.

Cluster Seeking Subset Generation

When covariance matrices are examined for equality, all parameters of description (the elements in the main diagonal and upper, or lower, triangle) resolve to a single, dichotomous, dimension—equality or nonequality. When dispersions differ, it seems reasonable to seek some summary indices rather than an exhaustive examination of elements in the main diagonal and upper triangle. Therefore we propose to parameterize the dispersions in a way that capitalizes on geometric concepts (as an interpretive aid) and not to consolidate these measures, but rather to consider them separately with some empirical guides for determining their relative importance. Other than size (the volume contained in a given hyperellipse of equal likelihood), which may be measured by generalized variance (determinant of the dispersion matrix) for dispersions that are otherwise equal, we propose two indices of dispersion:

---

[4]Although a quadratic boundary is, in general, optimal for the separation of such subsets, it may not necessarily perform much better than a linear one.

shape and orientation. We further propose that principal components analysis of the estimated within-group dispersion matrices may provide such a summarization.

Thus we propose to cluster groups into aggregates on the basis of greater similarity of dispersion within clusters than between clusters. The technique may therefore be described as cluster-seeking subset generation. The objective is to provide more appropriate pooling at the level of discrimination within the aggregates and to employ either linear or quadratic boundaries for discrimination between aggregates depending on earlier considerations.

In the setting of multivariate normal dispersions (with different centroids) that are equal except for rotations of their hyperellipses in measurement space, the most extreme dissimilarity would occur when the two major axes are orthogonal. The effect of pooling in this extreme situation would be to circularize the ccm. To the extent that the separate dispersions approach isotrophy, that is, as the separate dispersions approximate circularity evidenced by equal or near-equal eigen values, the pooling would do little harm. However, when the separate dispersions are strongly anisotropic, the potential error from pooling and consequent ccm circularization becomes more serious. In this way, anisotropy (shape) becomes an antecedent for characterizing similarity. That is, to the extent that the major axis of the hyperellipse is long relative to the minor axes, then the dispersions may be described, except for size, by the orientation (direction cosines) of the major axis. Consequently, similarity of dispersion may become similarity of orientation of major axes when the dispersions are strongly anisotropic. Similarity of orientation, in turn, is indexed by the cosine of the angle formed by any two major axes treated as p dimensional vectors.

If dispersions have been successfully clustered in this fashion, the effects of unequal size are easily dealt with by translating the decision boundary for discrimination either within or between clusters. The optimal decision rule for discrimination, when dispersions differ only in size, is obtainable from the log of the ratio of their generalized variances.

Principal components analysis serves two roles: a determination of anisotropy by the inequality of the eigen values of the within-group dispersion matrices; and description of the orientation of the major axis of the hyperellipse by its direction numbers, which are the elements of the eigen vector corresponding to the first eigen value (see appendix for mathematical discussion and simple numerical examples).

Principal Components Analysis

Principal components analysis is an orthogonal transformation that linearly combines variate values in the original coordinate system into new composite variables, called principal components, with the following properties: (1) The first principal component is the linear combination of coordinate values such that the resulting composite variable has maximum variance. (2) The second principal component is constrained to be orthogonal to the first; and, subject to that constraint, it is the linear combination with next largest variance. (3) Subsequent linear combinations, in turn, are mutually orthogonal with preceding ones, and they sequentially generate the next largest variance for each successive composite variable. (4) This procedure is continued until, at most, p linear combinations are formed, where p is the dimensionality of the measurement space. The definition ranks the variance obtainable with each linear combination in decreasing order. The transformation is distance preserving; therefore the total variance in either coordinate system is equal. The total variance is merely partitioned differently. Geometrically, the new variate values correspond to an interval scale on a new coordinate system which is an orthogonal transformation of the old system. If the variate values are centered about the origin, then the orthogonal transformation consists of rotation. The composite variate values geometrically correspond to the points of intersection of perpendicular lines from each point to the new axis. This set of numbers constitutes a new random variate with a mean of zero and a variance. The variance obtained is a function of the angle of rotation. The coordinate transformation desired is the one for which variance is maximized. If the samples are taken from a multivariate Gaussian population, the first principal component corresponds to the major axis of any hyperellipse that defines a locus of samples with equal likelihood. The first principal component so obtained is therefore the best univariate representation of the samples in measurement space (Figure 1).

Furthermore, the set of variances generated on the principal component may be used to index the shape of the "scatter diagram." Equal variances imply a circular dispersion or hypershpere of scatter. Unequal variances deform the scatter into elliptical shape. The former condition is called isotropic and the latter, anisotropic. The eigen values reported in this paper are a function of these variances (see appendix for details).

Other approaches to development of the principal components solution include the following: (1) Pearson approached the problem from the viewpoint of fitting an orthogonal subspace of q-dimensions to a swarm of n points in p-dimensional space where $q < p$. The criterion used was that the subspace should minimize the sums of squares perpendicular distances from the points to the subspace. The solution is the first q eigen vectors of the dispersion matrix. (2) Hottelling approached the problem from the random vector treatment in which the object was to find a dimensionality-reducing transformation matrix such that the transformed random q-vector is the best linear predictor of the original random p-vector where q<p. Again, the solution is the first q eigen vectors of the dispersion matrix (see Rao 1963 for further development).

The EEG Sleep-Staging Problem

Principal components analysis provides a description of shape and direction, especially the major axis, of the hyperellipse of equal likelihood for each multivariate swarm in measurement space. We propose that this information may direct the formation of clusters according to similarity of dispersion. This, in conjunction with the separability of these clusters in the measurement space, may provide a reasonable basis for deciding the use of cluster-seeking subset generation. It is important to note that separable clusters may not correspond to subsets of dispersion similarity. Likewise, dispersions may aggregate without corresponding to separable clusters of centroids as shown in Figure 2.

In the case of data from human subjects, the centroids were found to cluster well, as seen in Figure 3. These clusters, named DESYNC and SYNC on the basis of the gross appearance of the constituent EEG, were discriminated with linear boundary determined by BMD 07M after pooling groups W, 1, and REM of the training set into the DESYNC cluster, and pooling groups 2, 3, and 4 of the training set into the SYNC cluster. All test cases were correctly classified into one of these two subsets (Larsen and Walter 1970).

Although in this application the use of linear boundary for discrimination of clusters gave good results, this happy circumstance may not always

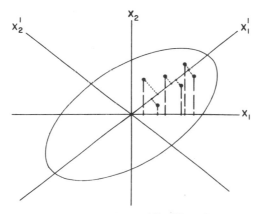

Figure 1. A bivariate Gaussian sample and equal-likelihood contour with original (x_1, x_2) and principal components (x'_1, x''_2) coordinates.

prevail. When linear boundaries yield poor results, at least two other strategies are possible. The one easier to implement is a conventional linear boundary constructed between the two border groups with classification of cases from other groups in the cluster by the border-group boundary. This strategy was successfully applied by us (Larsen et al. 1972 and 1973) with chimpanzee EEG sleep data. A more general but less widely available method would employ piecewise linear boundaries around one cluster. In this case some simplification is possible since the number of modes is known *a priori* (that is, the number of modes corresponds to the number of groups); therefore the order of the piecewise linear function is determined (Chang 1973) (Figures 4a, b, and c).

Although the centroids cluster, this alone cannot account for the improved classification results. According to earlier arguments, it is a necessary but not sufficient condition. The other condition is that the clusters must correspond to aggregates of groups with anisotropic dispersions and greater similarity of dispersion within aggregates than across aggregates as seen in Figure 4b.

Given the five-variate sleep-stage data (Larsen and Walter 1970), anisotropy may be determined by the variance on each principal component. We plot the eigen values as cumulative proportion of total dispersion for each group as shown in Figure 5.

Clearly, groups 2, 3, and 4 are strongly anisotropic with the first principal component of the covariance matrix containing over 95 percent of the trace for any of the dispersions. Groups W, 1, and REM, while less anisotropic than the others, are still dominated by the first principal component to extents ranging from 70 percent to 80 percent of the trace. In this setting inappropriate pooling could introduce substantial error if the dispersions are substantially different in orientation. Thus, the stage is set for characterizing similarity of dispersion by similarity of orientation of the separate first

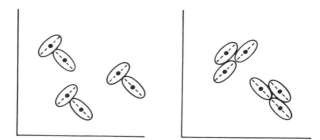

Figure 2. Left half of this figure illustrates clusters of centroids into three sets and aggregation of dispersions into two subsets. The disposition of centroids with the dispersion subsets makes them virtually unseparable. Right half illustrates two centroid clusters and two dispersion subsets that are separable.

Variable Original	Coefficients for Canonical Variable	
	1	2
1	0.05924	-0.01912
2	-0.18973	0.24574
3	-0.07564	-0.28936
4	1.90373	1.06857
5	-3.91635	-0.45981
6	-0.00008	0.00007
7	-0.00417	-0.01301
8	0.00939	0.01317
9	-0.07619	-0.05540
10	1.63194	-0.59304
11	0.00010	-0.00038
12	0.00147	0.00310
13	-0.00100	-0.00816
14	-0.00504	-0.00383
15	-0.00341	-0.02407
16	-0.02825	0.03771
17	0.01979	0.19271
18	-0.03453	0.05201
19	-0.13810	-0.04896
20	0.15389	0.04219

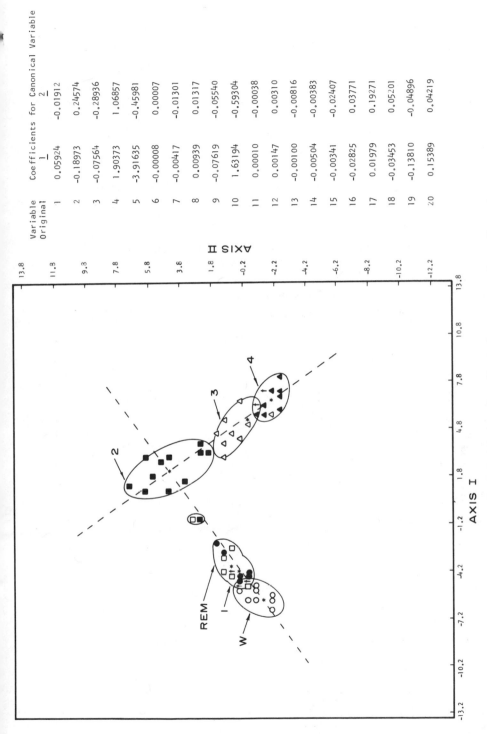

Figure 3. Plot of the six sleep stages in a discriminant space of two dimensions.

principal components. The object is to aggregate groups in such a way that the dispersions are similar within subsets and dissimilar between subsets.

The elements of the first principal component for each group are given in Table 2 after applying the constant multiplier, $k=100 \, |a_i| \, / \, \Sigma_i \, |a_i|$, to the weights. (This has the effect of removing absolute size.)[5,6]

Since these are also direction numbers, we may proceed to calculate direction cosines for each first principal component. Then similarity of orientation may be measured by the cosine of the angle between pairs of first principal components. This index is a coefficient of colinearity since colinear vectors are separated by an angle of zero degrees with an index of unity, while orthogonal vectors are separated by $\pi/2$ with an index of zero.

[5]Note that we are not using the raw first eigen vector. Rather we are using the first component that is a normalized and weighted version of the first eigen vector (see appendix for details).

[6]Removing absolute values obscures distributional properties of the loadings. However, we do not use these properties in present or later calculations. We do lose sight of the fact that eigen vectors associated with large eigen values will have more sampling variation in their loadings than vectors associated with smaller eigen values (Lawley 1963).

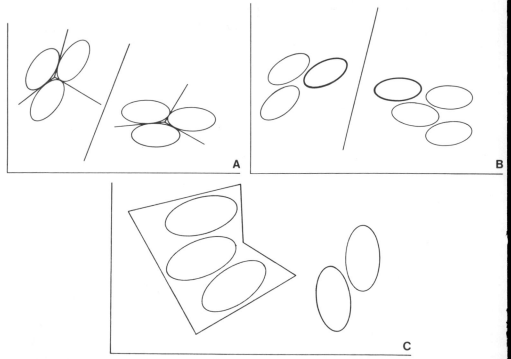

Figure 4. Illustration of separable dispersion subsets with linear separability within and between clusters. b: Discrimination of subsets by border groups (darkened). c: Discrimination of subsets by piecewise linear boundary.

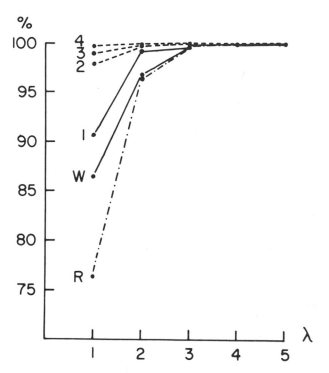

Figure 5. Plot of the eigen values of the six sleep stages as percentile values of the traces for each covariance matrix.

TABLE 2.
First Principal Component

Direction Numbers for Five Sleep Stages
and Waking on Five Variates

	W	1	R	2	3	4
1	6.25	40.65	41.30	74.50	95.30	95.95
2	26.25	46.60	34.00	8.85	3.11	1.985
3	61.70	6.55	18.65	4.27	0.99	0.10
4	0.29	4.50	0.389	0.70	-0.24	0.06
5	0.25	0.16	0.231	0.66	0.29	0.04

The cosine of the angle between two p-dimensional vectors is the sum of the products of their direction cosines. That is,

$$\cos \theta = \sum_{i=1}^{p} a_i \beta_i$$

where a_i and β_i are the direction cosines. Direction cosines are cosines of the angles the major axis makes with each coordinate axis. They are related to direction numbers, a_i, (the weights in the linear combination that provide the first principal component) as follows

$$a_i = a_i/c$$

where

$$c = \sqrt{\Sigma_i a_i^2}$$

The direction cosines for each first principal component are listed in Table 3. Simple inspection of direction cosines in Table 3 reveals that stages 2, 3, and 4 are similarly oriented in terms of their first principal component.

Among members of the DESYNC set, stages 1 and REM are more similarly oriented than either is to stage Wake. We will calculate the "coefficient of colinearity" for selected pairs of principal components as shown in Table 4.

Note that the orientation of the first principal component for stage Wake is rather unlike all other stages, but is most similar to stage REM.

On the basis of similarity of dispersion, it would appear that the groups 2, 3, and 4 should be aggregated into one cluster, named SYNC for the synchronous (slow, high-voltage) appearance of the EEG; whereas groups W, 1, and REM should be aggregated in another cluster, named DESYNC for the desynchronous (fast, low-voltage) appearance of the EEG. The groups in the SYNC subset have dispersions with principal components that are quite similar within subsets (the lowest being 2/4 = 0.994) and dissimilar between subsets (the highest being 1/2 = 0.741). The picture in the DESYNC cluster is not as clear; nevertheless, for each group the highest "coefficient" is still within the DESYNC set. The highest within-subset similarity being 1/R = 0.959, the lowest similarities are for those comparisons involving stage W. Yet the highest coefficient is for W/1 = 0.448, whereas the best comparison across subsets is still worse at 0.191 for W/2. In addition, not only the peak but also the average relationship is higher within subsets than across subsets.

It is interesting to compare the principal components for each group against the first component of the various pooled covariance matrices. We

TABLE 3.
First Principal Component

Direction Cosines for Five Sleep Stages and Waking

	W	1	R	2	3	4
$\Delta 1$	.093	.652	.728	.992	.999	.999
$\theta 2$	.390	.747	.601	.118	.033	.021
a_3	.916	.105	.329	.057	.010	.001
$\beta_1 4$	.004	.072	.007	.009	-.002	.001
$\beta_2 5$	.004	.003	.004	.009	.002	.001

TABLE 4.
Cosines Between Selected Pairs
of First Principal Components

$\cos \theta_{W/1} = 0.448$ $\cos \theta_{W/2} = 0.191$

$\cos \theta_{W/R} = 0.603$ $\cos \theta_{1/2} = 0.741$

$\cos \theta_{1/R} = 0.959$ $\cos \theta_{2/4} = 0.994$

begin with calculation of direction cosines for the following poolings: (1) combining all six groups into one common covariance matrix; (2) combining W, 1, and R into a DESYNC "common" covariance matrix; and (3) combining 2, 3, and 4 into a SYNC "common" covariance matrix. The direction cosines of the principal components for these 3 ccm are shown in Table 5.

Selected "correlations" are shown in Table 6.

It is plainly apparent that the groups that benefit most from segmentation by cluster-seeking subset generation are W, 1, and R. Their representation by the DESYNC ccm is much more realistic than is representation by the [D + S] ccm. It is also these groups in which error rates improve most after segmentation.

When we consider both orientation and shape, it becomes clear that clusters containing 2, 3, and 4 in SYNC, and W, 1, and R in DESYNC, provide a more reasonable basis for pooling than does the lumping of both subsets together. The dispersions of SYNC and DESYNC subset members are more similar within clusters than across clusters. We would expect pooling in the DESYNC cluster to be somewhat more damaging than pooling in the SYNC cluster because R is less anisotropic and W is different in orientation.

TABLE 5.
Direction Cosines of the First
Principal Component for
Various Poolings of
Covariance Matrices

	D+S	D	S
1	.999	.706	.999
2	.024	.684	.036
3	.006	.165	.001
4	-.004	.069	.008
5	.002	.028	.002

TABLE 6.
Cosines Between Selected First Principal Components
of Groups and Pooled Covariance Matrices

2/(D + S)	= 0.994	2/S	= 0.996		
W/D	= 0.484	1/D	= 0.994	R/D	= 0.980
W/(D + S)	= 0.099	1/(D + S)	= 0.665		

As an incidental observation, the direction cosines are of some inherent interest. Group W is closely oriented to the alpha axis (Table 3). Group 1 shows an important effect due to the theta range intensities in its orientation, whereas its delta effects are increased and alpha effects are decreased in comparison to W. Group REM has the second highest alpha direction in its orientation with relatively more delta and less theta effect than stage 1.

Conclusions

The use of multiple-group discriminant analysis as a parametric, supervised pattern-recognition machine depends on certain distributional assumptions in order to minimize misclassifications. One such parametric assumption is that the m groups correspond to samples from m multivariate Gaussian populations that differ only by their centroids; that is, the dispersion matrices are equal. Pattern-recognition studies of the EEG during sleep violate this assumption with the result that the linear boundary employed is not the optimum, nor is it the best linear boundary.

This situation can be improved when the differences in dispersions display the following characteristics: (1) the dispersions are anisotropic; (2) the dispersions may be aggregated into subsets so that there is greater similarity of dispersion within subsets than between subsets (as measured by the orientation of their first principal components); and (3) the aggregations correspond to separable clusters of groups.

The method makes use of principal components analysis to determine anisotropy and direction numbers of the major axis of the hyperellipse of equal likelihood. The cosine of the angle between pairs of first principal components allows aggregation of dispersions according to similarity, which, in the case of anisotropic dispersion, becomes similarity of orientation of first principal components.

If these subsets are separable, then a sequential decision process that classifies each case into first a cluster and then into a constituent group of the cluster is possible. This strategy would not result in an error rate improvement if the dispersions were equal, nor would it if the clusters did not correspond to aggregates based on greater similarity of dispersion within subsets than between subsets. The virtue of the sequential strategy lies in its use when the unequal dispersions are disposed as in items 1 through 3 above. Then the discrimination makes use of three common covariance matrices with more appropriate pooling at the second layer of the decision process than could be accomplished with a simple one-stage discrimination.

The above requirements for successful application of the parametric, sequential strategy will limit its generality. For this reason the method is a useful alternative to other strategies that operate in the setting of unequal dispersion matrices. It has the virtue of easy implementation with widely available programs. Lastly, the requirements are met to a useful degree in the EEG sleep-staging problem as previously described.

References

Anderson, T.W. 1963. Asymptotic theory for principal components analysis. *Ann. Math. Stat.* 34:122.

Anderson, T.W., and Bahadur, R.R. 1962. Classification into two multivariate normal distributions with different covariance matrices. *Ann. Math. Stat.* 33:420.

Chang, C.L. 1973. Pattern recognition by piecewise linear discriminant functions. *IEEE Transactions on Computers*, C-22 (9), p. 859.

Dixon, W.J. (ed.) 1968. *BMD Biomedical computer programs.* Health Sciences Computing Facility, UCLA School of Medicine, Los Angeles, California.

Johnson, L.C., Lubin, A., Naitoh, P., Nute, D., and Austin, M. 1969. Spectral analysis of the EEG in dominant and non-dominant subjects during waking and sleeping. *Electroencephalogr. Clin. Neurophysiol.* 26:361.

Larsen, L.E., Ruspini, E.H., McNew, J.J., Walter, D.O., and Adey, W.R. 1972. A test of sleep staging systems in the unrestrained chimpanzee. *Brain Res.* 40:319.

Larsen, L.E., Ruspini, E.H., McNew, J.J., Walter, D.O., and Adey, W.R., 1973. Classification and discrimination of the EEG during sleep. In P. Kellaway and I. Petersén (eds.), *Automation of Clinical Electroencephalography.* New York: Raven Press, p. 243.

Larsen, L.E., and Walter, D.O. 1969. On automatic methods of sleep staging by spectra of electroencephalograms. *Agressologie* 10 (special number):1.

Larsen, L.E., and Walter, D.O. 1970. On automatic methods of sleep staging by EEG spectra. *Electroencephalogr. Clin. Neurophysiol.* 28:459.

Larsen, L.E., Walter, D.O., McNew, J.J., and Adey, W.R. 1971. On the problem of bias in error rate estimation for discriminant analysis. *Pattern Recognition* 3:217.

Lawley, D.N., and Maxwell, A.E. 1963. *Factor Analysis as a Statistical Method.* London: Butterworths.

Rao, C.R. 1963. The use and interpretation of principal components analysis in applied research. Washington, D.C.: U.S. Office of Education Contract Report 2-10-065.

Rao, C.R. 1966. Discriminant function between composite hypotheses and related problems. *Biometrika* 53:339.

Appendix with Numerical Examples

Principal components analysis consists of a rotational transformation of coordinate axes with the object in mind that variance is maximized along the new axes. The set of new axes constitutes a set of normalized linear combinations (sum of squares of coefficients equal to unity) of the old coordinates. That is, in the population sense we have a p-dimensional random vector in the original coordinate system.

$$\underline{X} = \{x_1, x_2 \ldots x_p\}'$$

where $x_1, x_2 \ldots x_p$ are random variates.

The random p-vector has a mean of zero,

$$E(\underline{X}) = 0$$

and a dispersion matrix

$$E(\underline{XX}') = [\Sigma]$$

The linear combination is implemented by a p-dimensional column vector of coefficients

$$\underline{B} = \{b_1, b_2, \ldots b_p\}'$$

The linear combination is made by the following

$$U = b_1 x_1 + b_2 x_2 + \ldots + b_p x_p$$

$$U = \underline{B}'\underline{X}$$

The transformation $\underline{B}$ carries the random vector $\underline{X}$ into a random scalar variate U. The variance of U is

$$E(U)^2 = E(\underline{B}'\underline{X})^2$$

$$= E(\underline{B}'\underline{X}\underline{X}'\underline{B})$$

$$= \underline{B}'[\Sigma]\underline{B}$$

Thus, the variance of U depends on the coefficients of the combination and the dispersion matrix in the original coordinate system.

It is these variances, one for each set of coefficients, which are maximized subject to the condition that

$$\sum_{k=1}^{p} b_k^2 = 1.0$$

and that the sets are mutually orthogonal. That is, the inner products are zero.

$$\underline{B}^{(j)} \cdot \underline{B}^{(i)} = 0 \quad \text{for } i,j = 1,2, \ldots p$$

$$\text{and } i \neq j$$

or equivalently,

$$\sum_{k=1}^{p} b_k^{(i)} b_k^{(j)} = 0 \text{ where k indexes variates and i, j index sets of coefficients}$$

The column vectors of coefficients that maximize the above variances are found as the vectors that are invariant under the linear transformation $[\Sigma]$. That is, invariant vectors are those that are changed only by a scalar multiple with a given linear transformation

$$[\Sigma]\,\underline{B} = \lambda\underline{B}$$

where λ is a scalar constant. The invariant vector(s) are found by solving the following set of homogeneous equations:

$$[\Sigma]\underline{B} = \lambda\underline{B}$$

$$[\Sigma]\underline{B} - \lambda\underline{B} = 0$$

$$([\Sigma] - \lambda[I])\underline{B} = 0$$

A nontrivial solution exists when the coefficient matrix is singular. That is, when

$$|\Sigma - \lambda I| = 0$$

The values of λ which make the determinant zero are found by expanding the above determinant to produce a polynomial in λ, $\emptyset(\lambda)$, of degree p. The roots of $\emptyset(\lambda)$ are substituted separately into the coefficient matrix in order to find the corresponding $\underline{B}$. Thus, there are p sets of $\underline{B}^{(i)}$ where $i = 1, 2, \ldots$ p corresponding to the p roots of $\emptyset(\lambda)$. Furthermore, under the above conditions, the variance of composite, scalar variates $U^{(i)} = \underline{B}^{(i)}\underline{X}$ can be shown to be equal to the value of the corresponding root. That is,

$$E(U^{(i)})^2 = \lambda_i$$

If the roots of $\emptyset(\lambda)$ are ranked in decreasing magnitude, $\lambda_1 > \lambda_2 > \ldots > \lambda_p$, the first principal component, $\underline{B}^{(1)}$, makes the one linear combination with maximum possible variance. The variate values on this coordinate are covered by the random variate $U^{(1)}$ with variance of λ_1. Further, if $\underline{X}$ is from a multivariate normal population, the first principal component corresponds to the major axis at the hyperellipse of equal likelihood for the multivariate "scatter diagram."

Several additional features are of interest: (1) the roots of the characteristic polynomial $\emptyset(\lambda)$ are real and nonnegative; (2) the p sets of coefficients $B^{(i)}$ $i = 1, 2, \ldots$ p produce p random variates $U^{(i)}$, $i = 1, 2, \ldots$ p, which may constitute a random vector

$$\underline{U} = \{U^{(1)}, U^{(2)}, \ldots U^{(p)}\}$$

Similarly, the ordered set of column vectors $B^{(i)}$ may constitute a transformation matrix

$$\underline{U} = [B]\underline{X}$$

where $[B] = \begin{bmatrix} | & | & & | \\ \underline{B}^{(1)} & \underline{B}^{(2)} & \cdots & \underline{B}^{(p)} \\ | & | & & | \end{bmatrix}$

The transformation matrix is nonsingular and orthogonal

$$|B| \neq 0, \ [B]\ [B'] = [I] = [B']\ [B]$$

It carries the random vector $\underline{X}$ into the random vector $\underline{U}$. This matrix of normalized eigen vectors is known as a factor pattern matrix when the eigen vectors are multiplied by the square root of their corresponding eigen values

$$[A] = [B]\ [\Lambda^{\frac{1}{2}}]$$

where

$$[\Lambda^{\frac{1}{2}}] = \begin{vmatrix} \sqrt{\lambda_1} & & & \\ & \sqrt{\lambda_2} & & \\ & & \ddots & \\ & & & \sqrt{\lambda_p} \end{vmatrix}$$

Later presentation of the components analysis will be in terms of the factor pattern matrix since the squared length of the vector will then equal the corresponding eigen value and thus be an analog of variance on the component.

The random vector $\underline{U}$ in the new p-space has a dispersion matrix given by

$$E(\underline{U}\underline{U}') = [\Lambda]$$

where $[\Lambda]$ is

$$[\Lambda] = \begin{vmatrix} \lambda_1 & & & \\ & \lambda_2 & & \\ & & \ddots & \\ & & & \lambda_p \end{vmatrix}$$

That is, the dispersion matrix in the transformed space is diagonal with the eigen values of the characteristic equation down the main diagonal. The generalized variance is invariant. That is, the determinant of the two dispersion matrices are equal:

$$|\Lambda| = |\Sigma|$$

Lastly, the number of nonzero roots to $\emptyset(\lambda)$ depends on the rank of $[\Sigma]$. If $[\Sigma]$ is of full rank (rank equal to order) there are p nonzero roots to $\emptyset(\lambda)$. If the rank, r, is less than the order, p, then there are r<p nonzero roots to $\emptyset(\lambda)$; thus, there will be r coordinate axes to the new space.

This is one possible route to dimensionality reduction. Another route is to select the m largest roots of the dispersion matrix according to a criterion that most often operates on the notion that the p-m smallest roots are either indistinct (equal or nearly equal) or constitute an empirically unimportant proportion of the trace.

The variates are standardized (to have a mean of zero and a variance of unity) to simplify the figures and exposition. This has the consequence of making the covariance and correlation matrices equal. Furthermore, in the two-dimensional examples the principal component is constrained to make a 45-degree angle with the abscissa, either in quadrant I or II. The fact that unities are in the main diagonal means that the total variance to be modeled is p where p is the order of the matrix. In general, the components analysis solution is not invariant with normalization of variates. Also, distributional properties of eigen values and eigen vectors of correlation matrices are not as well treated as for the dispersion matrix (Anderson 1963).

Numerical Examples

Consider the following variance/covariance matrix $[S_1]$

$$[S_1] = [R_1] = \begin{vmatrix} 1.0 & 0.9 \\ 0.9 & 1.0 \end{vmatrix}$$

The eigen values are

$$\lambda_1 = 1.9$$

$$\lambda_2 = 0.1$$

Note that the sum of the eigen values equals the sum of the elements of the main diagonal, i.e., the trace of the matrix

$$\sum_{i=i}^{p} \lambda_i = \sum_{j=1}^{p} s_{jj} \text{ where p is the order of } [S].$$

The eigen vectors are

$$v_1 = [+0.70711 + 0.70711]'$$

$$[V] = v_1 \ v_2$$

$$v_2 = [-0.70711 + 0.70711]'$$

Note that these are normalized

$$\sum_{i=1}^{p} v_i^2 = 1.0$$

The factor pattern is

$$[A] = [V] \ [\Lambda^{\frac{1}{2}}]$$

$$[A] = \begin{bmatrix} 0.7071 & -0.7071 \\ 0.7071 & 0.7071 \end{bmatrix} \begin{bmatrix} 1.3748 & 0 \\ 0 & 0.3162 \end{bmatrix}$$

$$[A] = \begin{bmatrix} 0.9745 & -0.2234 \\ 0.9745 & 0.2234 \end{bmatrix}$$

If we take the columns of [A] as locating two vectors in a two-dimensional test space, we have the plot shown in Figure 6.

Note that the sign of s_{12} determines the quadrant in which the principal component will be. When s_{12} is positive, the first component will be in quadrant I. When it is negative, the first component will be in quadrant II. Furthermore, the squared lengths of vectors are equal to the eigen values. These, in turn, are proportional to the fraction of total variance explained on each axis. Given a bivariate normal scatter diagram, the ellipse encloses 1σ of variance on each axis as generated by the corresponding (new) composite variate. If the samples were from a bivariate Gaussian population, the first and second components would be the major and minor axes of any two-dimensional ellipse of equal likelihood. The high positive correlation (and equal variances) puts the major axis in quadrant I and implies a long major axis relative to the minor axis.

We may check the effect of sign on location of the first principal component by analyzing the following matrix:

$$[S_2] = \begin{vmatrix} 1.0 & -0.9 \\ -0.9 & 1.0 \end{vmatrix} = [R_2]$$

with $[S_1]$ for comparison

$$[S_1] = \begin{vmatrix} 1.0 & 0.9 \\ 0.9 & 1.0 \end{vmatrix} = [R_1]$$

The corresponding factor patterns are

$$A_1 = \begin{vmatrix} 0.975 & -0.223 \\ 0.975 & 0.223 \end{vmatrix}$$

$$A_2 = \begin{vmatrix} -0.975 & 0.223 \\ 0.975 & 0.223 \end{vmatrix}$$

The change in sign of covariance (correlation) moves the first principal component from quadrant I to quadrant II (Figure 7).

The effect of change from a high positive covariance (correlation) to an equally high negative correlation was to rotate the principal components coordinate system 90-degrees. The "shape" (ratio of lengths of major and minor axes) of the bivariate swarm is unchanged. Thus, the sign and values in the first column of $[A]$ determine the direction of the first principal component in the test space.

Components analysis also provides information concerning shape of the test space hyperellipse by way of the relative sizes of the eigen values. We noted before that a high correlation, regardless of sign, implies that the test

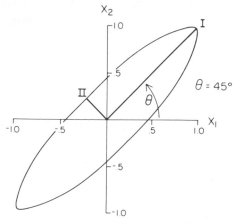

Figure 6. Major and minor axes of a bivariate Gaussian swarm with dispersion matrix S_1. (U.S. Army photograph)

space has a long major axis relative to its minor axis. However, once out of the bivariate case, it is more informative to consider the proportion of total variance generated or explained by each component as an index of relative dispersion along that axis. Thus we can determine something about shape of the multivariate swarm in measurement space. Consider a third two-dimensional example:

$$[S_3] = \begin{vmatrix} 1.0 & 0.5 \\ 0.5 & 1.0 \end{vmatrix} = [R_3]$$

The direction of its principal component is identical to the one for $[S_1]$. However, the shape of the ellipse is much rounder than before (Figure 8).

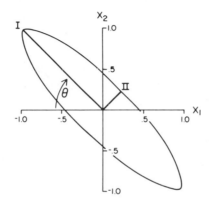

Figure 7. Major and minor axes of a bivariate Gaussian swarm with dispersion matrix S_2.

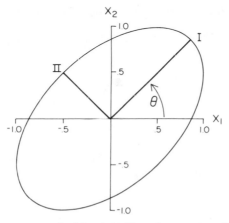

Figure 8. Major and minor axes of a bivariate Gaussian swarm with dispersion matrix S_3. (U.S. Army photograph)

This is in contrast to S_2 where shape was identical to S_1. We can summarize this information in a table or plot of eigen values as proportionate contribution to total dispersion as in Figure 9 and Table 7.

Let us consider two additional examples in three dimensions. Given the variance/covariance matrix $[S_4]$ written in upper triangular form,

$$[S_4] = \begin{vmatrix} 1.0 & 0.7 & 0.5 \\ & 1.0 & 0.9 \\ & & 1.0 \end{vmatrix} = [R_4]$$

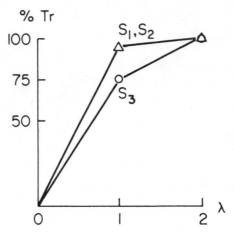

Figure 9. *A plot of the eigen values of S_1, S_2, and S_3 as percentage of the traces.*

TABLE 7.
Eigen Values for Three
Two-by-Two Dispersion Matrices

S_1: $\lambda_1 = 1.9\ (95\%)$ S_2: $\lambda_1 = 1.9\ (95\%)$

$\lambda_2 = 0.1\ (5\%)$ $\lambda_2 = 0.1\ (5\%)$

S_3: $\lambda_1 = 1.5\ (75\%)$

$\lambda_2 = 0.5\ (25\%)$

we have the following eigen values

$$\lambda_1 = 2.41\ (80\%),\ \lambda_2 = 0.524\ (18\%),\ \lambda_3 = 0.06\ (2\%)$$

The factor pattern is

$$[A_4] = \begin{vmatrix} 0.80 & -0.59 & 0.06 \\ 0.97 & 0.12 & -0.19 \\ 0.90 & 0.40 & 0.15 \end{vmatrix}$$

The direction of the first principal component and the shape of the distribution are seen in the test space as shown in Figure 10.

The relative shape is further illustrated in Figure 11 by plotting the cumulative proportion of total dispersion against the index i.

We form a second variance/covariance matrix by interchanging the third element of the second row and the second element of the first row. Thus,

$$[S_5] = \begin{vmatrix} 1.0 & 0.9 & 0.5 \\ & 1.0 & 0.7 \\ & & 1.0 \end{vmatrix} = [R_5]$$

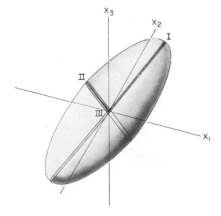

Figure 10. Axes of a trivariate normal swarm with dispersion matrix S_4.

The eigen values are unchanged from before, but the orientation of the factor score ellipse is slightly changed by rotation toward the X_1 axis (Figure 12). In the factor pattern the first and third rows have been interchanged.

$$[A_5] = \begin{vmatrix} 0.90 & 0.40 & 0.15 \\ 0.97 & 0.12 & -0.19 \\ 0.80 & -0.59 & 0.06 \end{vmatrix}$$

Thus, $[S_4]$ and $[S_5]$ do not differ at all in shape and only slightly in orientation. As a further index of similarity of orientation, we propose that the "coincidence" between the two principal components (as measured by the cosine of the angle between them) may be a useful guide when similarities of orientation are not obvious by inspection of the factor pattern.

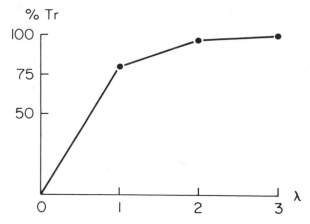

Figure 11. A plot of percentile eigen values for S. (U.S. Army photograph)

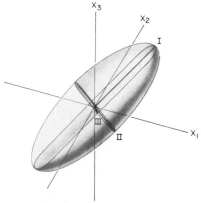

Figure 12. Axes of a trivariate normal swarm with dispersion matrix S_5 which is related to S_4 by interchanging elements s_{23} and s_{12}.

Given the coordinates of each first principal component $[\,l_1,\,l_2,\,\ldots\,l_p]$ or specifically

$\quad$ S_4: $[0.80,\ 0.97,\ 0.90]'$

$\quad$ S_5: $[0.90,\ 0.97,\ 0.80]'$

we convert these direction numbers, l_i to direction cosines a_i and β_i by dividing each with the constant C defined below:

$$C = \sqrt{\Sigma^p\ l_i{}^2}$$

where $\quad$ i=1, 2 ... p

Thus, $\quad$ $C = \sqrt{(0.80)^2 + (0.97)^2 + (0.90)^2}$

$\qquad\qquad$ $C = \sqrt{.64 + .94 + .81}$

$\qquad\qquad$ $C = \sqrt{2.39} = 1.546$

The direction cosines are

$\quad$ S_4: $[a_1,\ a_2,\ a_3]$

$\quad$ S_4: $\dfrac{0.80}{1.53},\ \dfrac{0.97}{1.53},\ \dfrac{0.90}{1.53} = [0.5174,\ 0.6274,\ 0.5821]'$

$\quad$ S_5: $[\beta_1, \beta_2, \beta_3]$

$\quad$ S_5: $\dfrac{0.90}{1.53},\ \dfrac{0.97}{1.53},\ \dfrac{0.80}{1.53} = [0.5821,\ 0.6274,\ 0.5174]'$

The cosine of the angle between these two vectors is given by the sum of the products of the direction cosines

$$\cos \theta = \sum_{i=1}^{p}\ a_i\beta_i$$

$\quad$ $= (0.5174)\,(0.5821) + (0.6274)\,(0.6274) + (0.5821)\,(0.5174)$

$\quad$ $= 0.2677 + 0.3936 + 0.3011$

$\quad$ $\cos \theta = 0.9624$

which confirms the impression that interchanging the two elements leaves the test space orientation of the first principal component essentially unchanged.

Acknowledgments

The computations reported herein were performed at the Division of Computer Research and Technology (DCRT) of the National Institutes of Health under an interagency liaison between Walter Reed Army Institute of Research (WRAIR) and DCRT. It is a pleasure to acknowledge the helpful review of this manuscript by D.B. Tang, Ph.D., senior statistician, Division of Biometrics, WRAIR. It is also a pleasure to acknowledge the patient typing and figure preparation provided by staff members of WRAIR and the Department of Neurophysiology, The Methodist Hospital, Houston, Texas.

digital systems

Harold W. Shipton, C. Eng., F.I.E.R.E.

Bioengineering Resource Facility
University of Iowa College of Medicine
Iowa City, Iowa

Historically, neurophysiological signal processing and analysis have been done by analog techniques. The biological preparation is living in real-time, and the essence of a physiological experiment is to isolate the variable under study and display it as a function of time. Thus the ubiquitous strip chart recorder is eminently suited for many of the more rudimentary forms of data display and presents the information in a form suitable for "eyeball" processing. It is rare for the neuroscientist to meet an integral sign where the independent variable is not time. For those interested in neural events the time unit is usually the millisecond; for the clinical electroencephalographer the hour is more appropriate. It is at the longer intervals of time that analog methods become very limited. For example, an analog integrator operating over a period of one second is an elegant and easily realized device: an analog integrator ranging over one hour is exceedingly cumbersome and cannot be realized to even a moderate degree of accuracy.

At the level of data analysis, a number of early devices were analog in nature. The first spectrum analyzers for the electroencephalogram (EEG) were of this type, and the earliest work on the auto and cross correlograms of the EEG were performed with drum analyzers working in an analog mode and relying on vacuum tube multipliers of exceedingly limited capability. It would be fair to say that up to the mid-1950s the only digital operation

193

routinely used by the physiologist was the operation of pulse counting in those few experimental techniques that made use of ionizing radiation. The trend to more quantifiable methods stems almost entirely from the efforts of the communication biophysics group at Massachusetts Institute of Technology. Their monograph, "Processing Neuroelectric Data" (Communication Biophysics Group of Research Laboratory of Electronics and William M. Siebert 1959), contains a great deal of relevant information and can be read with profit by anyone entering the area. The digital computer had been introduced into business and industry a few years before this but its cumbersome input/output devices and its extreme cost and complexity had discouraged its use as an on-line investigative tool except for a limited number of national defense applications where cost per unit of information was not regarded as significant constraint on the experimental design. Indeed, in its early days the digital computer was regarded more as a source of hypotheses about brain function than as a tool for their investigation. Superficial analogies between neuronal function as a binary mechanism and the digital computer enjoyed an enormous popularity, and it may well be that some of the loose statements about similarity between brain and computer turned off many serious investigators who might have looked at the value of digital techniques in their biological experiments.

Whatever the reason, it is true to say that prior to the work of the M.I.T. group the three major analytical processes in the investigation of the EEG were performed by on-line, real-time analog devices. Spectral analysis of a limited kind was performed by the wave analyzer described by Baldock and Walter (1946), correlation analysis by Barlow and Brazier (1954), and period analysis by Burch (1959). All these investigators used "home-grown" analog instruments. Averaging of evoked responses was just coming into vogue. It is of interest to note that Dawson (1954), who introduced this powerful technique to neurophysiology, used a combination of analog storage devices (capacitors) with mechanical switches which could in a sense be regarded as digital elements. Indeed, the block diagram of the original Dawson averager bears a remarkable resemblance to the block diagram of the digital devices, such as the Computer of Average Transients (CAT), that were commercially developed some years later and have become an apparently indispensable part of the neurophysiologist's armamentarium. The M.I.T. report referred to above described the elegant average response computer of Clark (1958), and this is the most clearly documented example of digital computer use in the 1950s.

Beyond question, the most important factor influencing the introduction of digital methods in neurophysiology was the design of the Laboratory Instrument Computer (LINC) developed by Wesley Clark and his associates (Clark and Molnar 1964). Since this computer was introduced, its speed has been progressively increased from the initial 8μ sec cycle time to 1.2μ sec in the currently available commercial machine while its cost has fallen by something approaching fifty percent. It should be remembered that an important part of the development effort of this machine involved considerations of economics. Part of the engineering specification included a statement that the machine should be (just) within the range of a well-established individual investigator. In any event, the machine has proved less costly than an electron microscope and many of them are used as dedicated instruments by single investigators or by small groups of investigators. The LINC has been extensively described in the literature, and here we will note only that its development was made possible by a close cooperative effort between members of the biological, engineering, and physical sciences. Such coordinated group activity is often tried but rarely successful.

In this paper we shall be primarily concerned with digital devices that are substantially less complex than the general-purpose digital computers of the LINC type, and we shall be particularly interested in devices that can be used in clinical and investigational laboratories to gather and process data from a wide range of preparations in varying psychophysiological states. This move toward special-purpose "black boxes" has been made possible in large part by the development of integrated circuits in which a substantial number of logical functions can be performed in the confines of one small plastic package. The sophistication of these devices has increased over the past few years while the price has fallen sharply. There is now a sufficiently wide range of components available to realize many devices exceedingly inexpensively. Moreover, the design process in digital systems differs from that commonly used by electronics engineers when producing physiological devices from analog components. Much of the reliability and repeatability of the digital circuit is engineered into the integrated circuit itself; thus, some of the responsibility for hardware and engineering has been transferred from the user to the device manufacturer. We shall be especially interested in instruments that embody such circuits because they are producible in quantity at prices so low that they can be widely used in clinical laboratories and thus enable a very large data base to be built up. Properly designed digital instruments are exceedingly docile and their operation is well within the range of operating personnel in hospital and clinical situations. It is central to the thesis of this paper that the development of such special-purpose devices will continue and will have major impact on the overall neurophysiological art. It is worth mentioning that the group who designed the LINC computer is now pursuing an aspect of computer design that may result in yet another breakthrough in the application of electronic techniques to physiology and medicine. In this concept the individual hardware components of computers are packaged in such a way as to permit programs to be written in hardware by the interconnection of a number of macromodules. While the wide use of these devices awaits large-scale production, the method is important enough to merit attention from anyone interested in the future of the digital computer art as applied to neurophysiology.

The principles of electronic circuits undoubtedly are well known to most readers of this volume and it would not be appropriate to attempt a full engineering discussion of all that is involved in the design of digital hardware. However, there are specific aspects of such systems, notably in the input and output sections, of which understanding is often less complete than desirable. Accordingly, I shall review these particular aspects briefly in order to put their problems and possibilities into a reasonable perspective.

The use of digital computation methods inevitably involves some process for converting the biological signal into a suitably scaled numerical value. This process is known as *analog to digital* (A/D) conversion and its principles are completely described in the literature. There are several possible techniques of varying complexity. The choice depends almost entirely on the time available to make a conversion (that is, on the data rate), and to some extent the speed of conversion is a nonlinear function of the dollar cost of the converter. Although the technology varies from system to system, all methods of conversion depend on making a comparison between a known value of voltage or current and the instantaneous value of the signal to be converted. Although the actual operation of comparing the sampled signal with a reference and adjusting the reference until equality occurs takes only a few microseconds, the sample must be stored in the computer and this storing operation, together with any other sequential operations the computer is undertaking, must be added to the total conversion time. Nevertheless, since conversion rates of the order of 10^4 conversions/second are readily obtained, these considerations are not usually too pressing for the neurophysiologist. The problems inherent in A/D conversion are somewhat less well understood in terms of overall accuracy. While, for many purposes, a conversion need only be effected to a relatively small number of bits (8 bits implying 1 part in 255), there are a number of factors that complicate the designer's choice of the actual word length to be employed. First, if the signal amplitude is allowed to exceed the reference voltage, then the conversion will be truncated at the maximum output value of the converter. Care must therefore be taken to see that overloads do not occur. At the other end of the scale, if the signal magnitude is small, then it will be represented by too few digits to permit its meaningful reconstruction. It is also necessary to consider the accuracy of A/D conversion in terms of the smallest step in the reference signal that can occur. If, for example, the reference voltage is of the order of 1 volt and an 8-bit converter is being used, then the converter can measure only to an accuracy of roughly 4 millivolts. It is therefore necessary to introduce a concept of "noise" into conversion systems that differs somewhat from the concept used in analog systems. Quantization noise, which is the term used to describe this particular phenomenon, is the difference between the real value of the signal at any instant and the measured value at that instant. This noise, of course, exists in addition to any other system noise introduced in the measurement and amplification chain. In many situations this latter noise is substantially greater than quantization noise. It should be remembered, however, that if a process such as averaging is being used to improve the signal noise ration of the biological signal, quantization noise will set the overall limit since signals below the quantization noise level cannot be recovered by an averaging process.

Perhaps the most difficult choice facing the designer and user of neurophysiological systems concerns the number of samples per unit time, that is, the sampling rate. While at first it might seem reasonable to make this rate as high as possible, this strategy will place unreasonably heavy demands on the storage capabilities of the computer or computerlike instrument since all samples must be stored and available for processing. Where the biological signal can be considered as band-limited, and this is usually the case, the problem can be tackled by recourse to the concepts of sampling theory. For all usual cases a sampling rate of twice the highest frequency present in the sample is both necessary and sufficient to define the signal. Considerations of sample interval are an important part of the study of information and have been exhaustively treated in the literature. Another important concept in the design of the system is the way in which the band width of the signal is limited prior to the A/D conversion. If the signal contains components at higher than the sampling frequency (for example, noise), it is possible for spurious frequencies to be produced by a process known as "aliasing." Suppose, as an example, that an EEG is being sampled at 32 samples per second to give, as in Bickford's compressed spectral array system, a spectrum of the signal in the range 0 to 16 Hz. Then a 60-Hz component present at the A/D converter would give rise to a signal at as much below the sampling rate as the interference is above it, and an entirely spurious signal at 4 Hz could be generated. It is thus necessary to consider extremely carefully the filtering of a signal before its application to an A/D converter. In the example cited above, the frequency response of the system must be flat from 0 to 16 Hz, but it should be attenuated to zero at frequencies above the sampling rate. Such filters are not easy to design and the engineer should be aware of the possibility of introducing spurious signal components at a point in the system following the input filter devices. In practice, the problem is not quite as formidable as it has been made to sound here since many signal-analysis systems are available that take into account the limitations implicit in the conversion process.

It should also be noted that when multichannel operation is required it is entirely feasible to use a single A/D converter and to feed the various channels of information to it successively by a multiplexing device. Such multiplexers are off-the-shelf components and are often combined in a single package with the hardware required to make a complete signal-conversion unit.

The processing of digital information almost always requires that data be stored in some form of *memory*. For very small systems a chain of bistable electronic devices (flip flops), that can be set to any desired initial state, often suffices as an adequate memory. Small hand-held electronic calculators use this type of storage. For large programmable computers the main memory has, until recently, depended heavily on magnetic systems. These memories are perhaps the best understood component of a total digital system; they will not be discussed further here except to note that once information has been entered into a magnetic memory system, it can be retained indefinitely, even if the power supply to the computer fails or the machine is switched off. Flip-flop storage depends on the maintenance of an adequate power supply at all times and is graphically described as "volatile" because of its propensity for losing data during small power interruptions.

In modern digital computers the main storage is almost always described as "random access." This property is in large part responsible for the speed and efficiency of modern digital machines. Typically, there is a plane of magnetic storage elements for each binary digit in the word, and information is written into or read from each of these planes in parallel. Early computers, which relied on magnetic drums for their main storage, perforce used serial entry and retrieval since location in the memory was represented by a physical location on the surface of a drum. Such serial memories are inherently slower and more awkward to use in general-purpose computers than are parallel machines. In recent years, however, very large flip-flop systems known as shift registers have become available that have many of the desirable properties of the magnetic drum without the impediments of extreme slowness and high cost associated with mechanical motion. These shift registers are comprised of binary elements and data can be entered into one end of the unit and retrieved at the other. Data are moved through the store by a series of clock pulses derived from the system timing. For many simple biophysical devices such memories are ideal, as it is often possible to enter data into the system digit by digit (or bit by bit), and for many physiological applications very high speed is not required. The bioengineering unit at the University of Iowa has recently been making a number of instruments that rely on this type of memory. Some of these have been described in the literature; others are still in the process of engineering development. Because of their utility to the neurophysiologist, a brief description of some of these instruments follows.

The use of any form of digital storage depends on the availability of appropriate hardware to perform arithmetical or logical operations on the data in storage. Almost all of the arithmetic functions can be performed by solid state units available on very small and inexpensive "chips." These have, in general, been designed for computer applications, and they usually perform their arithmetic on a word assembled in parallel.

Fortunately they are fast and operations may therefore be performed "on the fly." For general-purpose arithmetic this would be a cumbersome arrangement but for special-purpose machines it is entirely appropriate since the repertoire of operations is, generally speaking, limited.

An elementary example of a digital instrument for electroencephalography is the dual-channel on-line integrator described by Emde and Shipton (1974). In this device a pair of analog integrators is used for the initial signal processing. These have a short (circa 20 milliseconds) time constant and thus can be constructed reliably from inexpensive operational amplifiers. When a defined level of charge is exceeded, the integrator resets to zero and produces a short pulse. A digital counter totals these pulses over a preset time interval. At the end of this interval the contents of the counter are read out serially in binary coded decimal (BCD) by a simple marker pen on the EEG tracing. The appearance of a typical record is shown in Figure 1 which presents a comparison of the average amplitudes of two EEG signals. A number of features have been incorporated in this instrument to increase its utility, including a stimulus generator locked to the preset timer. Thus, pre- and poststimulus amplitudes may be directly compared.

01–A1

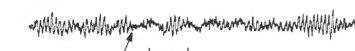

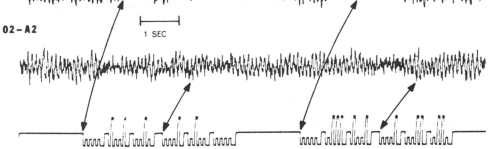

Figure 1. *Display of the relative voltage output of two EEG channels averaged over five-second intervals. The data are displayed in binary coded decimal from left to right. The relative amplitudes are thus 092, 140 during the first epoch and 079, 136 during the second.*

Over the years there have been many efforts to use the statistics implied by information theory as descriptors of EEG data. Many of the techniques are described by Saltzberg in this volume. Perhaps one of the simplest techniques is to produce something like the correlation function either of an ongoing signal with itself, with the signal from another topological area, or with an assumed "ideal" signal in the form of a template. Many computer programs can readily perform this operation and, as I have said in the introduction to this paper, early analog devices were used to compute correlation functions. A number of on-line real-time digital devices have been produced to compute these statistics, but many of them have been rather expensive and perhaps more elaborate than the nature of the biological signal justifies. This question of the "nature of the biological signal" is, of course, a thorny one, and it lies at the heart of many of the papers presented in this volume. So far as the surface EEG is concerned, we are forced to admit that our signal source is not easily accessible to our recording equipment. We know, for example, that the biochemical generators are linked to the electrodes by electrochemical circuits that have high, complex, and variable impedances. I believe that in the past we often made wrong decisions in handling EEG signals. We tended to borrow techniques from the information and communication engineers and thus to invest relatively large sums in hardware, much of which requires some degree of technical knowledge to operate and maintain. As a result, data were acquired on selected and relatively small groups of subjects, and perhaps one reason for their selection was their proximity to a computer-equipped laboratory. The intent of our division at Iowa, in producing special-purpose instrumentation, has been to enable the collection of a large clinical data base, and to insure the usefulness of some of the statistical techniques employed in the clinic.

The Iowa digital correlator has been described in the literature by Emde and Shipton (1972), and I shall refer in this paper only to its block diagram, Figure 2. It uses 65 integrated circuit packages and costs a little under $2000 in small quantities. It is docile and easy to use, although it must be admitted that the statistic that it computes departs from the ideal in at least one important respect: in the cross correlation mode, the signals are not normalized with respect to each other and therefore the device should most appropriately be considered as a co-variance computer. For the purposes of assessing the stability and stationarity of an EEG signal, this is of little consequence, but if attempt is made to operate on the output data, for example, to produce the power spectrum, the limitations of the instrument become immediately apparent.

As our last example we shall consider an instrument for a multichannel spectral analyzer that is currently undergoing development in our facility. Before we do so, it is necessary to consider some of the implications of

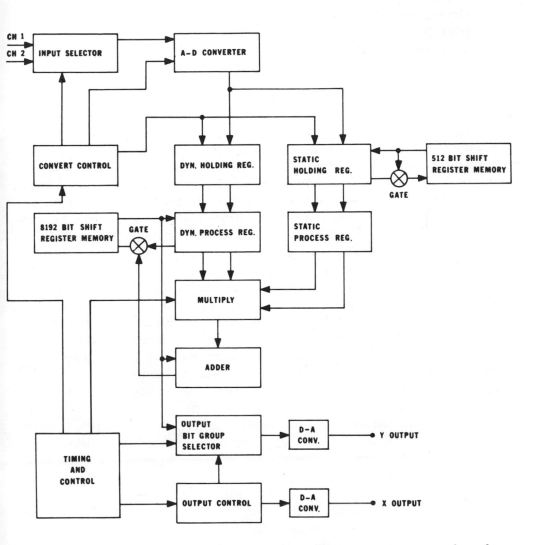

Figure 2. Overall block diagram of a digital on-line correlator. It can be seen that relatively complex circuitry is involved although, by the use of integrated circuits, it can be produced for a little under $2000. (Reproduced, by permission, from the Journal of Electroencephalography and Clinical Neurophysiology.)

spectral techniques as applied to biological signals. The treatment here differs from Saltzberg's in that it is directed to the mathematically unsophisticated and is necessarily less than precise. Spectral analysis may be used for two entirely separate purposes: as a model to gain insight into the nature of the physical processes that give rise to the signal, or merely to obtain a more quantifiable description of the EEG than is conveniently obtained from a verbal or written description of the primary record. For example, it may be easier to say that a waveform has a given amplitude with second and third harmonics of specified magnitude and phase relationship than to describe the pattern that is the combination of these frequencies. Because many of the spectral analyzers used for EEG do not give information about the relative phases of the components into which the signal is being broken, signal reconstruction from the output of such an analyzer is not possible. For this reason Grey Walter, in his early work, insisted that automatic analysis must be performed in substantially real-time and the analysis presented on the primary trace. The numerical output of the analyzer could then be considered in conjunction with the electroencephalographers' perceptions of pattern. Used in this way, analysis complemented but did not supplant the voltage/time EEG recording.

We must also discuss the way in which frequency analysis has been borrowed from other disciplines, especially the physical sciences. The physicist or engineer can assume *a priori* that there is a measure of stationarity in his signals. Stationarity means that a sample of given length characterizes the total record as effectively as any other sample of the same length. Since rotary or harmonic motion is involved in many physical systems, the physicist or engineer can also often predict the presence of repetitive components in the raw data. In these circumstances analysis is used to determine the magnitude and frequency of these periodic components. Given his assumptions, the more data the engineer analyzes the greater the precision of his results. In contrast, the electroencephalographer can make no assumptions about the stationarity of his data; the electrical signals are so lossely associated with underlying biochemical events that they must be regarded as epiphenomena. The validity of models of brain function derived from transforms of such data must not be accepted lightly.

In spite of these and other objections to spectral analysis, many variations of the method have been used and provide useful descriptors of EEG data. A concise and readily available outline of the various methods is given in a paper by Dumermuth and Flühler (1967), which also contains an excellent bibliography. These authors point out that because of the continuing development of analytic methods the general-purpose digital computer is an attractive instrument since it can be re-programmed as required. They also note that the use of a specialized algorithm (the fast Fourier transform, which is now almost ubiquitous) greatly reduces the time needed to compute spectra and indeed other time series statistics. Even so, the computational effort is substantial and, if multichannel operation is desired and if the computer must digitize the input signal and format and graph the output spectrum, the procedure cannot be done in real-time on most general-purpose laboratory computers.

The instrument being developed in our facility operates over the EEG frequency band, and it can simultaneously handle four channels of data. Provision is made to extend this to eight channels without excessive increase in hardware cost. Incoming signals are first filtered to lie within the frequency band of 1 to 25 Hz, and they are then multiplexed and converted to eight-bit digital data. The signals are then entered into a shift register store that accumulates samples for a period of four seconds. This is the analysis epoch and it has been chosen, first, because it needs the restrictions of the sampling theorem, and, second, because this analyzer is intended to be part of a clinical compressed spectral array (CSA) system. At the end of the epoch a number of logical switches operate so that the output of the shift register is connected to its input and the sample of data recirculates continuously. Ongoing signals are routed to a second identical register store. In the recirculating memory the clock rate is changed so that the signal now recirculates at 2048 times its input rate; accordingly, all components in the signal have been multiplied by this factor. This technique of frequency translation has been described frequently in the literature, and several commercial wave analyzers (for example, SAICOR-Honeywell) make use of the principle. In most available wave analyzers the stored sample is mixed with the output of a voltage-controlled oscillator that scans through the shifted frequency spectrum under consideration. The output of the shift register is usually converted to analog form before this mixing occurs. The output from the mixer is then demodulated and filtered. In our instrument the reference signal is obtained by examining the contents of a read-only memory that holds a table of values for the sines of angles between 0 and 180 degrees. After each pass through the read-only memory, a clock mechanism increments the speed at which the table is scanned and is so chosen as to multiply the incoming signal by the sine function at intervals that correspond to 0.25 Hz at the input. When the numerical value of each point in the spectrum has been computed, it may be passed through a square-root circuit and then converted to analog form for output display, or the square-root circuit may be bypassed. The output spectrum can thus represent either the amplitude spectrum or the more formally preferred power spectrum. At the time of writing, we have made no final decision on the form of output display to be supplied with this unit, but arrangements may be made either to write out the spectra simultaneously on a number of strip chart recorders (for example, spare channels of the EEG recorder), or the output may be displayed on a storage oscilloscope and combined with the necessary digital hardware to produce a compressed spectral array with the "hidden line" presentation described by Bickford. Since discrete increments of frequency are used in the multiplier table, the instrument produces a line spectrum rather than the continuous spectrum that is produced when the template signal is a sine wave swept over the entire frequency band. Accordingly, the analysis is not rigorous for highly stable signals, but for the EEG, in which signal stability is not high, the differences seem to be unimportant.

It may, of course, be argued that if there are short-term changes in the stationarity of an EEG, the analysis by a line spectrum device may be misleading. No defense is offered to this criticism: the design objective was to produce a clinical instrument, reliable and easy to use, that would permit such techniques as the compressed spectral array to be used routinely in the clinic. A four-channel version of this instrument would cost about $5000 in modest quantities. If to this were added the cost of a storage tube and a hard copy write-out device (for example, Tektronix 611), a total CSA system, exluding signal amplifiers, could be obtained for less than $10,000. Assuming an expected life of five years and taking the average EEG department's work load as 3000 records per year, the cost of adding this compressed spectral array facility is thus of the order of $0.75 per record. It may be that for many screening purposes the CSA will itself supplant the written strip chart record. This, however, awaits the results of extended clinical trials.

These few examples of digital hardware represent only a fraction of the aids to electroencephalographic research that are now feasible. There are signs that manufacturers are responding to demands for specialized systems in areas of clinical medicine in which sales volume is potentially high. For the smaller medical specialties such as electroencephalography, organizations such as the Bioengineering Resource Facility will continue to play an important role in the introduction of new methods.

Some important developments have not been discussed, partly because they do not fall within the limits of this volume and partly because they are developing so rapidly that a catalog is out of date by the time it is published. We have not, for instance, considered the important area of digital control of experiments, although such applications of the technology are blossoming. Microelectrodes are driven by digital motors controlled by digital circuits; animal behavior is modified by digital controllers whose dexterity and patience far exceeds that of the most dedicated research assistant. The list is long and growing daily. Nor have we described the range of logical and control functions that can be performed by readily obtainable integrated circuits. It is now possible, to give but one potentially significant case, to "build" an entire digital processor on a single, relatively inexpensive microcircuit chip. Memories are already available in integrated circuit packages and the cost of complex units has fallen rapidly to within the reach of the behavioral scientist. It is not at all unlikely that entire digital systems will be made small enough and rugged enough to be attached to free-roaming human beings. Although they lie well in the future, interfaces between brains and computers are already being considered. The implications to the study of electroencephalography and clinical neurophysiology are enormous. The computer will have become a true extension of the brain, and for the first time there will be meaningful large-scale man/machine interaction.

References

Baldock, G.R., and Walter, W.G. 1946. A new electronic analyzer. *Electronics Engineering* 18:339.

Barlow, J.S., and Brazier, M.A.B. 1954. A note on a correlator for electroencephalographic work. *Electroencephalogr. Clin. Neurophysiol.* 6:321.

Burch, N.R. 1959. Automatic analysis of the E.E.G. *Electroencephalogr. Clin. Neurophysiol.* 11:829.

Clark, W.A., Jr. 1958. Average response computer (ARC-1). *Quarterly Progress Report*, Research Laboratory of Electronics, Massachusetts Institute of Technology, p. 114.

Clark, W.A., and Molnar, C.E. 1964. The LINC: A description of the laboratory instrument computer. *Ann. N.Y. Acad. Sci.* 115:653.

Communication Biophysics Group of Research Laboratory of Electronics and William M. Siebert 1959. *Processing Neuroelectric Data.* Cambridge, Mass.: The Massachusetts Institute of Technology.

Dawson, G.D. 1954. A summation technique for the detection of small evoked potentials. *Electroencephalogr. Clin. Neurophysiol.* Supp. 4:26.

Dumermuth, G., and Flühler, H. 1967. Some modern aspects in numerical spectrum analysis of multichannel electroencephalographic data. *Med. Biol. Eng.* 5:319.

Emde, J.W., and Shipton, H.W. 1972. An on-line correlator for electroencephalography. *Electroencephalogr. Clin. Neurophysiol.* 33:527.

Emde, J.W., and Shipton, H.W. 1974. A dual digital integrator for EEG studies. *Electroencephalogr. Clin. Neurophysiol.* 37(2):185.

eeg analysis with hybrid computers

Jack R. Smith, Ph.D.

Department of Electrical Engineering
University of Florida
Gainesville, Florida

Perhaps a more accurate title for this article would be "Special-purpose Computers," since any digital computer analysis of the electroencephalogram (EEG) first requires converting continuous (analog) EEG signals into numbers (digits), and thus all computer analysis of an electroencephalogram is a hybrid computation. Many attempts at automated EEG analysis minimize the amount of analog processing and maximize the amount of processing done on a general-purpose digital computer. This can be inefficient or even limit the amount of data that can be analyzed. An automated system that mimics the electroencephalographer in analyzing EEG data (an anthropomimetic system) requires the capability to process simultaneously long epochs of several channels of data in real time, or faster. Today's general-purpose digital computers do not have this capability; but, if the data are first preprocessed with special-purpose instrumentation, it is possible to mimic closely some of the data-processing routines carried out by the electroencephalographer. This paper describes a Sleep Analyzing Hybrid Computer (SAHC) in order to demonstrate that with fairly inexpensive special-purpose instrumentation an increased amount of EEG data can be processed.

First, a definition of the different types of computers. A digital computer is so named because it operates on discrete numbers (digits). The abacus was one of the first digital computers. An analog computer operates on data that have a continuum of values and whose output also is a continuum of values. A slide rule is an example of an analog computer. A computer that uses both analog and digital data-processing is referred to as a hybrid computer. Computers can also be classified as general-purpose or special-purpose there are, for example, general-purpose analog computers and special-purpose hybrid computers. No clear distinction can be made between the two types of machines, but general-purpose normally refers to a computer in which the processing routine may be altered by programming, allowing the operator to control the different types of operations easily. A special-purpose computer is one designed for a limited number of tasks. In this system provisions do not have to be made for software manipulation, and more of the hardware may be devoted to the special purpose. Special-purpose computers are better able to carry out a limited number of tasks. The Walter EEG analyzer is an example of a special-purpose analog computer (Baldock and Walter 1946). Burch (1964) was one of the first to use a special-purpose hybrid system for EEG analysis. Minicomputers receive their names because they are relatively small general-purpose digital computers or "small, general purpose, stored program computers, capable of performing, on command, arithmetic, logical, and input/output operations" (Aupperle 1973). Add an analog-to-digital or digital-to-analog converter to a general-purpose digital computer and you have a hybrid computer.

Recent advances in microelectronics and integrated circuitry have made the design of special-purpose instrumentation economical and simple. In addition, the new minicomputers permit relatively easy interfacing of this instrumentation to a general-purpose machine, which is an important feature for editing and summarizing the processed data. Since EEG analysis requires analog amplification and filtering of the data, it is easy to perform additional processing of the data before the data are entered into a general-purpose computer. To illustrate this concept, several of the special-purpose routines used in processing human sleep data will be described. The rationale of our automated analysis procedures will be discussed in order to explain why we selected this particular computer architecture.

Automated Sleep EEG Analysis

The automated EEG analysis system attempts to imitate the procedures used by the electroencephalographer in analyzing the same data. This approach is motivated by an admiration for the way the human mind processes data; in most aspects human ability far exceeds that of any computer. The computer has an advantage mainly in carrying out repetitive operations in a well-defined situation. In the development of an anthropomimetic system a distinction must be made. Manual EEG analysis includes repetitive operations and operations that require intelligence to cope with unfamiliar data. I agree with Dreyfus (1972) that building artificial intelligence into present systems is impossible for several reasons. We need not decide whether or not it is theoretically possible; suffice it to say that today it is technically impossible. This observation provides an important guideline in formulating the system. We seek to identify instances in which the electroencephalographer performs repetitive operations, and instances in which he uses intelligence to cope with the uniqueness of the situation, and we then concentrate on developing automated processes for the repetitive tasks. One may deduce from these principles that the analysis of abnormal electroencephalograms is not a likely candidate for automation since in these records the electroencephalographer searches for abnormalities that are frequently manifested by spatial or temporal deviations from a norm and are not defined a priori. On the other hand, the analysis of sleep data is a good candidate for automation since it includes many repetitive operations to identify reasonably well-defined waveforms in the EEG. The sleep electroencephalographer recognizes delta, alpha, beta waves, sleep spindles, eye movements, and artifact or muscle activity. He does this not by scanning a single channel, but by scanning several channels of data simultaneously. Our anthropomimetic system tries to do the same. Such a system requires the capability of recognizing individual EEG patterns. Before discussing the complete system, I will describe a special-purpose hybrid system for recognizing waveforms in sleep EEG data.

Waveform Detection

We have tried several techniques for waveform detection—rectification, narrow-band filtering, threshold detection—and the so-called "optimal" technique of matched filtering (Smith et al. 1969). These procedures are unsatisfactory for several reasons. First, the optimal systems are optimal only in one sense. The criteria used do not include "false alarm" errors—the error of incorrectly stating that a waveform has occurred. Optimal filters are linear; for example, a matched filter may be designed to detect spindles in the EEG, but when large-amplitude events such as movement artifact occur, the spindle detector will incorrectly classify these as spindles (a type II error). Figure 1, A and B, illustrates this problem. In Figure 1A the output of a filter whose impulse response has been "matched" to the spindle waveform clearly indicates the presence of a spindle. Figure 1B presents an epoch of large muscle activity in the EEG. This signal also results in a large output from the matched filter. If peak detection is used, this large output will incorrectly denote a sigma spindle. Artifact detection may be used to reduce the number of false recognitions, but if most false alarms are to be eliminated many spindles will be missed (a type I error). Another reason the techniques men-

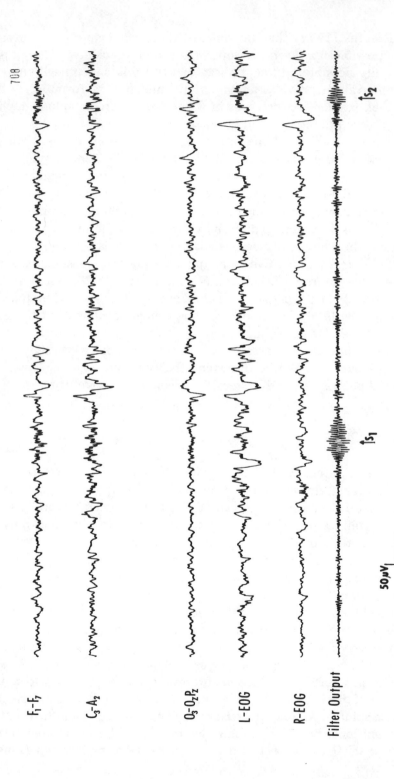

Figure 1A. The output of a "matched filter" used for spindle detection clearly indicates the presence of spindle activity in the frontal channel.

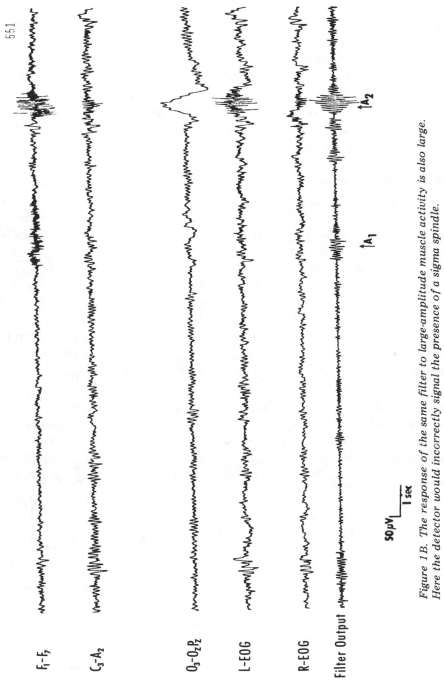

Figure 1B. The response of the same filter to large-amplitude muscle activity is also large. Here the detector would incorrectly signal the presence of a sigma spindle.

tioned are unsatisfactory is that the detection threshold must be changed for each subject (Smith and Karacan 1971). The criteria used by electroencephalographers for spindles, alpha, and beta activity do not include an amplitude criterion, while delta activity and rapid eye movements (REM) must exceed a preassigned criterion independent of the particular subject. Detection with matched filters does not correspond to the electroencephalographer's detection of phasic events.

The detector described here does not require threshold adjustments, but it does include an amplitude criterion for rapid eye movements and delta waveforms. A block diagram of the waveform detector is shown in Figure 2. It consists of a linear analog filter, an amplitude detector, a zero-crossing detector, a digital period discriminator, and a pattern recognizer. The operations subsequent to linear filtering could be performed fast enough by a minicomputer with an analog-to-digital converter, but since hardware and power supplies are needed for analog prefilters, it is cheaper to use hardware to implement the period and amplitude as well as the pattern-recognizing units. The purpose of the analog filter is to remove low- and high-frequency activity from the data to be analyzed without distorting the waveform of interest. A narrow-band filter centered around the waveform frequency is inadequate; such a filter will ring in response to large-amplitude, out-of-band signals and it also will distort the waveform. For example, if a 0.5- to 3.0-Hz bandpass filter is used as a delta prefilter, a single delta wave will be reduced in amplitude by about 50 percent because of the long filter rise time. For delta activity we use an analog filter bandwidth of about 0.1 to 8.0 Hz, leaving the more precise signal detection to the digital period discriminator. For bandpass filtering we use two filters illustrated in Figure 3. Each admittance Y_i is either a resistor or a capacitor, depending upon the frequency response desired. One filter is used for the low-frequency cut-off, one for the high-frequency cut-off. The operational amplifier used in the filter (μ—741)

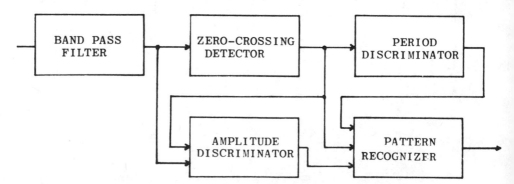

Figure 2. Simplified block diagram of a detector used to recognize phasic events in sleep EEGs.

costs less than $1, and each stage can be built with components costing about $2. Computer programs to determine the component values for the desired bandwidth are available (in Focal by Olsen 1972, and in Fortran by Ambuehl 1972). The zero-crossing detector (which can be built with a 710 comparator and 7400 nand gates for less than $2) generates a pulse each time the filtered input data cross baseline. For all activity except delta and rapid eye movement, every other zero-crossing is used because full-cycle detection is less sensitive to noise (Gondeck 1973). Since the analog prefilter cannot provide the necessary waveform period discrimination without distortion, the period discriminator in combination with the zero-crossing detector determines whether the wave period falls within the specified time window. A wave is defined as filtered EEG data between zero-cross detections (or alternate zero-cross detections for full-cycle detectors). We have used a digital counter and oscillator for this subsystem. The amplitude discriminator, used only for delta and REM activity, determines whether the wave meets the minimum amplitude criterion; it is constructed with a 711 dual comparator plus a J-K flip-flop. Information on whether or not each wave meets the amplitude and duration criteria is fed into the pattern recognizer which checks the input for a specified pattern. The pattern is empirically determined so that the waveform detector will be in close agreement with an electroencephalographer's interpretation of the same data. A pattern recognizer block diagram is given in Figure 4. The shift register is clocked at a constant rate. If a wave has met the amplitude and period requirements, a 1 will be entered into the shift register; if not, the entry is 0. The up/down counter registers how many 1s are in the shift register at any time. The clock rate and length of the shift register determine the memory time of the

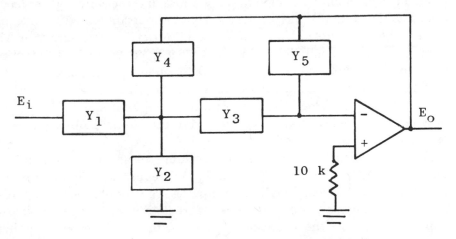

Figure 3. Schematic diagram of an inexpensive 12 db/octave filter for EEG activity. Each Y_i is either a capacitor or resistor depending on the type of filtering desired.

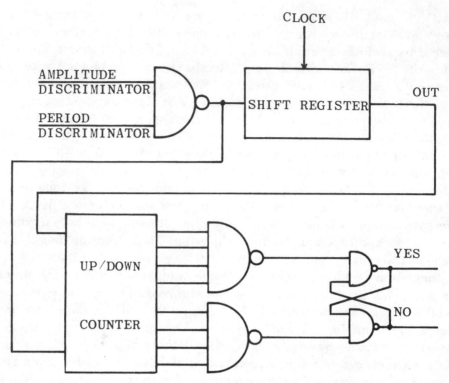

Figure 4. Pattern recognizer section of the waveform detector illustrated in Figure 2.

counter. For example, if the clock rate is 1 kHz and the shift register length is 1048 bits (MOS-2045), the memory is about one second long. For spindle, alpha, and beta waveforms, a satisfactory criterion is to require that 87.5 percent of a 0.42-second time window be occupied by inband detections (0.42 seconds or internal multiples of 0.42 are easily realized with this instrumentation). The period discriminator contains the duration of the last wave in digital form. When the pattern-recognizing unit states that a waveform is present, these data are accumulated to provide accurate information on the duration of the waveform.

These waveform detectors are an accurate means for detecting the important patterns in the sleep EEG, and they are now in daily operation as part of our Sleep Analyzing Hybrid Computer. The zero-crossing hysteresis and pattern requirements for each detector are determined empirically; after the initial calibration the detectors operate without adjustment for individual subjects, discriminating against artifacts, and yielding detection results that are in close agreement with those of the electroencephalographer.

Architecture of the Analyzer

The individual detectors are combined with a central processing unit (cpu) and a buffer memory for further analysis of the sleep data. The architecture of this system is shown in Figure 5. Each detector sends a signal to the central processing unit only when it has detected a waveform, and then it only sends data equivalent to the time of occurrence of that waveform. With this architecture a very simple central processing unit can be designed.

Another distinguishing feature of the system is that the REM detection criteria require the occurrence of eye-movement activity on both channels (Smith et al. 1970). This criterion is checked out on individual waveform detectors which also determine whether the eye movements are in or out of phase. The buffer contains the number of occurrences of individual waveforms and the length of time that activity has been present during the preceding minute. These measures are needed for sleep staging, but they also provide information for a more detailed analysis of the sleep data, and they are saved for later processing. The storing of these data could be in a mini-computer, but we use a digital cassette which, once each minute, records the length of time each waveform was present. The data are transferred to the cassette under the control of the cpu, and at the same time a limited quantity of data is printed out by a digital printer for immediate examination. Our system is able to process a sleep record either on-line in the sleep laboratory or 32 times faster off-line when it is recorded on magnetic tape. Arguments may be advanced to show that this amount of data processing cannot be done with a present-day digital computer and A/D converters alone; thus the special-purpose instrumentation has enabled us to gather much more information than could be obtained with general-purpose computing equipment. I will describe some of these data to illustrate the data-processing acquisition and editing capabilities of our approach.

Application Results

For the final processing the cassette data are entered into a mini-computer (PDP-8/e). The operator is able to select additional processing of the one-minute data summaries. Figure 6 shows a computer-generated plot of minute summaries of some of these data. The bottom portion of the plot contains the sleep-stage information. The plot above the sleep-stage plot illustrates how the minute summaries of delta time varied during the night; the alpha activity is shown directly above the delta plot. The top plot gives the number of spindle counts per minute during the night; the plot of the beta activity is immediately below the spindle plot. This plotting technique permits the investigator to obtain a more detailed and quantitative impres-

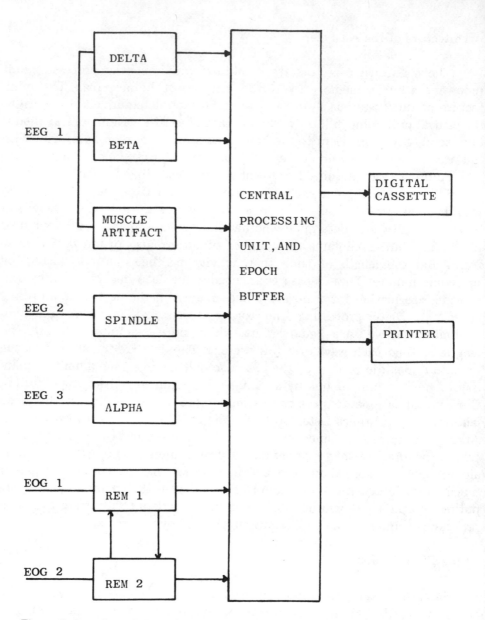

Figure 5. Overview of the architecture of the Sleep Analyzing Hybrid Computer.

sion of the night's sleep data than is feasible with a manual analysis of the EEG. This is an example of how special-purpose computer processing can assist the sleep researcher by providing objective quantitative data on the night's sleep of a subject. Figure 7 shows the effect of a mild hypnotic (Tranxene) on the sleep pattern using the delta activity as the quantitative indicator. The figure contains two plots of minute summaries of the number

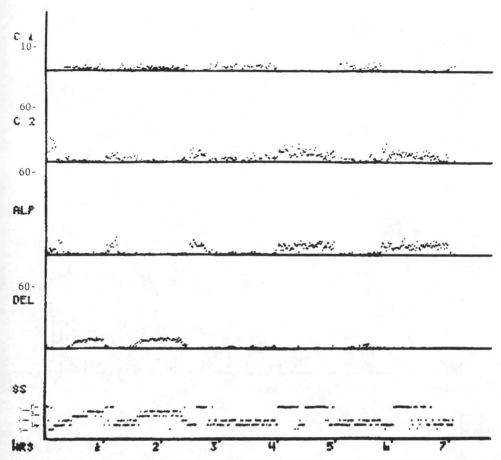

Figure 6. A computer (PDP/8e)-generated plot of the summary of one night's sleep data. The bottom plot is sleep stage (SS); directly above are the number of seconds of delta activity (DEL) and alpha activity (ALP) each minute. The top curve gives the number of sleep spindles, C1; C2 shows the minute summaries of beta activity.

of seconds occupied by delta activity during the entire night's sleep. The top plot is from a baseline night, and the lower plot, taken on the eighth night of drug administration, shows the marked reduction in delta activity (slow-wave sleep). Additional details on the effects of this drug on EEG delta activity have been presented elsewhere (Smith and Karacan 1973).

Conclusions

Special-purpose instrumentation and interfacing can greatly facilitate the extraction of quantitative data from the electroencephalogram. Although it requires the development of hardware, which is inexpensive compared to writing and using the software necessary to carry out similar tasks in a

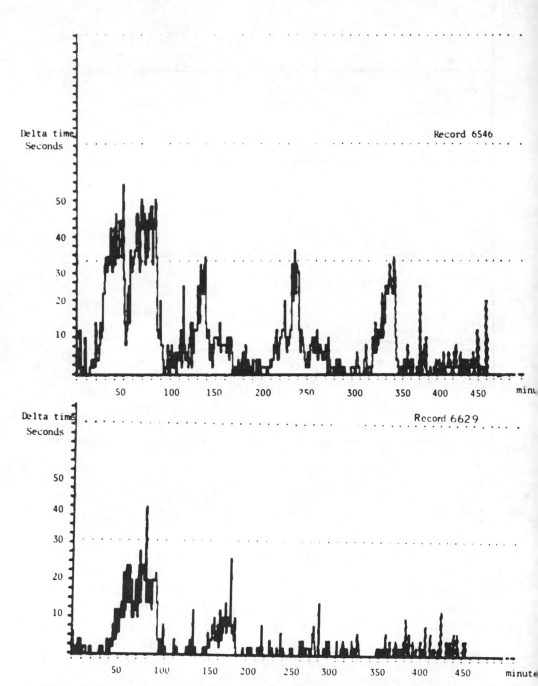

Figure 7. Minute summaries of the number of seconds of delta activity in the frontal channel. Record 6546 is a baseline night and Record 6629 is from the same subject on the eighth drug night.

general-purpose digital computer, the system provides for the acquisition of much information that cannot now be obtained with existing general-purpose computers.

Acknowledgment

This research was supported by research grant MH 16960.

References

Ambuehl, R.E. 1972. Computer aided design and evaluation of a special purpose computer. Master's thesis. Department of Electronic Engineering. Gainesville, Floriaa: University of Florida.

Aupperle, E.M. 1973. *Special Issue on Minicomputers.* Proceedings, Institute of Electrical and Electronics Engineers 61:1524.

Baldock, G.R., and Walter, W.G. 1946. A new electronic analyzer. *Electronic Engineering* 18:339.

Burch, N.R., Nettleton, W.J., Jr., Sweeney, J., and Edwards, R.J., Jr., 1964. Period analysis of the electroencephalogram on a general-purpose digital computer. *Ann. N.Y. Acad. Sci.* 115:827.

Dreyfus, H.L. 1972. *What Computers Can't Do.* New York: Harper & Row.

Gondeck, A. 1973. Quantification of the human sleep σ-spindle rhythm. Ph.D. dissertation, Department of Electrical Engineering, Gainesville, Florida: University of Florida.

Olsen, D.E. 1972. Speed active multipole filter design. *Electronic Design* 20(24):142.

Smith, J.R., Negin, M., and Nevis, A.H. 1969. Automated analysis of sleep electroencephalograms by hybrid computation. *IEEE Transactions on Systems, Science, and Cybernetics* 5:278.

Smith, J.R., Cronin, M.J., and Karacan, I. 1970. A multichannel hybrid system for rapid eye movement detection. *Comput. Biomed. Res.* 4:275.

Smith, J.R., and Karacan, I. 1971. Sleep staging by hybrid computation. *Electroencephalogr. Clin. Neurophysiol.* 31:231.

Smith, J.R., and Karacan, I. 1973. Quantification of the effects of a hypnotic-like drug on slow-wave sleep. In W.P. Koella and P. Levin (eds.), *Sleep.* p. 504. New York: S. Karger.

an interactive, developmental approach to real-time eeg analysis

Alan S. Gevins, and
Charles L. Yeager, M.D., Ph.D.

Langley Porter Neuropsychiatric Institute
University of California
San Francisco, California

In developing algorithms to combine multiple-channel electroencephalographic (EEG) spectral and transient analysis, interactive graphic display, and heuristic feature extraction in a single, integrated, real-time computer system, we have worked from the premise that an automated EEG analysis system should perform three major functions. It should be (1) an effective clinical tool; (2) a utile monitoring device during surgery, controlled drug studies, etc.; and (3) employable as a probing tool in research, capable of isolating relevant parameters in pilot studies. Computer analysis promises to overcome many of the limitations inherent in the traditional visual method of analysis by offering the possibility of standardized interpretation of EEG records and permitting the extension of research and diagnosis by the extraction of EEG features that are not apparent from visual analysis. In working toward these goals, it is vital that the advantages of the polygraph method over simplistic, automated analysis not be overlooked and eliminated. The traditional method affords a close relationship between the data collection and interpretive processes: the technician frequently adapts montage and other variables to suit conditions apparent during recording, thereby emphasizing features in the record that facilitate diagnosis and minimize costly reruns. In developing EEG analysis systems, we have kept in mind the benefits of not sacrificing this flexibility, and we have augmented automated decision-making with the available intelligence of both the technician and the diagnostician.

The Traditional Visual Method of EEG Reading

In the traditional method of electroencephalographic analysis, the value of an EEG record for interpretive purposes is determined, to a large extent, at the time of recording by adjustments made by the technician in the light of prevailing conditions including the patient's medical history and current condition, the characteristics of the EEG, and features of interest that appear during the progression of the test. It is advantageous for the clinician to be familiar with the technician's style of decision-making, as well as with the specifics of individual records. Once faced with a pen-written electroencephalogram, the clinician is charged with reducing an enormous quantity of information into a simple, interpretive statement. The main feature of this intricate process of data reduction is an individualistic, selective attitude toward the mass of data by means of which extracted features and patterns are compared in various ways to a body of internalized prototypes. Ability to classify and interpret these records accurately is obviously a subjective process, a function of cumulative experience. A severe limitation is placed on interpretation in that only visually detectable aspects of the waves can be utilized. Among the characteristics of wave-rhythm interaction that restrict interpretation based on visual analysis are masking, beats, waveform distortion, and difficulties in distinguishing the cause of modulation. The more complex the record, the more difficult the identification of the individual components; therefore, analysis of components must often be deemphasized in favor of a general interpretation of the overall pattern including amplitude, frequency, and group wave shape. Interchannel comparisons are essential to visual interpretation. Especially important are such major discrepancies in amplitude and wave shape as hemispheric asymmetry or focal activity. Evaluation of the total gestalt of the multichannel tracing also plays a major role in the interpretive process. Since the assessment is based on a complex of comparisons and extractions, it is inordinately difficult to define and quantify.

In "An EEG Reading Plan" (1972), the second author summarized the traditional method of analysis and interpretation of human EEG records in a four-step procedure: (1) initial record scan, noting electrode montage, time and amplification scales, and the age and condition of the subject; (2) secondary record scan, closely examining wave patterns characteristic of the dominant background, and noting the presence of transient or paroxysmal activity; (3) tertiary scan, determining the causes of variation from area to area and over time; (4) categorical summary of all features of the tracing that may be relevant to interpretation. An attempt is then made to relate these observations to known conditions of the subject.

The visual method of EEG analysis can never be totally standardized. During the acquisition process the many decisions the technician must make are subject to wide variability. During the process of interpretation the electroencephalographer selects relevant features, notes trends, and discriminates between them by means of qualitative comparisons based on personal experience and subject to great intra- and interindividual variation. The electroencephalographer has storage, retrieval, and pattern recognition abilities far beyond those of current computer systems. In evaluating a tracing he uses contextual cues distributed over the entire recording. He uses a large data base assembled over a long period of time and arrives at decisions in the presence of diagnostically irrelevant influences arising from extracerebral sources. Although it cannot now rival human interpretation and diagnosis, automated EEG analysis is useful for the standardization it imposes on data collection and analysis. In addition, potentially relevant features of the EEG are impossible to identify without mathematical analysis.

History of Automated EEG Systems

In traditional as well as in automated methods, information in the EEG record is abstracted in both the frequency and time domains (Burch 1959). If the coding unit is a standard interval, the result is measured as amplitude and the analysis is in the frequency domain. If, on the other hand, the coding unit is an amplitude relation (that is, the peak or baseline cross of a wave), the result is measured in the time domain (Burch, Greiner, and Correll 1955). If analysis is attained in one of these domains, it is accomplished at the cost of information in the other. Frequency domain methods have included the closed loop process described by Gibbs and Grass (1947), Knott (1953), and Shipton (1957), and the method of interval point coding, or analog-to-digital conversion, described by Shannon and Weaver (1949). Fourier transforms have been used virtually since the inception of electroencephalography (Grass and Gibbs 1938), but the application of spectral analysis based on the Fourier transform of the EEG was fully delineated by the work of Adey and Walter (Walter 1963; Walter and Adey 1963, 1965, 1966; Walter et al. 1966). The various implementations based on the Fast Fourier Transform (FFT) (Cooley and Tukey 1965) constitute the prime spectral domain techniques currently in use. The drawbacks of FFT-based EEG analysis—violations of the assumption of stationarity, insensitivity to transient events, and excessive computation time—naturally led to the investigation of other forms of analysis, including the entire class of orthonormal transforms that may be implemented with "fast" algorithms (Andrews and Caspari 1971). Since transforms like the Fast Walsh-Hadmard Transform (FWT) (Pratt, Kane, and Andrews 1969) and the Fast Haar Transform (FHT) (Andrews 1971) can be faster than the FFT by an order of magnitude or more, spectral estimates can be based on highly overlapped data, thus overcoming some of the drawbacks mentioned above. Bishop and Wilson (1972) presented an application of continuously overlapped Haar transforms to broad-band spectral analysis and transient detection of the EEG. Although not in connection with the EEG, Meisel (1972a) suggests the use of "custom" orthonormal transforms designed to match the salient characteristics of a particular signal. Unfortunately, it seems likely that, without remapping, results of an FWT of the EEG would present difficulties for human interpretation (Saltzberg 1973).

In the time domain, analysis is based on the selection of certain amplitude points for coding. Systems utilizing this method are peak point coding exemplified by the toposcope of Walter and Shipton (1951); baseline cross coding (or period analysis) advanced by Burch and Saltzberg (Burch, Greiner, and Correll 1955; Saltzberg and Burch 1959; Burch et al. 1964); wave shape coding devised by Buckley, Saltzberg, and Heath (1968); and the various uses of autocorrelation resulting from the original work of Wiener and Brazier (Wiener 1949, 1950; Brazier and Casby 1952; Barlow and Brazier 1954; Barlow, Brazier, and Rosenblith 1959). Other time domain analyses have either been based on such mathematical models as the autogressive series (Saltzberg 1968, Zetterberg 1969, Wennberg and Zetterberg 1971, Fenwick et al. 1971), or they have attempted to extract particular features of wave shape. Work in the latter category includes the three time domain descriptors of Hjorth (1970), the comparison of individual alpha waves (Hoovey, Heinemann, and Creutzfeldt 1972), and recognition of sharp waves and other transients (Buckley, Saltzberg, and Heath 1968; Carrie 1972a, 1972b, 1972c; Harper, Walter, and Kelly 1972). Straddling spectral and time domain approaches is the method of complex demodulation (Bingham, Godfrey, and Tukey 1967; Walter 1968; Naitoh et al. 1972), the collection of baseline cross information into spectral bins (Saltzberg and Burch 1971), and the applications based on the Haar transform (Bishop and Wilson 1972).

Several studies have been undertaken to compare representative techniques of quantitative EEG analysis among themselves and against the visual interpretive method. Saltzberg (1968) considered the fitting of autogressive models to the EEG, analysis based upon superposition of weighted square-wave trains, normalized even and odd scanning functions, and multichannel spectral analysis via Fast Fourier Transform. He determined that each method has its own utility, reflecting a compromise between resolution in time or frequency with considerations of processing implementation. In a series of experiments undertaken to compare the relative merits of automated period and frequency analysis with results obtained from the traditional visual method of evaluation of clinical electroencephalograms, Yeager and Heilbron (1972) concluded that, although for some purposes period analysis compared favorably with visual assessment and frequency analysis, the available methods are far from capable of handling the problems of clinical classification. The results of these studies emphasize that each of the automated methods focuses on an explicit feature or group of features of the signal, and, further, that such simple forms of analysis cannot by themselves provide descriptors with clustering unique enough to differentiate experimental groups that are not clearly distinguishable by visual analysis. Additional feature extraction is needed before classification can be attempted; for purposes of an integrated, general-purpose EEG analysis system the parallel use of several methods must be undertaken.

A survey of the literature (Cox, Nolle, and Arthur 1972) establishes two approaches toward automated EEG feature extraction, one mathematical (Mucciardi and Gose 1971), the other heuristic (Skuce, Cotman, and Thompson 1972). The mathematical approach extracts features and performs classification using various forms of multivariate analysis, namely clustering, regression, factor and discriminant analysis (Walter et al. 1966, Larsen et al. 1973). The heuristic approach attempts to mimic and standardize the human method of analysis. Both methods can use spectral or other forms of primary background analysis to preprocess the data. Although there have been some notable successes in classification and prediction, such as the seizure warning system of Viglione and his co-workers (Viglione, Ordon, and Risch 1970; Viglione 1973; Viglione and Martin 1973), results have not been generalizable. We believe that this situation results from the inadequate application of heuristic feature extraction after primary analysis, and before attempts at classification. Such feature extraction must be based on rudimentary electroencephalographic common sense. Alternatively, it is possible that when information theory methods and other mathematical feature extraction algorithms are developed for such problems as pattern recognition of visual images, the techniques will be applicable to EEG analysis.

Automated sleep-scoring systems deserve mention in the context of feature extraction and classification, since much effort has been focused on solving this clearly delineated problem. Period analysis has been applied to mimicking of sleep staging by Burch (Burch 1959, Burch et al. 1964) and by Fink and Itil (Fink, Itil, and Shapiro 1967; Itil et al. 1969). Lessard, Ford, and Hughes (1969) devised a method of feature extraction using multivariate linear discriminant analysis. Legewie and Probst (1969) combined period and amplitude analyses in their system. Hjorth (1970) created a time domain analyzer capable of automatic sleep staging that computed the variance of the EEG and its first and second derivatives. Viglione and his group (Viglione, Ordon, and Risch 1970; Viglione 1973; Viglione and Martin 1973) created a system using spectral analysis and electrooculographic (EOG) information. Heuristic methods have been used by several investigators endeavoring to extract such common features as the K-complex, alpha bursts, sleep spindles, and rapid eye movement (REM) bursts from the sleep record. These attempts have used both frequency and period analyses and recognition of events in the time domain. Smith and his colleagues (Smith, Cronin, and Karacan 1970; Bremer, Smith, and Karacan 1970) have, by one such method, successfully detected K-complex and REM activity. The lesson learned from sleep scoring has been that, even in such a clearly delineated area, there is not sufficient agreement among human scorers against which to compare the performance of automated systems. It would be helpful if a common set of data were used to evaluate all systems.

The forms of analysis described above are, for the most part, performed in several operations off-line or partially on-line, on large or small computers, using either analog or digital tapes as input. There are not many instances in the literature of integrated, real-time EEG analysis systems useful in the clinical EEG laboratory, where the overall activity of eight or more channels must be simultaneously analyzed. The system of Carrie and Frost (Frost 1969; Carrie and Frost 1971, 1973), is a refinement of a technique suggested by Legewie and Probst (1969). It is based upon a wavelength-amplitude summary and could probably be expanded for more flexible feature extraction from a greater number of channels. It is, however, restricted to a simple form of analysis and is not a true real-time, one-pass system.

The present state of computer analysis of the EEG is characterized by many isolated forms of analysis, each with its unique combination of effective algorithms and methods of feature extraction. Since most implementations were created for specific applications, or to expound particular methods of analysis, few generalized systems exist. The complexity of the EEG record, its interindividual variation and contamination by a wide variety of artifact, and the individualistic and largely nonquantifiable recognition methods of the electroencephalographer preclude the possibility that an automated system will replace the technician and the electroencephalographer in the near future. It is possible, however, to work toward the goal of automated classification and diagnosis while supplying the latest version of an evolving system to clinical and research personnel. Until an automated system can operate in isolation from human intelligence, it is sensible to call upon the attendant EEG technician to augment automated decision-making. Our method has been to implement primary feature extraction by spectral and transient analysis and display in a real-time, interactive systems environment. As more sophisticated feature-extracting capabilities are developed, they will be added to the present system and used to produce clinically useful results.

It might well be argued that the complexities of a real-time, interactive, developmental approach have an inhibiting effect on the creation of EEG analysis paradigms. Algorithm and system design, programming, and debugging are more abstruse, difficult, and time-consuming for real-time systems than for high-level language applications programs. However, if a system is eventually to replace the polygraph, the technician, and the electroencephalographer, it must, like the polygraph, be a real-time device. In addition, a real-time approach facilitates EEG analysis in such applications as patient monitoring during surgical procedures and for drug-response studies. The utility of a system designed for a particular set of clinical or research requirements is undermined by the subjective, individualistic approach of the clinician and the intricacy of the signal that defies simple processing. These considerations result in frequent alteration of method and display during the traditional analytic procedure. Automated, interactive systems should be similarly adaptable without the expense and tedious effort of reprogramming. Interactive alteration of analysis allows significant features to be isolated; it is important in research applications in which paradigms change frequently, as in pilot studies.

Overview of Real-Time EEG Analysis

Once the commitment to develop interactive, real-time systems has been made, the necessity for speed, efficiency, and generality imposes severe constraints on the choice of hardware and of analysis and software systems. Although the rapid evolution of computer technology has increased the power and capability of dedicated minicomputer systems, hardware considerations usually focus on making the most of the limited resources of a single laboratory. The choice of a real-time environment influences analysis algorithm design, since speed and memory allocation must be considered in addition to the characteristics of spectral estimators. Software systems must be optimized. Arithmetic precision should be no greater than is actually needed; algorithms that perform operations in place are preferable to those that require additional storage; and algorithms that permit interleaving of analysis processes should be used in preference to those based on linear, one-at-a-time operations. The overriding principle of software design is the use of a systems methodology that integrates hardware, mathematical algorithms, and software into a single functioning unit. This contrasts with a

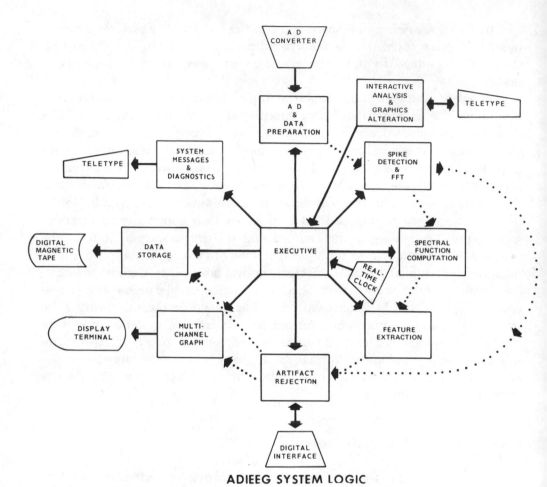

ADIEEG SYSTEM LOGIC
Solid lines indicate process control. Broken lines indicate data flow

Figure 1. Overview of an interactive, real-time EEG analysis and display system (ADIEEG). Program modules in rectangular boxes all reside in the minicomputer's memory and are executed in an interleaved manner by the multitasking executive. Odd-shaped boxes represent the various input or output devices.

design methodology that divides analysis into a series of discrete steps, each embodied in a separate program whose use is coordinated by the EEG operator. As is evident from Figure 1, in our version of a real-time interactive EEG analysis system, ADIEEG, the coordination and utilization of the individual process modules are supervised by the multitasking executive, while the technician or researcher alters analysis or display parameters and assists the processing system with pattern-recognition decisions. Each of the process modules will be discussed below. We will now consider effects of hardware and overall software design upon actual system implementation.

Hardware Considerations

Any specific statements made about computer hardware soon become obsolete as evolving technology permits more computation and peripheral capability for fewer dollars. For example, if the Fast Fourier Transform is used, the major portion of computing time is consumed by the transform itself, and little remains for the other necessary tasks shown in Figure 1. FFT processors on a single digital logic card have recently become available at costs moderate enough to justify their inclusion in an integrated, real-time EEG analysis system. Since the speed of special-purpose FFT processors may be up to several orders of magnitude greater than the fastest software FFT implementations, real-time constraints have been relaxed and central processor time freed for feature extraction and pattern recognition. Without such a special-purpose FFT processor, the present implementation of our system allows a real-time processing limit of eight channels of double precision integer power spectra and eight cross spectral and coherence pairs per second, with a resolution of from 1 to 64 Hz. Adequate central processor time remains for transient analysis and feature extraction as it is presently conceived. Such considerations as the amount of core memory, computer word length, availability of floating point arithmetic hardware, and speed and capacity of peripheral storage and display devices determine the actual limits of a real-time EEG analysis system in terms of the number of channels, spectral band width and resolution, variety and accuracy of other numerical functions computed, and flexibility of analysis and display. For example, a 12-bit, 8000-word computer without floating point hardware could not be expected to produce accurate spectral estimates and displays of eight coherence functions with band width to 64 Hz. For such a system a realistic limit would be four auto-spectra with band width of 1 to 32 Hz, or a greater number of channels if the spectra were only graphed and not used statistically.

The careful selection of peripheral devices is more crucial than the choice of a central processor. Transfers to industry-compatible magnetic tape should not limit the analysis capacity of the system. Interfacing tape drives with the central processor via a data channel, and having data transfer rates several times greater than the expected load ensure adequate facility. The choice of a graphics device is determined by speed and central processor drain. Traditionally designed X-Y plotters are typically too slow for real-time, multichannel spectral graphics, while faster electrostatic plotters offer fine resolution but are not easily viewed when used as monitoring devices or for interactive graphics. Fast-scan display devices, which require the computer to maintain and refresh the display, drain too much core space and central processor time, while economical displays containing their own refresh memory have not so far been quick enough, or could not maintain a suitably complex display. Storage tube devices meet other requirements, but they are inherently inflexible and usually not very bright. Aside from cost considerations, digital computer graphics processors, being fast, flexible, and bright, seem the ideal choice.

The hardware actually used in ADIEEG is a mixture of what was on hand and what was chosen. A 16,000-word PDP-15 computer, having an 18-bit word length and single precision integer arithmetic capability, is the central processor. It is configured with two 7-track, 45-inch per second industry-compatible magnetic tape units, two smaller digital tapes for program development, a Tektronix 4010 graphics terminal with 4602 hard copy unit, analog-to-digital converter, real-time clock, and digital interface with 10 bits of input and 4 bits of output. Sixteen thousand additional words of memory and a moving disk storage unit with 1.2 million word capacity are being added to implement additional feature extraction algorithms and permit time-sharing for program development. The disk controller, a PDP-11-05 computer, will perform ADIEEG analysis tasks in a multiprocessor configuration.

Software Design

The difficulty in implementing the sort of real-time system we have been discussing is in optimizing and integrating the software. Since they cause the computer to be idle while input or output transfers are taking place, linear programming procedures, such as those embodied in Fortran programs, are not efficient. General-purpose multiprogramming operating systems, although providing mechanisms to interleave analysis with input-output transfers, make excessive drains on computer resources in memory and time. A compromise between the two alternatives is a design incorporating a limited multitasking executive that performs the essential services of more complex operating systems, while taking advantage of the well-behaved characteristics of a dedicated EEG analysis system to keep overhead to a minimum. In this manner the various tasks shown in Figure 1 can be interleaved in a natural order of priorities with minimal drain on system resources by the executive.

The executive and most of the task modules must be coded in the assembly language of the computer because of the speed, compactness, and flexibility of assembly-language programming. Increased difficulty, extra cost, and prolonged development time must, in this instance, be borne, although some analysis and display task modules could be implemented with a reentrant, higher-level language. Unfortunately, assembly-language programming may also result in intricate, inflexible, idiosyncratic, and often undecipherable programming, suitable only for one unchanging purpose, if any. One must, therefore, design discrete program modules that can be executed independently in the environment of the multitasking system executive. General algorithms must be implemented in such a way that program variables can be computed rather than preset when the program is created. It will be possible, then, to completely reconfigure the analysis sytem in real-time by merely changing one or two parameters. These techniques also prolong program life, since the system may be adapted to different experimental paradigms without reprogramming. Whenever new forms of an analysis are needed, appropriate program modules may be added with relative ease.

System Operation

In addition to speed and flexibility, an important specification for a real-time EEG analysis system is ease of use by persons unfamiliar with computers and programming. Simple questions and answers should be used to enter the patient's or subject's identification data, so that technicians or researchers need not learn computer language or notation. It is also helpful if errors in entry cause the computer to type out a correct example. Further, it should be simple to change the parameters of analysis and display while the system is running. The system should keep track of time and montage, so that a predetermined sequence of operations may be undertaken without additional intervention. For example, one should be able initially to specify the collection of three minutes of eyes-closed spectra, followed by one minute each of hyperventilation and photic-driving. From then on the system should work by itself unless a change in protocol is desired. Auxiliary operations such as making hard copies from the graphics terminal should be automatic, and the system should inform the operator by typing a message or sounding a bell if something is amiss. Once the recording session has begun, interactions with the computer, such as temporarily suspending analysis or overriding artifact rejection decisions, should be rapid and performed remotely. For such purposes a small box with several push buttons, each having a predetermined use, may be connected to the computer's digital interface by a long cable.

The Multitasking Executive

The central function of the multitasking executive in a real-time EEG analysis system will now be described in detail. A real-time executive (RTE) is a body of program logic that allocates system resources in order to coordinate different phases of data processing with transmissions from and to real-time devices. In designing an RTE for physiological signal analysis systems, trade-offs may be made between generality of function and efficiency of operation. These trade-offs can be defined by considering present and projected requirements of the application environment, including the variability of application tasks, the speed with which the system must respond to internal and external events, the relation between user task modules and input-output (I/O) transfers, and the conditions imposed by the hardware configuration.

The simplest RTEs are embedded in particular applications programs, while more complex RTEs are separate program entities capable of performing a variety of background and I/O tasks in a multiprogramming environment (Gevins 1972). The notion that general-purpose RTEs outperform embedded control software in the execution of simple applications mistakes generality for efficiency by not considering the RTE's drain on system resources. Consider the uncomplicated task of digitizing, formatting, and storing 16 signal channels with a sampling rate of several kilohertz. A straightforward, interrupt-driven program with minimal control software could succeed at this task, while a complex, generalized RTE might fail. If the analysis paradigm involves more than five or so processes, and provision is made for such asynchronous operations as parameter alteration, a multitasking executive can coordinate acquisition, analysis, and output more efficiently than can implicit control software. The capabilities of an RTE for a projected system design should be defined as follows.

(1) Variability of applications programs: A single investigator wishing to process data from an experiment according to a fixed analysis plan does not need an RTE. For his purpose, data may be stored on analog or digital magnetic tape, and analyzed off-line using programs written in a higher-level language such as Fortran or Algol. If several investigators share a dedicated computing facility and need real-time data collection and analysis, use of a general RTE to manage I/O, task scheduling, and execution enables them to implement analysis paradigms with minimal knowledge of the complexities of real-time systems. Somewhere in between these extremes are dedicated EEG analysis systems, such as the one described here, that offer as options some of the commonly used forms of analysis and display. *(2) Data rate and response time:* The higher the overall data rate, and the lower the response time necessary to service an external event, the greater the need to optimize system resources by tailoring the RTE to the application. *(3) Conditions imposed by the hardware environment:* It is assumed, of course, that an RTE is designed to use the features of a particular computer model. If priority-interrupt hardware is present, problems associated with reentrant device

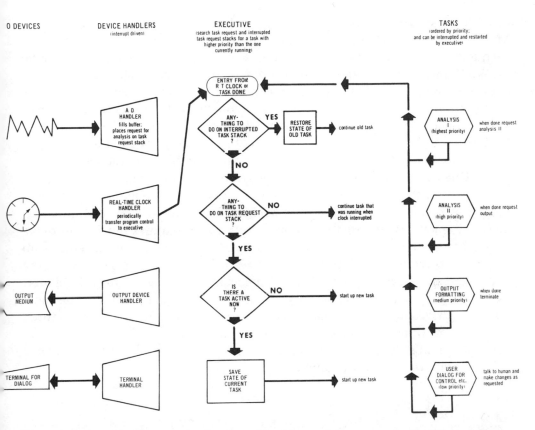

Figure 2. Schematic diagram of a simple multitasking real-time executive (RTE) as used in an interactive EEG analysis and display system. Not all of the program modules or input-output devices are shown. A program task module is assigned a priority and is executed in turn when a request for it is placed on an ordered list (task request stack). Pulses from the real-time clock cause the task request stack to be searched for the program task module with the highest priority. If a task of lower priority is currently active, its machine state is saved on interrupted task stack so that it can be continued at a later time. The operation of device handlers is asynchronous with program task module execution.

handlers are minimized. Adequate byte- and bit-manipulating instructions facilitate multiple use of a single storage location. General-purpose registers may be used to pass parameters to a task, while hardware push-down stacks simplify executive design.

A simple multitasking executive as presented schematically in Figure 2 is used in our EEG analysis system. Task scheduling is facilitated through a task request stack (queue), an ordered list of elements containing the priority and starting address of tasks waiting to be executed. Another stack, the interrupted task stack, is used to save the program state of a priority level that has been suspended in order to run tasks of higher priority. An interrupt from a real-time clock periodically causes the executive to scan the task request stack for a task having a higher priority than the currently active task. If one is found, the program state of the current task (machine state and reentrant locations) is saved and the new task is initiated. The new task may either run to completion, returning control to the executive, or it may be suspended when its time slice is consumed, so that a task of higher priority can be initiated. If entrance to the executive is from a completed task, the interrupted task stack is scanned, as is the task request stack.

Queues can be structured contiguously with one entry following another in adjacent core locations (Figure 3a), noncontiguously with each entry being joined by forward and backward pointers (Figure 3b), or circularly (Figure 3c). Reordering a contiguous queue requires moving all of its elements by removing the top entry and pushing all the remaining entries up by one. Reordering noncontiguous queues involves changing pointers in the next and the previous entry without physically removing an entry. Similarly, reordering circular queues is only a matter of changing pointers. The most basic multitasking RTE we have discussed uses two contiguously structured queues, of which the interrupted task stack is of fixed length. In more complex RTEs the number of queues is greater, and dynamically allocatable structures save a significant amount of space.

REAL TIME DATA STRUCTURES

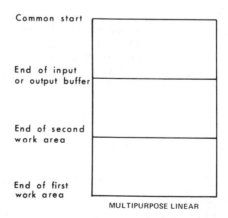

Figure 3a.

Figure 3. Five representative data structures used in an interactive, real-time EEG analysis and display system. Hybrid forms are commonly used. (See text for detailed explanation.)

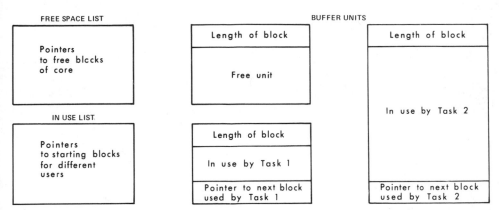

FREE SPACE LIST

Pointers
to free blocks
of core

IN USE LIST

Pointers
to starting blocks
for different
users

BUFFER UNITS

Length of block

Free unit

Length of block

In use by Task 1

Pointer to next block
used by Task 1

Length of block

In use by Task 2

Pointer to next block
used by Task 2

DYNAMICALLY ALLOCATED NON-CONTIGUOUS (LINKED LISTS)

NOTES:

1. Allows very flexible use of available core when various tasks do not use fixed amounts of space, or when the number of user tasks cannot be determined beforehand, as in a general purpose multitasking real time executive.

2. Has very high overhead.

3. Many variations are possible, such as backward as well as forward pointers, space allocation based upon amount of space needed and size of block, etc.

4. Can also be used for space allocation on mass storage devices.

Figure 3b.

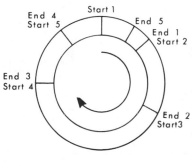

End 4
Start 5

Start 1

End 5
End 1
Start 2

End 3
Start 4

End 2
Start3

CIRCULAR (RING)

NOTES:

1. Used when transactions on a buffer are of variable length and occur at irregular times, as in conversational input, or when input-output occurs asynchronously with processing as in communications with a remote processor.

2. Has greatly increased overhead.

Figure 3c.

The overhead incurred by an RTE depends on the frequency with which it is used. This should be as infrequent as possible, while still responding to the needs of the processing enviroment. An easily changeable parameter, governing executive use, may be set empirically.

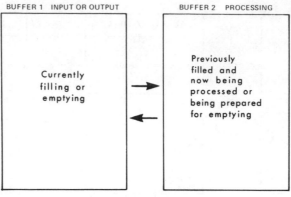

PAIRED LINEAR

NOTES:

1. Allows input or output concurrent with analysis.
    When input or output is completed on Buffer 1, Buffer 1's
    data will be processed, while Buffer 2 will by then be ready
    for input or output.

2. It is possible to have a set of N buffers for complicated
    analysis tasks.

Figure 3d.

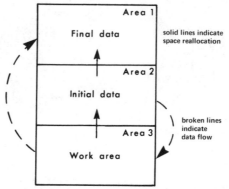

DYNAMICALLY ALLOCATED LINEAR

NOTES:

1. As values from Area 2 are transferred to Area 3, freed core locations
    from Area 2 are appended to Area 1. Eventually Area 3 can also be
    added to Area 1.

2. Used when core space is limited and many operations are made on a
    data set, changing the amount of space occupied by the data.

Figure 3e.

Error Detection and System Stability

A variety of anomalous conditions may cause multitasking analysis systems to crash unpredictably and randomly. A core dump at such a time is generally of little value, since all that can be seen is the chaos of perhaps several million operations following the onset of the anomalous condition. Even if the cause can be found, it provides little solace to the individual who has lost several hours' work. Fortunately, when well-maintained hardware supports a fully debugged multitasking analysis system, these anomalous conditions rarely occur. Unless it occurs at a particular vulnerable time, such as when an executive stack is altered, the rare processor anomaly is unnoticed. Simple checks on address and parameter ranges at the crucial system junctures can prevent serious damage by causing unreasonable requests to be discarded. The data associated with the time frame in which the anomaly occurred is likewise discarded, internal indicators are reset, the problem is reported with an appropriate message on the terminal, and processing continues. The net effect of a detected anomaly, then, is a small hole in the ongoing analysis.

The temporary unavailability of an output device, or parity errors in transmission, have serious effects on real-time analysis systems, since there is no provision for more than momentary internal data storage, and it is not possible to back up the patient's record and reenter the signal that has been lost. Real-time error recovery algorithms must then minimize data loss by rapidly restoring the normal data flow. If parity errors occur during transmission to magnetic tape, a portion of the tape may be skipped to bypass areas of uneven oxide, or a standby I/O device may be activated. Finally, human intervention may be required and message alarms must be sounded. There is no limit to the amount of error detection and recovery logic that can be built into a system. The degree of effort in this area must match the application of the system and the weaknesses of its hard and soft components. For pilot experimental studies, extensive error detection and correction are unnecessary. But, if the results of analysis are to be used during surgical procedures, system realiability is vital. For routine clinical and experimental use, a modicum of error detection and recovery logic will permit continuous analysis, except during gross failure of major systems components.

Real-Time Data Buffer Structures

If core memory were effectively unlimited and real-time constraints did not exist, EEG analysis would not require data buffer structures more complex than simple contiguous lists. To meet the constraints of space and time, various data structures must be implemented. In Figure 3a, a simple extension of the contiguous list is described as a multipurpose, linear buffer in which an area of core is set aside for more than one purpose. In a multitasking environment the use of such buffers must generally be restricted to a single priority level so that a higher-priority process will not destroy the data area of a lower-priority process. An important exception is one in which data are transferred from task to task and level to level through such multipurpose areas. For example, the buffer used for an FFT could then be used to compute spectral estimates by a lower-priority process. A familiar extension of the simple or multipurpose linear buffer is the paired linear buffer, which is commonly used to interleave input-output transfers with other processing (Figure 3d). The constraint imposed by this arrangement is that the time course of the slower process must, in the case of double buffering, be shorter than the period of the faster process minus the length of the faster process; otherwise, a buffer will not be free when the faster process is activated again. As noted in Figure 3d, one may allow for more than double buffering when the complexity of processing between input and output is sufficiently complex. Unfortunately, increasing the depth of buffering will allow a task requiring more than real time to run only for a limited time.

When the circular or ring buffer structure shown in Figure 3c is used, the overhead per transaction is greatly increased by the need for checking the physical end of the buffer each time a pointer is advanced. This is so because the last location of a contiguous section of core is followed logically by the first location of that section. When the results of EEG analysis are transmitted to a remote computer for additional processing, a ring buffer structure can be advantageously used. The primary processor will make entries into the communications buffer whenever the need arises, while the secondary processor will empty the buffer asynchronously. Buffer space will then be made immediately available to the primary processor as data are accepted by the remote processor.

Frequently the size of a data set varies as a series of operations are performed on it. If memory locations are limited, the effective size of an area may be increased by dynamically reallocating locations as they become unoccupied. As shown in Figure 3e, which illustrates the preparation of spectral data for graphics display, a portion of the spectra representing a single EEG channel will be transferred from Area 2 to Area 3, the work area. Eventually, values from the work area will be packed into Area 1, and then transferred to the graphics device. As this process goes toward completion, Area 1 will grow while Area 2 will shrink. As the last channel is processed, the work area itself may be made part of Area 1. The cost of this juggling is the overhead of changing the end point of the various buffers, and checking that this limit is not exceeded.

A more general form of buffer structure is the noncontiguous linked list shown in Figure 3b. Space is allocated for a particular data set from the free space list which consists of pointers to blocks of free memory. For each data set there is an entry in an in-use or directory list that points to the first unit occupied by that set. Since each data buffer unit contains a pointer to the next (and perhaps also to the previous) buffer unit for that set, a threaded list may be traced once the starting address of a data set is known. The obvious advantage of such a structure is its flexibility: data sets can expand and shrink and do not require the reservation of space for the maximally expanded state of each set. If the minimum size of a buffer unit is relatively large, the considerable overhead of noncontiguous linked list structures decreases as references to lists of free space become less frequent. In a dedicated, real-time EEG analysis system, this form of data structure can be efficiently used for the allocation of space on a random-access, mass-storage device.

We have outlined in schematic form several of the possible data structures used in real-time signal analysis systems. In practice, hybrid forms are devised to meet the needs of the application.

Mass Storage

The problem of storage may be expressed as the process of deciding what not to store. For pre-pilot experimental studies and for most routine clinical purposes the various spectral and feature-oriented graphs are sufficient to guide decisions, and only minimal numerical output is needed for statistical treatment. Lengthy research programs require more output, and the original data should be kept in some form. As a back-up, one can retain analog tapes, or digital tapes containing either raw data or orthogonal transform coefficients. It is more difficult to determine the limits of real-time processing as preparation for off-line statistical analysis. One can keep all spectral bins and transient indices, or proceed with further data-pruning by retaining only selected portions of averaged results. The former method often results in the somewhat arbitrary discarding of entire channels, epochs, and runs because the execution of multivariate statistical analysis on large computers is expensive. Excessive real-time pruning and averaging can also lead to arbitrary discarding of data. For a real-time, feature-extracting, and ultimately feature-classifying EEG analysis system, industry-compatible digital magnetic tape and disk storage procedures provide a reasonable amount of output for further statistical analysis, demonstrate the system's current level of feature-extracting performance, and facilitate the assembly of a feature-oriented, clinical data base. Tapes of spectral estimates and time domain indices are optionally processed with off-line data editing programs that format selected data in response to dialog-specified parameters. In this way limited, but immediate, statistical processing such as multiple regression, factor analysis, or analysis of variance may be performed.

Real-Time Algorithms For Time-Series Analysis

We will not review the intricacies of time-series analysis using Fast Fourier Transform. The topic has been covered by Bendat and Piersol (1966), Jenkins and Watts (1968), and more recently by Otnes and Enochson (1972) from the point of view of actual computer implementations. In addition, many workers have reviewed time series analysis of the EEG (Walter and Adey 1963, 1965, 1966; Adey 1970; Walter 1963; Walter et al. 1966; Dumermuth and Flühler 1967; Dumermuth 1968; Dumermuth and Keller 1973; Kleiner et al. 1970). We will only mention here those aspects of time-series analysis that are applicable to the limited memory and central processor capabilities of real-time implementations on dedicated minicomputers.

The digitizing rate applied to the EEG signal should be as low as possible without losing potentially useful information, and without incurring signal aliasing. A single, fixed-frequency, analog low-pass filter does not meet the requirements of an on-line alterable sampling rate, while digital low-pass filtering algorithms generally require excessive computation time. An interim solution, which we have adopted, is to use three sets of sharp cutoff, analog low-pass filters with three dB points at 25, 50, and 100 Hz. The appropriate filter channels are then program-selected when the sampling rate is altered to 64, 128, and 256 Hz respectively. If special studies call for higher or lower sampling rates, appropriate filters may be plugged in.

The sampling and digitizing operation implicitly multiplies the data by a square window equal to one during the sampling interval, and equal to zero outside it. As is well known, the Fourier transformation of such a window is a function of shape, $\frac{\sin(\pi fT)}{(\pi fT)}$ where T is the time window and f is the frequency. These undesirable spectral side lobes may be reduced by multiplying the time series by a different data window prior to transformation, or by applying a spectral window to the raw periodograms. Of the many functions whose Fourier transformation has lower side lobes than does the implicit square window, a raised cosine bell window of form $\cos^2(\pi t/T)$, while not having optimal resolution, is efficient computationally since only the first and last 10 percent of the data points for each epoch are affected. With reference to the method of ensemble averaging of spectra, Otnes and Enochson (1972) describe a spectral window having better side-lobe rejection properties, although the implementation is more costly computationally. Even with short transform epochs of 0.5 to 2.0 seconds, there are appreciable trends in the EEG. These are represented in the frequency domain as large components in the first several spectral bins; they often contaminate frequencies of interest above 1 Hz, especially when a spectral window is applied. Nonzero mean and trend can be removed before the application of a data window, and the first one or two frequency bins may be discarded before spectral smoothing (Gevins and Yeager 1972).

There are various implementations of the FFT (Cooley, Lewis, and Welch 1967), some using mixed radix algorithms (Singleton 1969), others based on matrix operations (Andrews 1972). We have streamlined a fixed-point, radix two-assembly language FFT obtained from a computer users' group (DeBoer and DeJongh 1970). By adding program logic to transform and unscramble two EEG channels at a time (Gevins 1973), a transform rate of about 0.5 milliseconds per point is obtained. This is sufficient to provide continuous double precision (36-bit) spectral estimates of eight autopower channels and eight cross spectral and coherence pairs, with usable spectral resolution to 48 Hz in 1-Hz steps. Sufficient idle time remains to permit the functioning of the various transient-analysis and feature-extraction algorithms described below.

The use of a 0.5- to 2.0-second transform window length reflects a fortunate convergence of EEG characteristics with restrictions imposed by limited core capacity. However, even for short epochs, there is evidence that the EEG is nonstationary (Dumermuth et al. 1971, Huber et al. 1971), suggesting that studies of the moment-to-moment changes in spectral values may yield parameters useful for characterizing the background EEG. Since processes of shorter duration than the transform epoch are averaged together, and phase shifts occurring during the sampling window result in the cancellation of spectral activity in the bin around which the shift is occurring (Walter 1968), other forms of analysis must be used to achieve finer resolution. Some of these are complex demodulation (Bingham, Godfrey, and Tukey 1967; Walter 1968; Levine et al. 1972; Naitoh et al. 1972), autocorrelation (Brazier and Casby 1952; Barlow and Brazier 1954; Barlow, Brazier, and Rosenblith 1959; Barlow 1961), and other forms of time domain analysis (Fenwick et al. 1971; Saltzberg, Lustick, and Heath 1971; Wennberg and Zetterberg 1971; Maynard 1972). It must be noted, however, that an increase in resolution in the time domain is obtained at the expense of resolution in the frequency domain. Alternatively, one could overlap the FFT or another more computationally efficient orthonormal transform (Andrews 1971) by large amounts, noting changes in the bins of interest (Bishop and Wilson 1972). For real-time systems, spectral estimates are conveniently produced by ensemble averaging short transforms as outlined by Welch (1967) for autopower spectra. We have also applied this method to compute cross spectral estimates, using double precision integer arithmetic. If spectral values are to be used statistically, one must consider the extent to which the fine grain of the EEG signal should be destroyed by spectral smoothing or ensemble averaging in order to improve the reliability of the estimates. The answer to this question obviously depends on the phenomena under investigation. If the aim is to characterize the background EEG during the eyes-closed state, it is not unreasonable to ensemble average 60 or more one-second transforms. If the problem is to monitor the immediate EEG changes induced by intravenous administration of a psychoactive drug, one may wish to look at unsmoothed, unaveraged periodograms, temporarily deferring considerations of statistical reliability. By allowing the ensemble averaging constant to be an on-line parameter, experimentation with the various alternatives is possible.

Transient Analysis

Orthonormal transforms, such as the FFT, used with nonoverlapping windows of one second or more, characterize the average background of the EEG and are not uniquely sensitive to such transient activity as the sharp paroxysmal waveforms (spikes and sharp waves) associated with epilepsy. Since the appearance of a sharp transient in a polygraph tracing is modified by background activity, the decision to identify a particular wave as clinically significant cannot be based on a universal set of precisely defined criteria. Electroencephalographers often agree as to the characterization of a record in terms of overall absence or presence of sharp paroxysmal transients, while differing as to the identification of individual waves (Gose 1974); this situation has made the development of automated systems difficult. Regardless of the form of implementation, the purpose of such systems has been to match clinical judgment on a wave-by-wave basis. The extraction of primary features has been emphasized, while the classification problem remains largely untouched. Classification must be based on both the totality of individual decisions for each wave, and comparison with data derived from a normal population. Our initial efforts have been directed at improving sharp transient wave recognition by developing heuristic algorithms based on the contextual criteria of clinical electroencephalography (Gibbs and Gibbs 1952, Kooi 1971, Maulsby 1971). Additionally, we have attempted to demonstrate the feasibility of performing such transient analysis in parallel with real-time spectral analysis and display in a dedicated minicomputer.

One of the early reported attempts to automate seizure detection (Bickford 1959) employed amplitude and frequency as the discriminating parameters. While useful for detecting the occurrence of seizures, amplitude criteria failed to distinguish isolated spikes and sharp waves from artifact, or from large-amplitude EEG phenomena. Buckley, Saltzberg, and Heath (1968) implemented a more efficient system that used curvature-at-the-peak criteria and correlated activity on several channels. However, since this system was developed to detect only the very large spikes found in depth electrode recordings, it would not necessarily detect sharp waves or low-amplitude spikes mixed in the same recording. It could also mistake a continuous train of sharp alpha waves for spikes, since it could not adapt its decision threshold to the context of the ongoing signal. Carrie (1972a) subsequently used decision criteria based on the ratio of a parameter's current value to its moving average, thus allowing adaptation to changing EEG characteristics. Eventually the filtered second derivative was selected as a suitable parameter (Carrie 1973). In addition, a sequential decision procedure was employed to locate spike and wave complexes (Carrie 1972b); however, it is not sensitive to mixed patterns. While differing in algorithms and implementation, other attempts at detecting sharp transients support the conclusion that further development is needed before such systems can be of general clinical use. Smith (1974) reported a device using rise time and curvature as parameters, while Saltzberg (Saltzberg et al. 1971) and Zetterberg (1973) used matched digital filtering. Goldberg et al. (1973), using combinations of high-pass filtering, amplitude, period, and context as a method of feature extraction, found that a minimum of three spikes per minute had to be found before comparisons between visual and computer detection could be made. Ebe and Homma (Ebe et al. 1973, Homma et al. 1973) report the development of a small comprehensive system, but clinical evaluation is not presented. Hill and Townsend (1973) attempted to estimate the mean rate of spike firing in laboratory rats, using unsupervised training methods to determine the cutoff point for spikes in a bimodal distribution of peak angles. While only applicable to clinical electroencephalography in cases of prolonged spiking, the work is exemplary in that an additional analysis is applied beyond primary feature extraction.

The transient detection algorithms to be described here form a single module in the ADIEEG system (Figure 1) capable of operating either alone or in parallel with spectral analysis and display. For computational purposes the EEG is treated as two distinct signals, a source of background EEG and a source of transient waveforms, to which signal conditioning and digitizing rates are individually applied. For the real-time analysis, up to eight transient channels are low-pass filtered at 50 Hz, sampled 128 or 256 times per second, and digitized to 11 bits. The limit of eight channels reflects the methodology of the Langley Porter Institute EEG laboratory rather than restrictions imposed by computational considerations. For playback of analog tapes at speeds greater than real time, appropriately higher low-pass cutoff frequencies and sampling rates are used. Peaks are identified by locating a change in sign of the signal's first derivative, $X^\bullet(t)$. The curvature is computed in the region of the peak $C(t) = X''(t)/ [1 + X'^2(t)]^{3/2}$, where $X''(t)$ is the second derivative at time t. In the region where $X'(t)$ is zero, the equation simplifies to $C(t) = X''(t)$. In order to introduce the electroencephalographer's bias toward higher amplitude but less sharp transient waveforms (sharp waves), the weighted curvature, $S(t)$, is computed $S(t) = C(t) + k_1 X(t)$, where k_1 is an empirically determined amplitude weighting factor having a base value of 0.063. This might appear to contradict the work of Townsend and Hill (1973) and comments made by Glaser (1973) who argued for the normalization of sharpness measures by amplitude. However, decisions here are based on comparisons with moving averages; thus the parameters are in effect normalized. In preliminary work we found that the use of an absolute measure of sharpness favors the discrimination of small, high-frequency waves of nonpathogenic origin over the larger, but not as sharp, clinically significant sharp transients.

The weighted curvature is compared with a sharpness index, $\bar{S}(t)$ characterizing the immediately preceding N EEG samples,

$$\bar{S}(t) = \frac{(N-1) \cdot S(t-1) + S(t)}{N}.$$

This index is a moving average of the weighted curvature, $S(t)$. $\bar{S}(t)$ is the updated moving average of the weighted curvature at time t, and N is the moving average window length, typically 128. When the ratio of the weighted curvature, $S(t)$, to the current value of the moving average $\bar{S}(t)$ exceeds a threshold value, k_2, typically 2.5, an entry is made in a table of sharp transient events of potential clinical significance. A candidate kernel containing corroborative data such as $S(t)$, $\bar{S}(t)$, and the spikiness index $S(t)/\bar{S}(t)$ on all channels is also saved for further processing.

Data on a patient's clinical history are used in a rudimentary manner to set transient analysis parameters which discriminate between extracerebral artifact and potentially significant sharp transient events. At present, two sets of default parameters for the various constants and thresholds are used, one for persons with known epileptogenic EEG patterns, and one for "normals," reflecting use of the system for either measuring the effects of anticonvulsant therapy, or screening an unknown population. Several criteria are then applied to the potentially significant waveforms as represented in the candidate kernel. The magnitude of the spikiness index is compared with an upper bound for acceptable transients, k_3. If this threshold is exceeded, the waveform is assumed to have been oversharp, and an artifact routine is invoked to discard the kernel, momentarily inhibit data collection, and attend to various other housekeeping functions including storage of time, and location and cause of artifact. Sharp transients which occur frequently or have excessive spread over the scalp are also rejected, unless the parameters are set up for seizure scoring.

Once the candidate data kernel is temporarily assumed not to have been artifact-generated, further characterizations are extracted, based on the pattern of activity on adjacent channels, phase reversals (bipolar recordings), and polarity of the first component of multiphasic waveform (monopolar montage). Channels anatomically adjacent to the one containing the waveform of interest, the hypothetical focus, are required to exhibit a peak whose spikiness index meets a reduced criterion, typically 0.75 of k_2, within 50 milliseconds. If this adjacency is not detected, the candidate data kernel is assumed not to have clinical significance and is discarded. After the final component of a multiphasic waveform (triphasic, polyspike, etc.) is identified and adjacent channels have been examined, a search is undertaken for a slow wave (defined as a waveform of low curvature with respect to the background spikiness index). This search, lasting up to 500 milliseconds, is undertaken with a lowered analog-to-digital sampling rate, typically 16 samples per second, to reduce contamination by high frequency components.

At this time, weights characterizing the degree of match with empirically determined EEG criteria are assigned as follows (Celesia 1974): (1) 75 percent of all clinically significant sharp transients are associated with a slow wave, (2) in monopolar recordings about 90 percent of all clinically significant sharp transients have a first component which is surface-negative. The candidate waveform's data kernel, together with the weights assigned as a result of the previously detailed analysis, is compared with a table of parameters and weights derived from sharp transient events that have been detected and accepted during the course of the analysis session. This final matching criterion is designed for long recording and for system use in measuring the effects of anticonvulsant therapy. The weight given the pattern-matching criterion is increased as a function of the number of waveforms so far detected. Obviously, this biases the detection of waveforms having characteristics similar to those already detected. Since the matching pattern is continuously updated, however, adaptation to the ongoing activity compensates somewhat for this defect. Further studies will determine the effectiveness of this procedure in developing a template to be used as a matched digital filter.

If the sum of the accumulated weights exceeds a threshold criterion, k_7, the candidate waveform is declared to be a clinically significant sharp transient event, and an "S" is printed on the relevant portion of the current spectral graph. When used as a stand-alone sharp transient detection system, the report will print the time of occurrence of sharp transients and their characteristics. Additionally, data characterizing the waveform, including the candidate's data kernel, and the weights and thresholds in use at the time of the event, are saved on a mass storage device. At the conclusion of the analysis run, a histogram showing sharp transient counts vs. time is produced from the stored data. When sufficient clinical data have been accumulated, clustering techniques will be applied.

If, in the opinion of the attending operator, the decision of the analysis system is in error, a control button may be depressed causing the amplitude-weighted sharpness and the final decision thresholds, respectively k_2 and k_7, to be adjusted by a fixed increment in the appropriate direction. This is at best an interim procedure and works only when the various weights given to the heuristic factors are already closely aligned with the characteristics of an individual's recording. In order to evaluate performance, a subsystem has been developed to compare prescored EEG recordings with system detections. It types out "+", "-", or "?" for a correct identification, a missed event, or an unscored event respectively. Further development of this facility is planned to serve as a means of automatically adjusting the weights and thresholds to match a particular clinician's judgment.

It is difficult to make direct comparisons across individuals when using transient detection algorithms that are based upon weighting and thresholding procedures, because the thresholds vary continuously. However, if progress is made at automatic adjustment of weight and thresholds, comparisons similar to those now made visually will be possible. Although systems such as the one described here may be tweaked to produce a reasonable degree of agreement with the results of visual analysis for selected portions of recordings from selected subjects, further development is needed before generalized testing may be performed in a clinical environment. Among other EEG phenomena, artifact, vertex sharp waves, and spikey alpha rhythms can create false positive identifications during the initial feature-extracting process. For purposes of classification, use of the patient's clinical history and comparison with a broad clinical data base must be performed after the initial feature extraction.

Artifact Rejection

It is no trivial task to devise algorithms that distinguish, in a general way, cortical electrical activity from nonbrain artifact produced by physiologic and instrumental sources. The problems are even more formidable if artifact rejection decisions are to be made in real time. Some artifacts, like those arising from eye movements, may be recorded with extra electrodes, and either electrically subtracted from the contaminated EEG electrodes

(Girton and Kamiya 1973) or used to discard entire segments of the time history. Gross body motion artifacts may be recognized by very high spectral values compared to the previous analysis history. One may even have the subject generate artifacts during a calibration period to determine character-istic time- and spectral-domain artifact parameters, which can then be used to discard artifact during the subsequent analysis session. Unfortunately, no matter how cleverly one tries to eliminate artifact, some of its remains, and valid EEG is also mistakenly discarded. An interim solution, adopted in order to facilitate real-time EEG analysis, is to supply the EEG technician with a means of informing the system that it has either missed an artifact or has mistakenly identified EEG as artifact. The feedback can be of immediate use in improving artifact-rejection performance by causing decision thresh-olds to be altered. Although we have not yet implemented such a program, one may store and analyze the artifact-rejection decisions so that experience gained from many subjects may be incorporated in the heuristics in a more general manner.

Interactive Graphics

Many forms of display have been applied to the electrical potentials recorded from the scalp, of which the polygraph is the most familiar. The toposcope of Walter and Shipton (1951) is a dynamic display, while the topograms of Rémond (1961) and the contour displays of spectra by Walter (1963) are more static. In choosing a display for our own spectral-oriented system, a compromise between dynamic and static forms was sought to facilitate interpretation by electroencephalographers. The chosen form of graphics is a compressed spectral array (Bickford, Fleming, and Billinger 1971; Bickford et al. 1973) consisting of contour plots of frequency with overlapping lines suppressed. In this display the abscissa represents frequency in Hertz, while the ordinate represents both amplitude (the height of each individual line) and time (each successive line starting at the bottom is the ensemble average of the next set of Fourier transforms). Figure 4 is a typical display, used to characterize the background EEG over the entire scalp. Eight channels are shown, the top four representing the left frontal (LF), left central (LC), left temporal (LT), and left occipital (LO) areas first with eyes closed, then with eyes open. The bottom four channels represent the same montage, except that they are taken from the right side of the scalp. The frequency scale in this case extends to 32 Hz, while each spectral line repre-sents five seconds of activity. This graph demonstrates the learned ability of the subject to maintain his alpha rhythm during the eyes-open state, in the frontal as well as the occipital electrodes. A slight asymmetry of amplitude and frequency between homologous placements is evident.

Aside from processing efficiency, the utility of a real-time EEG analysis system is manifest in the interaction of the clinician in the recording process. By fine-tuning the analysis and display, an individual's characteristic brain wave activity may be revealed. Use of the graphics capability can make differences in electrophysiological state surprisingly clear, even to those unfamiliar with the EEG. Figure 5 shows a spectral graph derived from a patient with severe temporal lobe epilepsy; it clearly reveals an abnormal amount of low-frequency activity, especially in the temporal area. Figure 6 shows the same patient after surgical intervention. The reappearance of the alpha rhythm and the reduction of the slow temporal activity is evident, although a marked asymmetry in amplitude between homologous occipital electrodes is evident.

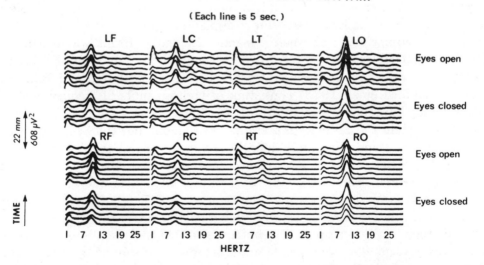

Figure 4. Typical example of an eight-channel power spectral display produced in real time. Computer-drawn frequency, amplitude, and time scale labels have been redrawn by artist for clarity. Frequency scale graphed extends to 32 Hz, while stored frequency components extend to 48 Hz. Each line represents the ensemble average of five 1-second Fast Fourier Transforms.

It is often desirable to depict changes occurring over a relatively long period of time. Figure 7 represents 30 minutes of EEG recorded from a patient with hypoglycemia; it shows the extreme slowing induced by insulin. When significant changes are barely discernible in the background spectral graphs, expanding one or two channels with a very narrow spectral bandwidth can make such detail apparent. Figures 8 and 9, which show EEG changes occurring during a course of electroconvulsive therapy (ECT), are enlarged so that only the theta and alpha activity from the two occipital leads is shown. The upper half of Figure 8 shows the normal baseline alpha, while in the lower half the alpha has slowed by more than one-half cycle per second. In the upper half of Figure 9 the slowing is more prominent 24 hours after the fourth ECT treatment, while in the lower half a double alpha peak is seen as the normal alpha activity begins to reappear one week after

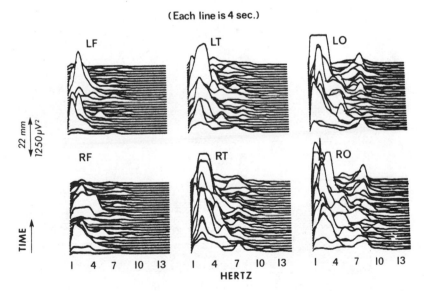

TEMPORAL LOBE EPILEPSY,
PRE SURGERY

(Each line is 4 sec.)

Figure 5. Six channels of power spectra from a patient with severe temporal lobe epilepsy prior to surgical intervention. Large amount of abnormal low-frequency activity in temporal and occipital leads is apparent.

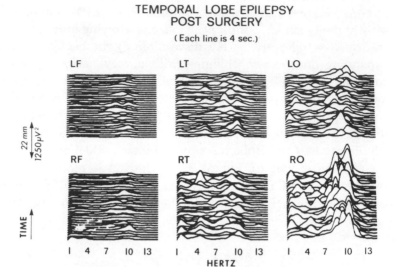

Figure 6. Six channels of power spectra following surgical intervention. Slow temporal activity has been reduced while asymmetrical occipital alpha peaks have appeared.

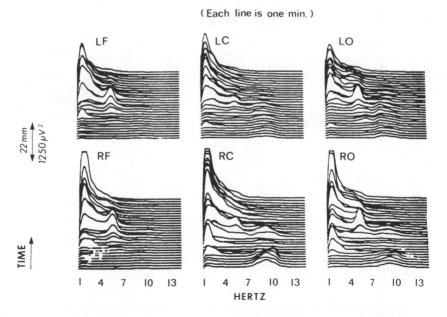

Figure 7. Thirty minutes of power spectra, 30 minutes after administration of insulin. Gradual increase of slowing is evident.

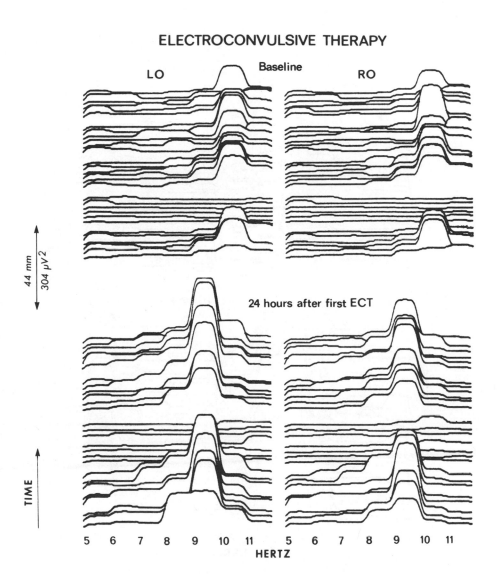

Figure 8. Expanded view of 5- to 12-Hz activity from occipital leads before and 24 hours after the first electroconvulsive treatment. Slowing of alpha rhythm is apparent.

ELECTROCONVULSIVE THERAPY

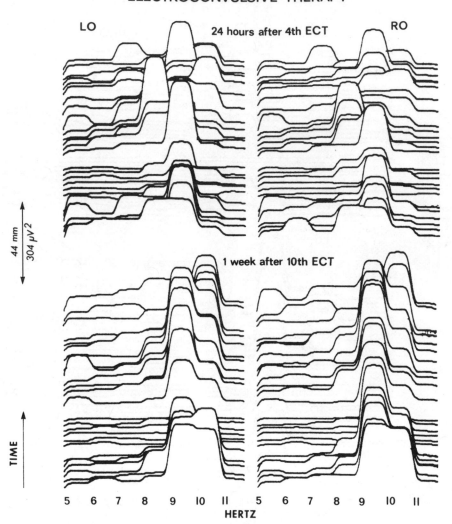

Figure 9. Continued view of the course of electroconvulsive treatment. Twenty-four hours after the fourth treatment there is additional slowing; one week after the tenth treatment a double alpha peak is present.

the last treatment. Spectral functions other than autopower are often revealing. In Figure 10 a composite picture of a malignant glioma with a right frontal focus shows both autopower and coherence spectra. The widely distributed coherence peaks in the leads bridging the focus are evident.

The possibilities are manifold: transforms such as square root and arc tangent can compress or expand the differences between peaks of varying height; the appearance of the graphs can be changed by decreasing the amount of spectral smoothing, thus stressing the distinctions between adjacent frequency bins; spacing between lines can be increased to allow finer discrimination of individual spectra; spectral lines can be offset to allow looking behind peaks into the valleys; or a floating level can be introduced to show only spectra above a significant value.

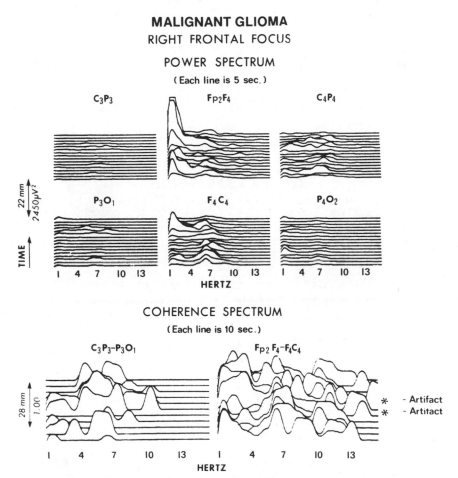

Figure 10. Power and coherence spectra from a patient with a malignant glioma. Note slow activity in right frontal lead. Coherence spectrum bridging the focus shows high peaks across the spectrum.

INTERACTIVE MODIFICATION
OF REAL TIME ANALYSIS AND DISPLAY

A*D*I*E*E*G
ANALYSIS PARAMETERS

CLOCK RATE	512	ENTER: 256
# TICKS PER SAMPLE	4	
A/D CHANNELS	0 1 2 3 4 5 6 7	
X SPECTRAL PAIRS	0 1 2 3 4 5 6 7	
# POINTS PER FFT	128	
TAPE OUTPUT PATTERN	11 13 2 7 4	
ANALOG TAPE	N	ENTER: Y<ES>
# PERIODS IN RUN	0	
PROTOCOL	6	ENTER: 6 6 6 6 3 3
MAGTAPE OUTPUT	N	ENTER: Y<ES>
PULSE WIDTH	128	

A*D*I*E*E*G
GRAPHICS PARAMETERS

FUNCTION	P	ENTER: C<OHERENCE>
ENSEMBLES	4	
POWER CHANNELS	0 2 4 1 3 5	
COHERENCE PAIRS	0 1 2 3 4	
MAX FREQUENCY	20	ENTER: 100 <HERTZ>
MIN FREQUENCY	0	ENTER: 1 <HERTZ>
POWER SCALING	9	
DISPLAY THRESHOLD	0	ENTER: 4
SMOOTHING	3	
VERTICAL SPACING	8	
HI FREQ MUL FACTOR	0	
MULT CUTOFF FREQ	15	
HIDDEN LINES	Y	ENTER: N<O>

Figure 11. Menu for interactive parameter alteration. Cross-hairs are used to select the parameter to be modified, while alpha numeric characters are used for an entry. Abbreviations are normally used to enter parameter values.

Parameter Modification

In the context of real-time signal analysis the term, interactive graphics, refers to alteration of the form and parameters of display from a live source rather than from a previously stored data base. In our system, ADIEEG, the form of display is currently fixed to compressed spectral arrays, while the interactive aspect concerns the selection of various combinations of spectral function, EEG channels, frequency band width, and various other associated parameters. Parameters are modified by using the graphic input and alphanumeric modes of the Tektronix 4010 terminal. Positioning a cursor, the user first selects the parameter to be modified from a menu, and then enters a stereotyped English or numeric phrase to effect the change, as shown in Figure 11. To minimize interference with ongoing data collection, analysis, and storage, system graphics and interactive parameter alteration modules are mostly asynchronous. For example, the display may be changed from two to six channels without disrupting an eight-channel data flow to the mass storage device. Certain crucial parameters, such as the real-time clock or sampling rates, may only be modified when the system is quiescent, since they necessitate manual adjustment of the clock and recomputation of the entire buffer structure.

Error Detection

At initialization time the user enters the subject's name, age, handedness, diagnosis, and other pertinent information. Errors made at this time elicit an example of the correct input form, and the entry can then be corrected. When parameters are modified interactively, a higher level of competence on the part of the user is assumed and error correction is relatively passive. If a typographical error or illogical entry is made, an error signal is given and the entry must be repeated. By not indicating the class of error, large ASC11 buffers devoted to error messages are eliminated and increased space is available for data. Of course, if a combination of parameters, not one of which is incorrect, creates an impossible condition such as a lack of adequate buffer space, the user is informed explicitly and advised to reconfigure the analysis.

The Process of Feature Extraction

We have described a programming system that derives spectral function estimates and transient indices and performs interactive graphics in real time. If the only purpose of such a system were to present power spectral displays, much of the generality and many of the time-consuming refinements of spectral estimation could be dispensed with. A simpler design would write raw spectral coefficients and time-domain indices on digital tape, while graphing rough estimates of the power spectrum. In an evolutionary approach, spectral and transient analysis and display are the first stage of a systems development that aims ultimately at classification and diagnosis. Numerical classification methods are restricted to problems of relatively low dimensionality (Nilsson 1965, Mendel and Fu 1970, Andrews 1972, Meisel 1972b, Chen 1973). Often arbitrary decisions must be made to meet the imposed constraints, resulting in the deletion of much of an EEG recording session. In addition, premature application of classification procedures often results in decision rules based on descriptors that have little intersubject generality. The procedures to be considered attempt to eliminate some of this arbitrariness by allowing more flexibility in data-pruning decisions through the use of additional processing prior to attempts of classification.

Real-time feature extraction of the EEG is conceived in two parts, simple combining and heuristic pruning. By using means and standard deviations of computed spectral and transient values, simple combining results in the extraction of indices and feature complexes that are clinically useful. Such features are organized by frequency band, period of occurrence, and topological area; they include normalized power, coherence based on bins with significant amounts of auto- and cross-power, symmetry ratios based on power and coherence, and number, location, and time of occurrence of transient phenomena. For conditions associated with obviously aberrant EEG patterns, including in general the epilepsies, brain tumors, and degenerative diseases, these simple features should be sufficient for EEG screening and routine clinical examination.

Traditional EEG interpretation and manual feature extraction using the interactive facility of the analysis system have generated some guidelines for automated algorithms. Some examples of this process have been presented in the sections on transient analysis and interactive graphics. The second part of the feature-extraction process proposed here consists of programming the decision process, so that storage and the future course of analysis can be based on heuristic rules derived from clinical experience. Such criteria include "gross" differences in amplitude across homologous areas, "high" incidence of spikes, and "abnormal" focal sites of activity. To effect such decisions, an analysis-directing executive must be added to the basic system configuration (Figure 1). The analysis-directing executive will supervise the logical flow of data, including choice of analysis and parameters, in direct analogy with the multitasking executive which schedules and executes task modules. By endowing the real-time analysis system with the ability to organize its processing flexibility, emphasizing the overall and specific characteristics of an individual's EEG, the machine will be performing, in its own terms, the initial stages of an integrated approach to EEG interpretation. This does not mean that the technique is applicable to other than trivial cases of classification, since the attempt to construct electroencephalographic automatons to perform classification and diagnosis does not seem to be fruitful. It is hoped, however, that these techniques will produce compacted data sets that have more intersubject generality when mathematical pattern-classification algorithms are applied.

Summary

An integrated systems approach to real-time EEG analysis has been outlined, with stress on the evolutionary nature of development. Overall design considerations for hardware and software systems have been presented; aspects pertaining to real-time paradigms, including multitasking executive and data structure design, have been described in detail. Spectral and transient analysis and artifact-rejection algorithms suitable for real-time implementations have been presented. A discussion of interactive analysis and graphics has stressed the need for generality and flexibility in systems design. Finally, the next stage of development, heuristic feature extraction, has been suggested as a necessary prerequisite to attempts at automated classification and diagnosis.

Acknowledgments

Appreciation is expressed to the following individuals who helped develop the system described in this paper: Stephen Diamond, systems programmer, for work done on transient analysis and interactive graphics; Adi Gevins, research associate, for technical writing support; Joseph Henderson and Mary Martis, EEG technicians, for assistance with data collection; Douglas Livingston, research technician, for assistance with data collection, program development, and hardware maintenance; Mary McNicholas, secretary, for manuscript preparation; Fred Oehler, electronics specialist, for design and implementation of computer interfaces and computer systems maintenance.

Systems development is supported by the National Institutes of Health Grant NS-10471.

References

Adey, W.R. 1970. On-line computation in behavioral neurophysiology. In J.P. Schadé and J. Smith, *Progress in Brain Research: Computers and Brains* (23), p. 23. New York: Elsevier.

Andrews, H.C. 1971. Multidimensional rotations in feature space. *IEEE Transactions on Computers* C-20:1045.

Andrews, H.C. 1972. *Introduction to Mathematical Techniques in Pattern Recognition.* New York: John Wiley.

Andrews, H.C., and Caspari, K.L. 1971. Degrees of freedom and modular structure in matrix multiplication. *IEEE Transactions on Computers* C-20:133.

Barlow, J.S. 1961. Autocorrelation and crosscorrelation techniques in EEG analysis. *Electroencephalogr. Clin. Neurophysiol.* suppl. 20:31.

Barlow, J.S., and Brazier, M.A.B. 1954. A note on a correlator for electroencephalographic work. *Electroencephalogr. Clin. Neurophysiol.* 6:321.

Barlow, J.S., Brazier, M.A.B., and Rosenblith, W.A. 1959. The application of autocorrelation analysis to electroencephalography. *Proc. 1st Nation. Biophysics Conf.*, p. 622. New Haven: Yale University Press.

Bendat, J., and Piersol, A.G. 1966. *The Measurement and Analysis of Random Data.* New York: John Wiley.

Bickford, R.G. 1959. An automatic recognition system for spike-and-wave with simultaneous testing of motor response. *Electroencephalogr. Clin. Neurophysiol.* 11:397.

Bickford, R.G., Brimm, J., Berger, L., and Aung, M. 1973. Application of compressed spectral array in clinical EEG. In P. Kellaway and I. Petersén (eds.), *Automation of Clinical Electroencephalography*, p. 103. New York: Raven Press.

Bickford, R.G., Fleming, N.I., and Billinger, T.W. 1971. Compression of EEG data by isometric power spectral plots. *Electroencephalogr. Clin. Neurophysiol.* 31:631.

Bingham, C., Godfrey, M.D., and Tukey, J.W. 1967. Modern techniques of power spectrum estimation. *IEEE Transactions on Audio and Electroacoustics* AU-15:56.

Bishop, A.O., Jr., and Wilson, W.P. 1972. Computer analysis of the clinical EEG. *Electroencephalogr. Clin. Neurophysiol.* 31:117.

Brazier, M.A.B., and Casby, J.U. 1952. Crosscorrelation and autocorrelation studies of electroencephalographic potentials. *Electroencephalogr. Clin. Neurophysiol.* 4:201.

Bremer, G., Smith, J.R., and Karacan, I. 1970. Automatic detection of the K-complex in sleep electroencephalograms. *IEEE Trans. Biomed. Eng.* BME-17:314.

Buckley, J.K., Saltzberg, B., and Heath, R.G. 1968. Decision criteria and detection circuitry for multiple channel EEG correlation. *IEEE Region 3 Convention Record* 26:1.

Burch, N.R. 1959. Automatic analysis of the electroencephalogram: A review and classification of systems. *Electroencephalogr. Clin. Neurophysiol.* 2:827.

Burch, N.R., Greiner, T.H., and Correll, E.G. 1955. Automatic analysis of electroencephalograms on an index of minimal changes in human consciousness. *Fed. Proc.* 14:23.

Burch, N.R., Nettleton, W.J., Jr., Sweeny, J., and Edwards, R.J., Jr. 1964. Period analysis of the electroencephalogram on a general-purpose digital computer. *Ann. N.Y. Acad. Sci.* 115:827.

Carrie, J.R.G. 1972a. A technique for analyzing transient EEG abnormalities. *Electroencephalogr. Clin. Neurophysiol.* 32:199.

Carrie, J.R.G. 1972b. A hybrid computer technique for detecting sharp EEG transients. *Electroencephalogr. Clin. Neurophysiol.* 33:336.

Carrie, J.R.G. 1972c. A hybrid computer system for detecting and quantifying spike and wave EEG patterns. *Electroencephalogr. Clin. Neurophysiol.* 33:339.

Carrie, J.R.G. 1973. The detection and quantification of transient and paroxysmal EEG abnormalities. In P. Kellaway and I. Petersén (eds.), *Automation of Clinical Electroencephalography*, p. 217. New York: Raven Press.

Carrie, J.R.G., and Frost, J.D., Jr. 1971. A small computer system for EEG wavelength amplitude profile analysis. *Biomedical Computing* 2:251.

Carrie, J.R.G., and Frost, J.D., Jr. 1973. Wavelength-amplitude profile analysis in clinical EEG. In P. Kellaway and I. Petersén (eds.), *Automation of Clinical Electroencephalography*, p. 65. New York: Raven Press.

Celesia, G.G. 1974. Paper presented at *West and Central EEG Society Meeting*, Denver, Colorado, April, 1974.

Chen, C. 1973. *Statistical Pattern Recognition*. Rochelle Park, N.J.: Spartan Books.

Cooley, J.W., Lewis, P.A.W., and Welch, P.D. 1967. *The Fast Fourier Transform Algorithm and its Applications*. Research Paper RC-1743. Yorktown Heights, N.Y.: IBM Watson Research Center.

Cooley, J.W., and Tukey, J.S. 1965. An algorithm for the machine calculation of complex Fourier series. *Mathematical Computing* 19:297.

Cox, J.R., Nolle, F.M., and Arthur, R.M. 1972. Digital analysis of the electroencephalogram, the blood pressure wave, and the electrocardiogram. *IEEE Proceedings* 60:1137.

DeBoer, E., and DeJongh, H.R. 1970. *Ultra-fast Fourier Transform*. Decus Program Library No. 15-2. Maynard, Mass.: DECUS.

Dumermuth, G. 1968. Variance spectra of electroencephalograms in twins. A contribution to the problem of EEG background activity in childhood. In P. Kellaway and I. Petersén (eds.), *Clinical Electroencephalography of Children*, p. 119. New York: Grune & Stratton.

Dumermuth, G. and Flühler, H. 1967. Some modern aspects in numerical analysis of multichannel electroencephalographic data. *Med. Biol. Eng.* 5:319.

Dumermuth, G., Huber, P.J., Kleiner, B., and Gasser, T. 1971. Analysis of the interrelations between frequency bands of the EEG by means of the bispectrum. *Electroencephalogr. Clin. Neurophysiol.* 31:137.

Dumermuth, G., and Keller, E. 1973. EEG spectral analysis by means of Fast Fourier Transform. In P. Kellaway and I. Petersén (eds.), *Automation of Clinical Electroencephalography*, p. 145. New York: Raven Press.

Ebe, M., Homma, I., Ishiyama, Y., Suzuki, T., Ogawa, T., Shiono, H., Nakamura, T., and Abe, Z. 1973. Automatic analysis of clinical information in EEG. *Electroencephalogr. Clin. Neurophysiol.* 34:706.

Fenwick, P.B.C., Michie, P., Dollimore, J., and Fenton, G.W. 1971. Mathematical simulation of the electroencephalogram using an autoregressive series. *Biomedical Computing* 2:281.

Fink, M., Itil, T.M., and Shapiro, D.M. 1967. Digital computer analysis of the human

EEG in psychiatric research. *Compr. Psychiatry* 8:521.

Frost, J.D., Jr. 1969. Wavelength analysis of the EEG—the alpha profile. *Electroencephalogr. Clin. Neurophysiol.* 27:702.

Gevins, A.S. 1972. Real time executive design in signal processing systems. *Decus Proceedings,* Fall, p. 165.

Gevins, A.S. 1973. Doubling the speed of Fourier transformation of real data. *Decuscope* 12:24.

Gevins, A.S., and Yeager, C.L. 1972. EEG spectral analysis in real time. *Decus Proceedings,* Spring, p. 71.

Gibbs, F.A., and Gibbs, E.L. 1952. *Atlas of Electroencephalography, Volume II: Epilepsy.* Reading, Mass.: Addison-Wesley.

Gibbs, F.A., and Grass, A.M. 1947. Frequency analysis of electroencephalograms. *Science* 105:132.

Girton, D.G., and Kamiya, J. 1973. A simple on-line technique for removing eye movement artifacts from the EEG. *Electroencephalogr. Clin. Neurophysiol.* 34:212.

Glaser, E.M. 1973. Comments on "semiautomatic quantification of sharpness of EEG phenomena." *IEEE Trans. Biomed. Eng.* 20:313.

Goldberg, P., Samson-Dollfus, D. and Grémy, F. 1973. An approach to automatic pattern recognition of the electroencephalogram: background rhythm and paroxysmal elements. *Meth. Inform. Med.* (3):155.

Gose, E.E. 1974. Computerized EEG spike detection. *13th Annual San Diego Biomedical Symposium Abstracts,* p. 57.

Grass, A.M., and Gibbs, F.A. 1938. Fourier transform of the electroencephalogram. *J. Neurophysiol.* 1:521.

Harper, R.M., Walter, D.O., and Kelly, D.S. 1972. On-line classification of neurophysiological wave forms. *Decus Proceedings,* Fall, p. 65.

Hill, A.G., and Townsend, H.R.A. 1973. The automatic estimation of epileptic spike activity. *Biomedical Computing* (4):149.

Hjorth, B. 1970. EEG analysis based on time domain properties. *Electroencephalogr. Clin. Neurophysiol.* 29:306.

Homma, I., Ebe, M., Ishiyama, Y., Suzuki, T., Ogawa, T., Shiono, H., Nakamura, T., and Abe, Z. 1973. Automatic analyzer of clinical EEG in 12 channels-recording. *Digest of the 10th International Conference on Medical and Biological Engineering,* Dresden, p. 121.

Hoovey, Z.B., Heinemann, U., and Creutzfeldt, O.D. 1972. Inter-hemispheric synchrony of alpha waves. *Electroencephalogr. Clin. Neurophysiol.* 32:337.

Huber, P.J., Kleiner, B., Gasser, T., and Dumermuth, G. 1971. Statistical methods for investigation of phase relations in stationary stochastic processes. *IEEE Transactions on Audio and Electroacoustics* AU-19:78.

Itil, T.M., Shapiro, D.M., Fink, M., and Kassebaum, D. 1969. Digital computer classifications of EEG sleep stages. *Electroencephalogr. Clin. Neurophysiol.* 27:76.

Jenkins, G.M., and Watts, D.G. 1968. *Spectral Analysis and its Applications.* San Francisco: Holden Day.

Kleiner, B., Flühler, H., Huber, P.J., and Dumermuth, G. 1970. Spectrum analysis of the electroencephalogram. *Computer Programs in Biomedicine* 1:183.

Knott, J.R. 1953. Automatic frequency analysis. *Electroencephalogr. Clin. Neurophysiol.* suppl. 4:17.

Kooi, K.A. 1971. *Fundamentals of Electroencephalography.* New York: Harper & Row.

Larsen, L.E., Ruspini, E.H., McNew, J.J., Walter, D.O., and Adey, W.R. 1973. Classification and discrimination of the EEG during sleep. In P. Kellaway and I. Petersén (eds.), *Automation of Clinical Electroencephalography,* p. 243. New York: Raven Press.

Legewie, H. and Probst, W. 1969. On-line analysis of EEG with a small computer (period-amplitude analysis). *Electroencephalogr. Clin. Neurophysiol.* 27:533.

Lessard, C.S., Ford, G.E., and Hughes, H.M. 1969. Decomposition and variability of EEG information during sleep. *IEEE 12th Midwest Symposium on Circuit Theory Conference Record* 5:7.

Levine, D.A., Elashoff, R., Callaway, E., III, Payne, D., and Jones, R.T. 1972. Evoked potential analysis by complex demodulation. *Electroencephalogr. Clin. Neurophysiol.* 32:513.

Maulsby, R.L. 1971. Some guidelines for assessment of spikes and sharp waves in EEG tracings. *American Journal of Electroencephalograph Technology* 11:3.

Maynard, D.E. 1972. Separation of the sinusoidal components of the human electroencephalogram. *Nature* 236:228.

Meisel, W.S. 1972a. Personal communication.

Meisel, W.S. 1972b. *Computer-Oriented Approaches to Pattern Recognition.* New York: Academic Press.

Mendel, J.M., and Fu, K.S. 1970. *Adaptive, Learning and Pattern Recognition Systems.* New York: Academic Press.

Mucciardi, A.N., and Gose, E.E. 1971. A comparison of seven techniques for choosing subsets of pattern recognition properties. *IEEE Transactions on Computers* C-20:1023.

Naitoh, P., Nute, C., Hord, D., and Johnson, L.C. 1972. Comparisons of complex demodulation with spectrum in detailed analysis of the alpha rhythm. *Western EEG Society Annual Conference,* University of California, San Diego Neurosciences seminar.

Nilsson, N.J. 1965. *Learning Machines: Foundations of Trainable Pattern-Classifying Systems.* New York: McGraw-Hill.

Otnes, R.K., and Enochson, L. 1972. *Digital Time Series Analysis.* New York: John Wiley.

Pratt, W.K., Kane, J., and Andrews, H.C. 1969. Hadamard transform image coding. *IEEE Proceedings* 57:58.

Rémond, A. 1961. Integrated and topological analysis of the EEG. *Electroencephalogr. Clin. Neurophysiol.* suppl. 20:64.

Saltzberg, B. 1968. *Evaluation of Digital Computer-Analysis of the EEG.* Prog. Report, Grant NBO 4705, National Institute of Neurological Diseases and Blindness.

Saltzberg, B. 1973. Personal communication.

Saltzberg, B., and Burch, N.R. 1959. A rapidly convergent orthogonal representation for EEG time series and related methods of automatic analysis. *IRE Wescon Convention Record* 8:39.

Saltzberg, B., and Burch, N.R. 1971. Period analytic estimates of moments of the power spectrum: a simplified time domain procedure. *Electroencephalogr. Clin. Neurophysiol.*

30:568.

Saltzberg, B., Lustick, L.S., and Heath, R.G. 1971. Detection of focal depth spiking in the scalp EEG of monkeys. *Electroencephalogr. Clin. Neurophysiol.* 31:327.

Shannon, E.E., and Weaver, W.W. 1949. *The Mathematical Theory of Communication.* Urbana: University of Illinois Press.

Shipton, H.W. 1957. An improved electrotoposcope. *Electroencephalogr. Clin. Neurophysiol.* 9:182.

Singleton, R.C. 1969. An algorithm for computing the mixed radix Fast Fourier Transform. *IEEE Transactions on Audio and Electroacoustics* AU-17:93.

Skuce, D.R., Cotman, J., and Thompson, C.J. 1972. A realistic approach to determining clinically useful features of the EEG. *Decus Proceedings*, Fall, p. 59.

Smith, J.R. 1974. Automatic analysis and detection of EEG spikes. *IEEE Trans. Biomed. Eng.* 21:1.

Smith, J.R., Cronin, M.J., and Karacan, I. 1970. A multichannel hybrid system for rapid eye movement detection (REM detection). *Comput. Biomed. Res.* 4:275.

Viglione, S.S. 1973. Comments on pattern recognition. In P. Kellaway and I. Petersén (eds.), *Automation of Clinical Electroencephalography*, p. 287. New York: Raven Press.

Viglione, S.S., and Martin, W.B. 1973. Automatic analysis of the EEG for sleep staging. In P. Kellaway and I. Petersén (eds.), *Automation of Clinical Electroencephalography*, p. 269. New York: Raven Press.

Viglione, S.S., Ordon, V.A., and Risch, F. 1970. *A Methodology for Detecting Ongoing Changes in the EEG Prior to Clinical Seizures.* MDAC Paper WD 1399 (a). McDonnel Astronautic Company, Western Division, Huntington Beach, California.

Walter, D.O. 1963. Spectral analysis for electroencephalograms: mathematical determination of neurophysiological relationships from records of limited duration. *Exp. Neurol.* 8:155.

Walter, D.O. 1968. The method of complex demodulation. Advances in EEG analysis. *Electroencephalogr. Clin. Neurophysiol.* suppl. 27:53.

Walter, D.O., and Adey, W.R. 1963. Spectral analysis of electroencephalograms recorded during learning in the cat, before and after subthalamic lesions. *Exp. Neurol.* 7:481.

Walter, D.O., and Adey, W.R. 1965. Analysis of brain waves as multiple statistical time series. *IEEE Trans. Biomed. Eng.* 12:8.

Walter, D.O., and Adey, W.R. 1966. Linear and non-linear mechanisms of brain-wave generation. *Ann. N.Y. Acad. Sci.* 128:772.

Walter, D.O., Rhodes, J.M., Brown, B.S., and Adey, W.R. 1966. Comprehensive spectral analysis of human EEG generators in posterior cerebral regions. *Electroencephalogr. Clin. Neurophysiol.* 20:334.

Walter, W.G., and Shipton, H.W. 1951. A new toposcopic display system. *Electroencephalogr. Clin. Neurophysiol.* 3:281.

Welch, P.D. 1967. The use of FFT for the estimation of power spectra. *IEEE Transactions on Audio and Electroacoustics* AU-15:70.

Wennberg, A., and Zetterberg, L.H. 1971. Application of a computer-based model for EEG analysis. *Electroencephalogr. Clin. Neurophysiol.* 31:457.

Wiener, N. 1949. *Extrapolation, Interpolation and Smoothing of Stationary Time Series.*

New York: John Wiley.

Wiener, N. 1950. *Extrapolation, Interpolation and Smoothing of Stationary Time Series with Engineering Applications.* New York: John Wiley.

Yeager, C.L. 1972. *An EEG Reading Plan.* NIH Grant Application NS-10471-01.

Yeager, C.L., and Heilbron, D.C. 1972. *Computer Classification of Clinical Electroencephalograms.* Progress Report, Grant Navy No. 00-14-70C-0248.

Zetterberg, L.H. 1969. Estimation of parameters for a linear difference equation. *Mathematical Biosciences* 5:227.

Zetterberg, L.H. 1973. Spike detection by computer and by analog equipment. In P. Kellaway and I. Petersén (eds.), *Automation of Clinical Electroencephalography*, p. 227. New York: Raven Press.

electroencephalographic studies of withdrawal from addiction in the papio papio

Keith F. Killam, Ph.D., and
Eva King Killam, Ph.D.

Department of Pharmacology
University of California School of Medicine
Davis, California

This report focuses upon the Senegalese baboon, *Papio papio*, as an appropriate subject for the study of drug dependence, specifically opiate dependence. Further, in the description of the process of the development of tolerance to morphine and of the subsequent withdrawal syndrome, it might be possible to shed additional light on the nature of the photomyoclonic syndrome that seems to be prevalent in the *Papio papio*.

Killam and Deneau (1973) have studied differences among four species of subhuman primates over the full spectrum of opiate dependence including the development phase, the degree of established tolerance as measured by the response to antagonists, and the characteristics of the withdrawal syndrome following abrupt cessation of the intake of morphine. The four species studied were the Senegalese baboon, *Papio papio;* the rhesus monkey, *Macaca mulatta;* the bonnet monkey, *Macaca irius;* and the sooty mangabey, *Cercocebus fuligunosis.* Since the subhuman primate of reference to date has been the rhesus monkey, the major yardsticks have been those developed by the group at the University of Michigan (Irwin 1954), with the original clinical description of Himmelsbach and Small (1937) and Kolb and Himmelsbach (1938) serving as reference criteria. The baboon compared favorably with the rhesus monkey as an appropriate model of human opiate dependency; in a few instances, the case could be made that the syndrome in the baboon more closely resembled that in man.

Of particular interest was the infiuence of the states of dependency and withdrawal on the underlying photomyoclonic syndrome of the baboon. The particular baboon under study, the *Papio papio*, has been under intensive investigation in the laboratory of Robert Naquet and in our own laboratories since 1966, when we uncovered a marked proclivity for epileptic seizures in this species. In response to flashing light this baboon shows progressive clonic seizure activity starting in periocular musculature and spreading to face, neck, and whole body followed by either rapid, clonic convulsive movements or "ensalve"-isolated, myoclonic jerks. The seizure elicited in this fashion have been shown to resemble those seen in man in distribution of spike-wave followed by high-voltage EEG activity, in distribution of potentials evoked by single light flashes, and in response to pharmacological agents increasing and/or controlling seizures in epileptic man. At aperiodic intervals during the stabilization and establishment of tolerance to 16 mg/kg per day intramuscularly (i.m.) of morphine sulfate, four baboons showing mild, limited seizure responses were tested for their response to intermittent light stimulation. The photomyoclonic syndrome abated in all cases during this time. Further, during withdrawal initiated either by nalorphine or by abrupt cessation of the injection schedule, no evidence of clinical epileptiform seizure activity compounded the sequelae of withdrawal. These studies were carried out in animals without implanted electrodes, thus precluding a detailed analysis of brain-wave changes concomitant with the changes in dependence, tolerance, and withdrawal states.

This report will describe the electroencephalographic events associated with the establishment of opiate dependence and acute withdrawal in the baboon. The baboons used were in the colony for more than one year before the initiation of this study. They were free of intercurrent diseases and were maintained on standard diets and other handling procedures, except that no Ketamine, or Sernylan, or dietary supplements of isoniazid for prophylactic control of tuberculosis were permitted. Over the past 18 months these subjects were monitored biweekly to establish their individual patterns of response to flashing light and, hence, the stability of the photomyoclonic syndrome. In all cases the animals selected exhibited predictable but not maximal patterns of response. The usual response to intermittent light stimulation was twitching about the eyes which spread to the face, with occasional but not regular body involvement. These animals were selected on the premise that the hyperexcitability often seen during withdrawal may enhance the underlying epileptic syndrome.

The electroencephalograms were recorded by means of stainless steel screw electrodes set into the skull over areas corresponding to the international protocol of human encephalography of the Ten-Twenty system.

Epoxy-coated wires connected electrodes to a receptacle which was affixed in turn to the skull of the animal. All EEG recordings were made using hard-wire connections with cables made of Microdot Mini-noise cable. A Grass Model IV electroencephalograph served as the primary amplifying system. The signals were recorded both on paper and on multichannel FM magnetic tape. The latter was achieved with appropriate patching to an Ampex FR 100 B. A time-code generator using IRIG-B BCD coding indexed both the paper and tape records. The EEG recordings were subjected to spectral analysis on the LINC II computer using programs described by Joy, Hance, and Killam (1971).

The drug regimen consisted of daily injections at 0800, 1600, and 2400 hours over a period of about 2½ months. The initial dosage was 2 mg/kg per i.m. injection. After some tolerance developed this was followed by 4 mg/kg i.m. injections and finally by 6 mg/kg i.m. injections. During the establishment of the tolerance the regimen was held static for at least one week before moving to the next dosage level to avoid some earlier specific neural toxicities which had been reported (Irwin 1954). The animals were then held at the 6 mg/kg unit dosage level (18 mg/kg/day) for at least one month before withdrawal studies were initiated.

During the long-term recordings the animals were placed in chairs with hip and arm restraints rather than the conventional pillory-like restraining devices. When the restraints are properly fitted and there is little distracting traffic, the animals seem to adjust well to this form of restraint. Such an arrangement allows continuous recording over long periods of time.

To study the development of tolerance, electroencephalograms were recorded regularly throughout the 2½-month chronic injection period. Times selected for such monitoring were the day before the first dose, the day preceding and the day of each dose increment, and finally days spaced similarly through the longer period of constant dosage (6 mg/kg) before withdrawal.

Animals were placed in chairs well before the dose scheduled at 1600 hours. Recordings were begun at 1530 hours (7½ hours after the previous morphine dose) and continued for at least 30 minutes following drug administration at 1600 hours.

Initial doses at 2 mg/kg led to semistuporous behavior. After two to three doses no signs of gross depression were observable. With each increment of dose there was a return of semistuporous behavior similar to that seen initially. In addition, as tolerance developed animal care personnel reported that the animals became more tractable, and specific attentive responses were elicited by the investigator approaching with syringe and needle in hand.

Electroencephalograms taken during the establishment of tolerance showed changes that recurred with each dosage increment and then faded with repeated drug administration. The slowing of the EEG at frequencies in the range of one cycle per 2 to 3 Hz indicated only maximal behavioral depression and was short-lived. Other changes in power over the classical ranges of frequencies were found most predictably in parieto-occipital and anterior lateral parietal derivations.

As can be seen in Figure 1, a pronounced peak appeard at 10 Hz following the 2 mg/kg i.m. injection in the parieto-occipital area. This peak decreased and was replaced by a peak at the 7-Hz range when drug dosages were increased to 4 and 6 mg/kg.

The more lateral derivations exhibited a reduction in the peak at 13 to 15 Hz with each increment of morphine (Figure 2). As can be seen in the

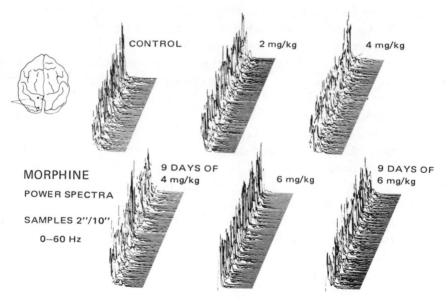

Figure 1. Power spectra from corticograms derived from the parieto-occipital area of a **Papip papio** *before drug administration and following chronic administration of morphine sulfate intramuscularly.* **Upper** *set: Control denotes serial spectra for 20 to 40 minutes without drug. Two mg/kg represents spectra after the initial dose of morphine sulfate. Four mg/kg represents spectra after nine days of administration of morphine sulfate at 2 mg/kg three times a day and a new dose increment at 4 mg/kg on the tenth day.* **Lower** *set: Left—spectra on the ninth day of serial injection of morphine sulfate at 4 mg/kg. Middle—spectra from the tenth day of 4 mg/kg and first of 6 mg/kg. Right—spectra from the ninth day at 6 mg/kg three times a day. The derivation is indicated by the phantom. The power spectra are calculated over 0 to 60 Hz. Each spectrum represents two seconds of original data. The time between spectra is eight seconds.*

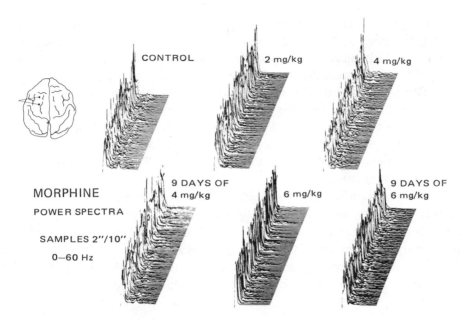

Figure 2. Power spectra from corticograms derived from laterofrontal areas of a **Papio papio** before drug administration and following chronic administration of morphine sulfate intramuscularly. See Figure 1 for details.

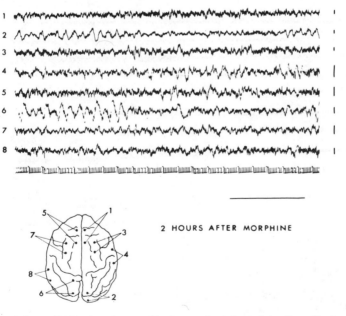

Figure 3. Electroencephalogram from a **Papio papio** *tolerant to the effects of morphine sulfate. Animal has been maintained at 18 mg/kg/day of morphine sulfate i.m. for two months. Record taken two hours after last drug administration. Time line represents five seconds and amplitude lines represent 100 μvolts.*

panels representing spectra determined after nine days of 4 mg/kg and of 6 mg/kg, the peak at 13 to 15 Hz returned. Thus, as the behavioral depression associated with morphine administration abates, the EEG changes seem to normalize. These semichronic effects have been replicated in three animals.

The remainder of the data to be described comes from a baboon recorded continuously for five consecutive days. The animal had been stabilized on morphine sulfate at 18 mg/kg per day for two months. The first two days of the recording session represent monitoring during the routine injection schedule at 0800, 1600, and 2400 hours. The final three days were recorded during withdrawal.

Two hours after morphine injection, sporadic runs of slow waves appeared in parieto-occipital derivation (cf. leads 2 and 6) (Figure 3). With time this activity spread to include lateral parietal regions. Four to 4½ hours after morphine, spindle trains appeared with minimal changes in behavior (Figure 4). The frequency of these spindles was at 7 Hz rather than 10 Hz, the characteristic record of this animal's undrugged state.

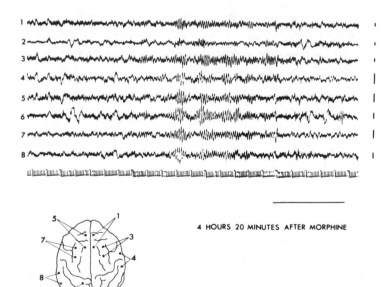

4 HOURS 20 MINUTES AFTER MORPHINE

Figure 4. Electroencephalogram from a **Papio papio** *tolerant to the effects of morphine sulfate. Animal has been maintained at 18 mg/kg/day of morphine sulfate i.m. for two months. Record taken 4 hours and 20 minutes after the last drug administration. Time line represents five seconds and amplitude lines represent 100 µvolts.*

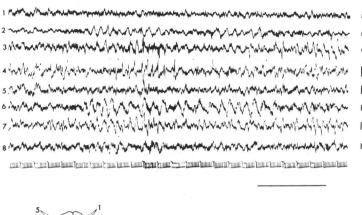

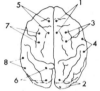

7 HOURS AFTER MORPHINE

*Figure 5. Electroencephalogram from a **Papio papio** tolerant to the effects of morphine sulfate. Animal has been maintained at 18 mg/kg/day of morphine sulfate i.m. for two months. Record taken seven hours after the last drug administration. Time line represents five seconds and amplitude lines represent 100 μvolts.*

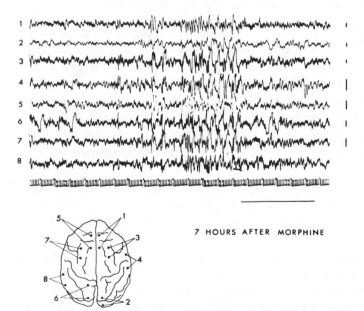

*Figure 6. Electroencephalogram from a **Papio papio** tolerant to the effects of morphine sulfate. Animal has been maintained at 18 mg/kg/day of morphine sulfate i.m. for two months. Record taken seven hours after the last drug administration. Time line represents five seconds and amplitude lines represent 100 μvolts.*

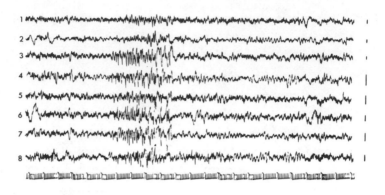

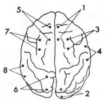

7 HOURS 23 MINUTES AFTER MORPHINE

Figure 7. Electroencephalogram from a **Papio papio** *tolerant to the effects of morphine sulfate. Animal has been maintained at 18 mg/kg/day of morphine sulfate i.m. for two months. Record taken 7 hours and 23 minutes after the last drug administration. Time line represents five seconds and amplitude lines represent 100 μvolts.*

The foregoing were the quasi-abnormal characteristics of the daytime segment of 0800 to 1400 hours. Frank periods of paroxysmal activity in the 1400-2400-0800-hour segment are illustrated in Figures 5, 6, and 7. Note that the activity may be aperiodic as in Figure 5, or related to spindle activity as in Figures 6 and 7. Similar patterns of activity have been reported for the untreated but maximally sensitive baboon during nocturnal sleep (Bert and Collomb 1966; Killam, Killam, and Naquet 1967; Balzano 1968). Following morphine injection the paroxysmal activity abated for about two hours.

Ten to 12 hours after the withholding of the usual dosage of morphine in the tolerant animal, there appeared signs of major autonomic disturbances. Salivation, retching, and vomiting were common. The animal's hands and feet sweated. Interspersed with these episodes were long runs of the waveform patterns already illustrated. The retching and vomiting gave way to vocalization and nonaggressive yawning.

Beginning about 16 hours after the last morphine injection, there appeared a phase of hyperreflexia and hyperresponsiveness to light and sound. Bouts of so-called "wet dog" shakes appeared. One bout is illustrated in Figure 8. Note the lack of accompanying paroxysmal EEG activity. It might be that the "wet dog" shake phenomenon is exaggerated shivering, subject to

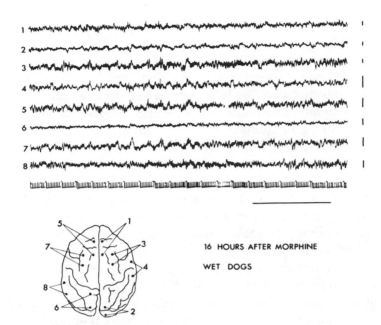

Figure 8. Electroencephalogram from a **Papio papio** *in withdrawal from morphine dependence. Record taken 16 hours after the last drug administration. Time line represents five seconds and amplitude lines represent 100 μvolts.*

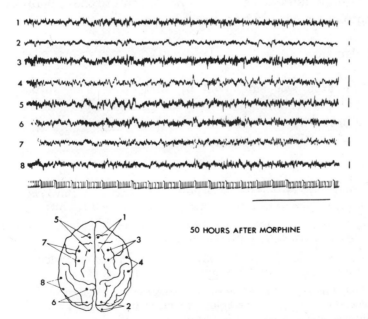

Figure 9. Electroencephalogram from a **Papio papio** *in withdrawal from morphine dependence. Record taken 50 hours after the last drug administration. Time line represents five seconds and amplitude lines represent 100 μvolts.*

segmental modification and representation rather than involving cortical processes. During this phase the slow and paroxysmal EEG activity gave way to nonsynchronized activity with few dominant spectral characteristics.

These EEG signs lasted through the next phase of 36 to 72 hours after the last morphine injection. We have termed this phase a "pseudotranquilization" phase. The animals became tractable and appeared to be in generalized discomfort. Stroking or rubbing by the experimenter was affectionately received and encouraged by the animal. The EEG throughout this phase, as well as in part of the former and part of the next phase, is typified by Figure 9.

The succeeding phase was characterized by the animal's hyperresponsiveness and hyperirritability in a behavioral sense. The EEG showed signs of normalization during this period, with total recovery about 96 hours after the last dose of morphine.

While it is tempting to generalize from findings in this one animal, such generalization must await further replication. The observations during induction of tolerance have been replicated, lending hope that the total process in the Senegalese baboon may follow the characteristics described.

It seems possible that the neuronal systems subserving the photomyoclonic syndrome of the baboon may be modified by the state of tolerance to morphine, but the two are not mutually interdependent. Further, the withdrawal syndrome does not appear to be additive to the epileptiform process of the photomyoclonic syndrome or its expression.

Acknowledgments

The research was supported by MH17471. The authors gratefully acknowledge the technical assistance of Douglas Lytle, Edwin Budd, and Mauricette Broco.

References

Balzano, E. 1968. Étude polygraphique du sommeil nocturne du *Papio papio* (Babouin du Sénégal). Thesis. Faculté des Science de Marseille, Université d'Aix-Marseille.

Bert, J., and Collomb, H. 1966. L'électroéncephalogramme du sommeil nocturne chez le babouin. Étude par télémétrie. *J. Physiol.* 58:285.

Himmelsbach, C.K., and Small, L.F. 1937. Clinical studies of drug addiction. II. Rossium treatment of drug addiction. *Public Health Report Supplement* 125.

Irwin, S. 1954. Characteristics of depression, antagonism and development of tolerance, physical dependence and neuropathology to morphine and morphine-like agents in the monkey *(Macaca mulatta). Dissertation Abstracts* 14:686.

Joy, R.M., Hance, A.J., and Killam, K.F., Jr. 1971. Spectral analysis of lung EEG samples for comparative purposes. *Neuropharmacology* 10:471.

Killam, K.F., and Deneau, G.A. 1973. A study of morphine dependence in four species of subhuman primates. *Proc. West. Pharmacol. Soc.* 16:1.

Killam, K.F., Killam, E.K., and Naquet, R. 1967. An animal model of light sensitive epilepsy. *Electroencephalogr. Clin. Neurophysiol.* 22:497.

Kolb, L., and Himmelsbach, C.K. 1938. Clinical studies of drug addiction. III. A critical review of the withdrawal treatments with method of evaluating abstinence syndromes. *Am. J. Psychiatry* 94:759.

period analysis of the electroencephalogram of subhuman primates

H.L. Altshuler, Ph.D., and
Neil R. Burch, M.D.

Texas Research Institute of Mental Sciences
Houston, Texas

Since the electroencephalogram has become widely used in studies of the effects of drugs on the central nervous system, a method has been sought to allow the recognition of drugs based on the EEG patterns produced by each drug (Fink et al. 1968, Killam and Gehrmann 1972). A promising technique derived from the period-analytic methodology of Burch (Burch, Greiner, and Correll 1955; Burch 1959; Burch et al. 1964) is being developed in our laboratory. It is proving useful in distinguishing among drugs that produce similar behavioral effects. The discrimination is based on the pattern of changes in the three period-analytic descriptors of the EEG, the major, intermediate, and minor periods. The pattern of changes for one drug can be compared with those for other drugs in evaluating similarities and differences among compounds.

The study reported here was designed to demonstrate that the period-analytic methodology is sufficiently sensitive to drug effects to allow ready differentiation between such closely related drug pairs as cocaine and *d*-amphetamine. In addition, the study was undertaken to determine whether period analysis can be employed to develop an efficient, inexpensive, and sensitive method of summarizing the effects of a drug on the mammalian central nervous system. We believe this strategy may become a useful tool in studies of acute and chronic drug effects on the EEG and in the evaluation of mechanisms of drug action on the central nervous system.

Methods

Six male rhesus monkeys ranging in weight from 4 to 6 kilograms were used in these studies. All animals had been previously involved in other behavioral and biomedical experiments, but not for one year prior to the beginning of this program. The animals' health was monitored by weekly blood counts, monthly physical examinations and tuberculosis tests, and quarterly herpes B virus screenings.

Stainless-steel screw electrodes were implanted in each animal according to a standard stereotaxic montage (Table 1) based upon the Ten-Twenty system. The stainless-steel screw electrodes were connected to an Amphenol electronic plug and the screws, electrode wire, and plug cemented onto the monkey's skull with dental acrylic cement. Sodium pentobarbital (30 mg/kg i.v.) was used as the surgical anesthetic.

Postoperative care of the animals consisted of daily penicillin G injections (300,000 units i.m.), daily white blood counts, weekly complete blood counts, and other diagnostic laboratory procedures as necessary. On days in which experiments were conducted, the animals were brought to the EEG recording area about 40 minutes before the beginning of the recording session. They were allowed to sit quietly in primate restraining chairs so that their cardiovascular and respiratory parameters stabilized and they acclimated to their surroundings.

The protocol for all drug or saline vehicle experiments is given in Table 2. Drug injections were given for 60 seconds into the superficial saphenous or cephalic veins, and the EEG recorded for 90 minutes following the drug dose.

Data Collection and Analysis

The electroencephalogram was amplified through a Beckman Type TE clinical electroencephalograph. An analog tape of the EEG was recorded simultaneously with the paper record, and the signal passed through period encoders and a data logging system as described previously (Burch et al. 1964). The digitized and coded data were then written on digital tape with a Digi-Data Model 1400 FM digital tape recorder. The digital tapes containing the encoded EEG signal were processed by an IBM 360-50 computer which performed data analysis and summarization using a program of our design. For analytic purposes each experiment was divided into seven ten-minute segments by the conditions imposed by the protocol. Each of the ten-minute epochs was further subdivided into three three-minute epochs and, further, into one-minute epochs. The summarized data from each one-minute epoch were averaged to provide a mean summary for the three-minute epoch, and

TABLE 1.
Stereotaxic Coordinates of Placements of
Skull Electrodes with Stainless Steel Screws in
Macaca Mulatta (4 to 6 kg)

Electrode Number	Anterior - Posterior	Right - Left
1	A47	0
2	A30	R10
3	A20	R10
4	A7	R10
5	APO	R10
6	P25	R10
7	P35	R10
8	APO	R16
9	P9	R16
10	A8.5	R28
11	A1.5	R28
12	A30	L10
13	A20	L10
14	A7	L10
15	APO	L10
16	P25	L10
17	P35	L10
18	APO	L16
19	P9	L16
20	A8.5	L28
21	A1.5	L28
22	P3	0
23	P25	0

Eight channels of EEG are recorded and analyzed on-line in a "monopolar" montage of left-right frontal, parietal, occipital, and temporal leads. The experimental protocol utilized in this preliminary work is outlined in Table 2.

TABLE 2.
Protocol for Recording Sessions

Time (min)	Recording
0-10	Spontaneous EEG
11-20	EEG during photic stimulation
21-30	Spontaneous EEG
Intravenous drug dose	
31-40	Spontaneous EEG
41-50	EEG during photic stimulation
51-60	Spontaneous EEG
61-70	EEG during photic stimulation
71-80	Spontaneous EEG
81-90	EEG during photic stimulation
91-100	Spontaneous EEG
101-110	EEG during photic stimulation
111-120	Spontaneous EEG
121-130	EEG during photic stimulation
131-140	Spontaneous EEG

the three-minute summaries were averaged to provide a ten-minute summary. In the experiments reported here, four or more animals were considered together as a group and the mean response used for data summarization.

The three parameters computed with the period-analytic methodology, major period (baseline crosses), intermediate period (first derivative), and minor period (second derivative), were used to evaluate the acute effects of drugs. Several other possible computations derived with period analysis, such as spectral distribution of period counts and period analysis of the photically driven EEG, were also studied during these experiments but will not be reported here.

Results

The data generated by these studies reveal significant and easily delineated differences between the drugs evaluated. Figures 1A through 4C summarize the changes in period-analytic descriptors following intravenous doses of chlorpromazine, pentobarbital, d-amphetamine, and cocaine, comparing them to responses following intravenous doses of saline. It should be noted that the responses to intravenous saline doses varied only slightly over the course of the 90-minute experiment. Significant differences between drugs may be observed in the temporal aspects, direction, and magnitude of the changes.

As can be seen in Figures 1A through 4C, the large amounts and types of data obtained by this method require further reduction of the data base to allow more direct comparison between drug effects. Tables 3A through 3D illustrate one method of reduction that allows such a comparison. Each table compares the effects of the four drugs on each of the four brain areas. The most valid comparisons can be made between the most closely related compounds studied, that is, pentobarbital versus chlorpromazine and cocaine versus d-amphetamine.

Table 3A summarizes the effects of the four drugs on the frontal area of the monkey brain. Comparing the two central nervous system depressants, chlorpromazine and pentobarbital, it can be observed that chlorpromazine decreased major and intermediate period counts after the 1.0 mg/kg dose and the 10.0 mg/kg dose. The minor period counts changed little. The major period response to the 2.0 mg/kg dose of pentobarbital was characterized by an increase in baseline crosses (counts), reflecting the behaviorally excitatory effect of that dose. The intermediate and minor period counts were unchanged following the 2.0 mg/kg dose of pentobarbital, but the 20.0 mg/kg dose decreased major, intermediate, and minor period counts. The effect of the 20.0 mg/kg dose of pentobarbital on the EEG corroborates the drug's behavioral effect of sedation. The principal differences observed between chlorpromazine and pentobarbital were that the 1.0 mg/kg dose of chlorpromazine decreased major period counts, while the 2.0 mg/kg dose of pentobarbital increased them. The intermediate period response patterns differed from the major period patterns. The 1.0 mg/kg dose of chlorpromazine decreased intermediate period counts and changed minor period counts only slightly. The 2.0 mg/kg dose of pentobarbital, on the other hand, altered neither intermediate nor minor period counts significantly. The 10.0 mg/kg dose of chlorpromazine and the 20.0 mg/kg dose of pentobarbital resulted in a decrease in major and intermediate period counts. Only pentobarbital decreased the minor period counts in the frontal area.

Comparisons of the effects of d-amphetamine and cocaine on the frontal area revealed several clearly defined differences between the drugs. The 0.5 mg/kg dose of d-amphetamine slightly decreased major and intermediate period counts but did not significantly change minor period counts. The responses to cocaine in the frontal area represented quite a different pattern. Both the 2.5 mg/kg and the 5.0 mg/kg doses of cocaine decreased major period counts, but only the 2.5 mg/kg dose decreased the intermediate period counts. The 5.0 mg/kg dose of cocaine did not significantly change the intermediate and minor period counts, nor did the 2.5 mg/kg cocaine dose alter the minor period counts. It can be seen, therefore, that the brain responds quite differently to these two pairs of behaviorally similar drugs when the electrical changes are summarized and compared on the basis of period-analytic descriptors.

The differences between the effects of d-amphetamine and cocaine on the central area (Table 3B) were more subtle. Major period responses to both d-amphetamine and cocaine were characterized by increased baseline crosses. The 5.0 mg/kg dose of cocaine, however, caused a transient decrease in major period counts preceding the increase. The 2.5 mg/kg dose of cocaine caused a similar biphasic response.

The intermediate period summaries of the central area responses illustrate the marked differences between the two drugs. The 0.5 mg/kg dose of d-amphetamine did not change intermediate period counts and the 2.5 mg/kg dose increased the counts only slightly. In contrast, the 2.5 mg/kg (low) dose of cocaine caused slight increases in intermediate period counts, and the 5.0 mg/kg (high) cocaine dose resulted in quite marked intermediate period count increases. The minor period summary reflects similar differences. The lower doses of either drug caused little change in the minor period counts from the central area. The 2.5 mg/kg dose of d-amphetamine caused a slight but significant decrease in minor period counts but little change was seen following the 5.0 mg/kg cocaine dose.

The period-analytic descriptors of EEG responses recorded from the temporal area are summarized in Table 3C. The differences observed between the closely related compounds (chlorpromazine versus pentobarbital; d-amphetamine versus cocaine) can be characterized by both differences in direction and magnitude of change. For example, the 20.0 mg/kg dose of pentobarbital caused highly significant decreases in major and intermediate period counts, but the 10.0 mg/kg dose of chlorpromazine was less effective. The d-amphetamine:cocaine differences were both in direction and in magnitude of change. The major differences in the temporal area following the lower doses of these compounds were in the major period, as distinguished from the response patterns of the central area. The differences in central area response patterns were in all three periods and the biphasic nature of the responses to cocaine.

Table 3D summarizes the responses recorded from the occipital area following the four drugs. The differences between the closely related compounds were both in direction and in magnitude of change. The chlorpromazine:pentobarbital distinctions observed in the major period summary were primarily those of magnitude of change. The 1.0 mg/kg dose of chlorpromazine significantly decreased major period counts, and the 2.0 mg/kg dose of pentobarbital slightly increased major period counts. The 10.0 mg/kg dose of chlorpromazine slightly decreased major period counts, while the 20.0 mg/kg dose of pentobarbital significantly decreased major period counts. The d-amphetamine:cocaine comparison was primarily one of magnitude of response, and was quite marked in the different major and minor period responses to the higher doses of both drugs. It is interesting that the drugs which are profound CNS stimulators have such marked effects in the occipital area. The mechanisms of these changes are currently under investigation.

There were striking differences in response patterns to the drugs. For example, the differences in the responses between cocaine and d-amphetamine were primarily that the magnitude of the cocaine responses was greater than that for d-amphetamine in the frontal area; the cocaine responses were biphasic in the central area, but d-amphetamine responses were not. The differences between d-amphetamine and cocaine in the temporal and occipital areas were slight but distinct: the major period cocaine responses were characterized by a decrease in baseline crosses, or a biphasic response, while the amphetamine responses were not. The occipital area differences were also primarily differences in magnitude. The occipital area responses to cocaine were represented by increases in counts for all descriptors and doses, but the d-amphetamine responses were more variable.

The most striking differences between chlorpromazine and pentobarbital were related to the differential effects of the low and high doses of pentobarbital. Even for the high doses, however, differences between the drugs were apparent, such as the significant decrease in frontal, central, and temporal area minor period counts following the high dose of pentobarbital but not chlorpromazine. In addition, both the low and high doses of pentobarbital had more pronounced effects on minor period counts from all brain areas than did either dose of chlorpromazine.

Figures 1A, 1B, and 1C. Summary of period analytic descriptors following two doses of chlorpromazine when compared with saline doses. Note that the major period (baseline cross), intermediate period (first derivative), and, to a lesser extent, minor period (second derivative) counts are reduced following chlorpromazine.

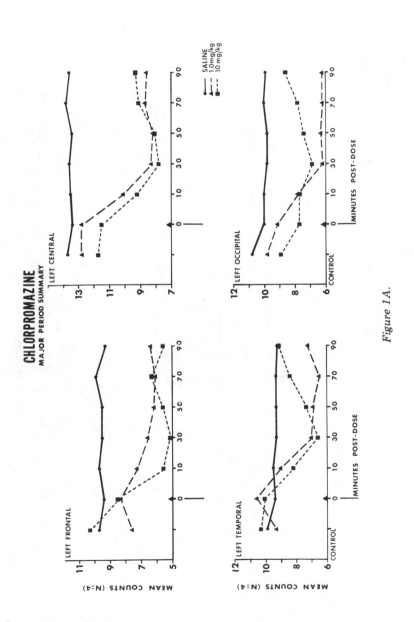

Figure 1A.

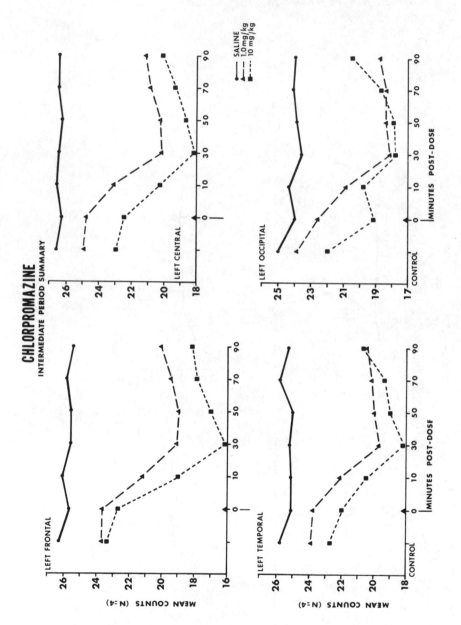

Figure 1B.

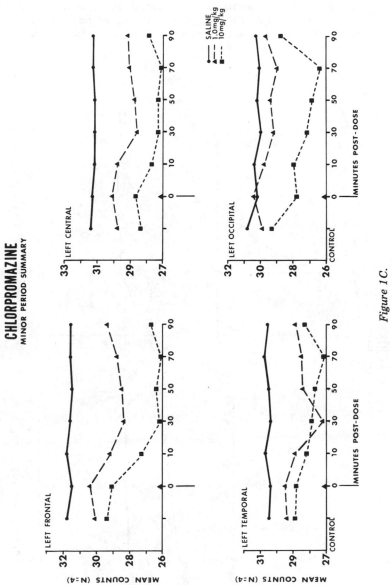

Figure 1C.

Figures 2A, 2B, and 2C. Summary of period-analytic descriptors following intravenous pentobarbital. Note that the two doses selected for comparison with saline illustrate two diverse effects of barbiturates. The low dose, 2 mg/kg, is often associated with behavioral excitation, and the higher dose, 20 mg/kg, is a strong hypnotic. Similarly, the EEG changes observed in the major period demonstrate an increase in major period counts following the low dose of pentobarbital and a dramatic decrease in major period counts following the 20 mg/kg dose. The low-dose stimulant effect was less pronounced in intermediate and minor periods, but the high-dose decrease in counts was still observed in intermediate and minor period summaries.

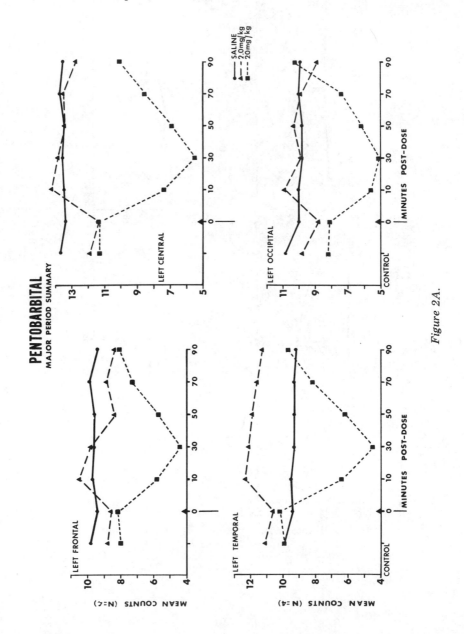

Figure 2A.

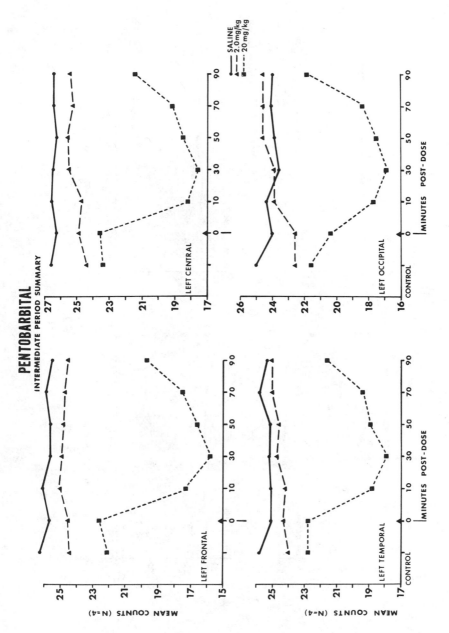

Figure 2B.

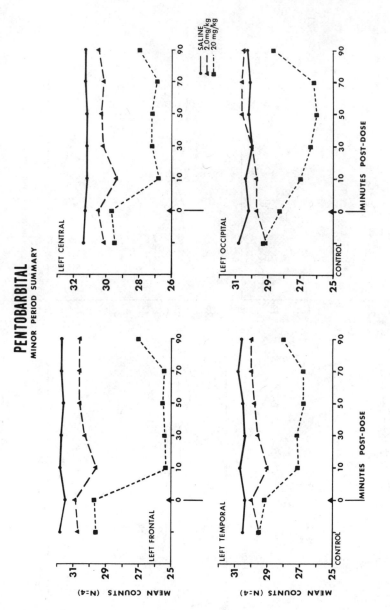

Figure 2C.

Figures 3A, 3B, and 3C. Period analytic descriptors for intravenous d-amphetamine. Intravenous doses of this compound exhibit marked brain area specificity. Note the pronounced increase in counts in major period, intermediate period, and minor period summaries of the EEG obtained from the occipital area.

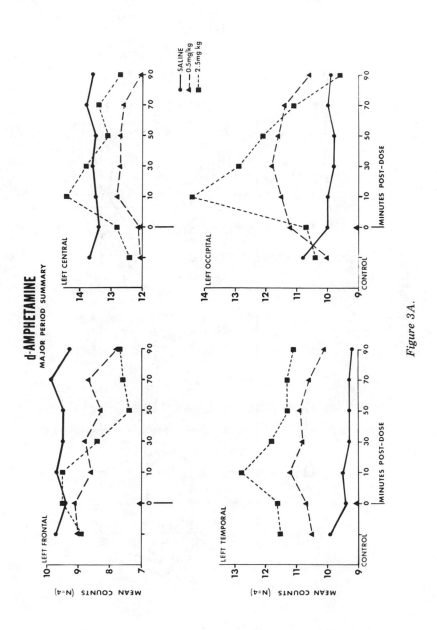

Figure 3A.

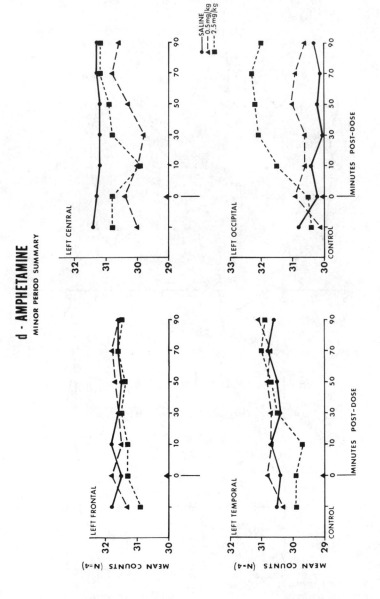

Figure 3B.

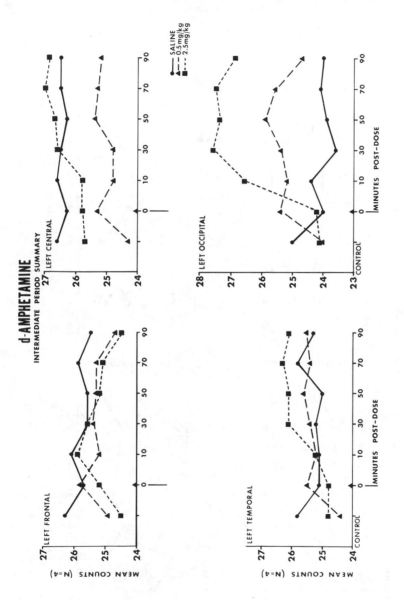

Figure 3C.

Figures 4A, 4B, and 4C. Period-analytic descriptors for intravenous cocaine. Note that the effects of cocaine were generally seen to be biphasic with a transient initial decrease in counts, especially in the major period, representing hypersynchrony of the EEG. Pronounced increases in intermediate and minor period counts were seen in the occipital area, and biphasic changes were seen in the other three areas.

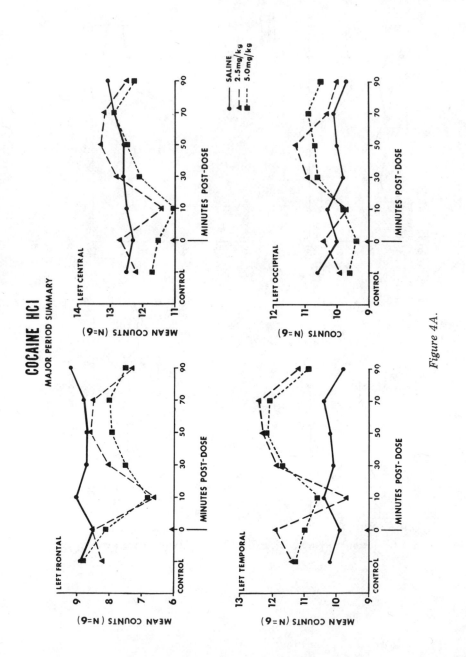

Figure 4A.

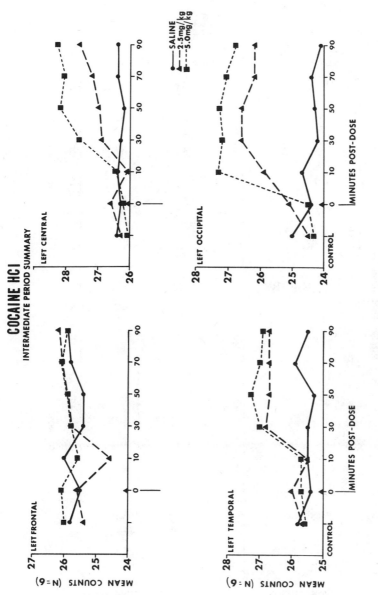

Figure 4B.

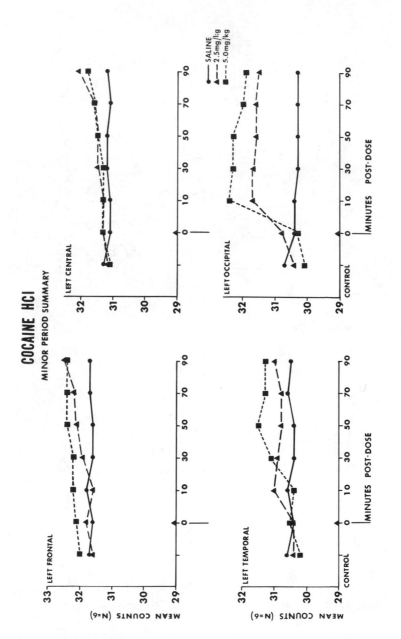

Figure 4C.

Tables 3A, 3B, 3C, and 3D. Characteristic period-analytic responses of chlorpromazine, pentobarbital, *d*-amphetamine, and cocaine recorded from four brain areas. The four tables are a summary of the differential responses (changes in period counts) of two doses each of four drugs in the frontal, central, temporal, and occipital areas of the primate brain. Note the manner in which each drug seems to have a characteristic pattern based on direction of change, period-analytic descriptor, and dosage relationship. This characteristic change seems useful in determining the template response for that drug, which can then be compared to other drugs, and which provides a useful, quantifiable tool for distinguishing drugs on the basis of their electroencephalographic characteristics.

The designations in Tables 3A, 3B, 3C, and 3D represent the following changes: increase—greater than two counts; decrease—greater than two counts; slight increase—less than two counts; slight decrease—less than two counts; marked increase—greater than three counts; marked decrease—greater than three counts; no change—less than one count.

TABLE 3A.
Summary of Direction of Period-Analytic Responses to Four Drugs
Frontal Area

Period	Dosage	Chlorpromazine	Drug Pentobarbital	d-Amphetamine	Cocaine
Major	low	decrease	increase	slight decrease	transient decrease
	high	decrease	decrease	decrease	transient decrease
Intermediate	low	decrease	no change	no change	transient decrease, then slight increase
	high	decrease	decrease	increase	no change
Minor	low	slight decrease	no change	no change	slight increase
	high	no change	decrease	no change	no change

TABLE 3B.
Summary of Direction of Period-Analytic Responses to Four Drugs
Central Area

Period	Dosage	Chlorpromazine	Drug Pentobarbital	d-Amphetamine	Cocaine
Major	low	decrease	increase	no change	slight decrease, then slight increase
	high	decrease	decrease	increase	slight decrease, then slight increase
Intermediate	low	decrease	no change	slight increase	slight increase
	high	decrease	decrease	slight increase	increase
Minor	low	no change	no change	no change	no change
	high	no change	decrease	transient decrease	no change

TABLE 3C.
Summary of Direction of Period-Analytic Responses to Four Drugs
Temporal Area

Period	Dosage	Chlorpromazine	Drug Pentobarbital	d-Amphetamine	Cocaine
Major	low	decrease	transient increase	no change	transient decrease
	high	slight decrease	marked decrease	transient increase	slight decrease, then slight increase
Intermediate	low	decrease	no change	slight increase	slight increase
	high	decrease	marked decrease	increase	slight increase
Minor	low	slight decrease	no change	no change	no change
	high	decrease	decrease	slight increase	slight increase

TABLE 3D.
Summary of Direction of Period-Analytic Responses to Four Drugs
Occipital Area

Period	Dosage	Chlorpromazine	Drug Pentobarbital	d-Amphetamine	Cocaine
Major	low	decrease	slight increase	slight increase	increase
	high	slight decrease	decrease	marked increase	increase
Intermediate	low	decrease	slight increase	slight increase	increase
	high	decrease	decrease	marked increase	marked increase
Minor	low	no change	no change	no change	increase
	high	slight decrease	slight decrease	increase	marked increase

Discussion

The search for an electroencephalographic method sensitive enough to allow discrimination between drugs has included the requirement that the technique be fairly inexpensive and used easily by neuropharmacological laboratories possessing a minimum amount of equipment. Period analysis has been used for clinical electroencephalography for many years. The technique was developed with several goals in mind, among which were compatibility with the large computer facilities available at most research centers, since such compatibility eliminated the need for dedicated computer equipment and real-time operations. Period analysis provided these advantages by digitizing and coding the EEG signal on-line using relatively inexpensive, special-purpose encoders. This method of EEG analysis was, therefore, a logical choice for meeting the demands of a busy experimental and clinical EEG laboratory (Burch 1959, Burch et al. 1964).

It is surprising that period analysis has remained primarily the domain of human experimentation. The work of Fink, Itil, and their coworkers (Fink and Itil 1965; Fink et al. 1968; Fink 1969), and Burch (Burch, Whisenand, and Dossett, in press), and Straw (Straw and Sauer 1973) represents the relatively few studies in which the period-analytic system has been used for neuropharmacological and neurophysiological studies in animals. The experiments reported here represent the first time the technique has been systematically applied to pharmacological studies in conscious subhuman primates.

The data reported here demonstrate that period analysis can be successfully used in experiments involving the automatic analysis of the conscious subhuman primate EEG. In addition, the data demonstrate that the method is exceedingly sensitive to very small differences in the effects of closely related drugs on the EEG.

Period analysis is a high-resolution technique; by its very nature it is capable of recording sizable second-to-second fluctuations in the EEG. The averaging technique we employed in these experiments was intended, among other things, to attenuate such fluctuations without masking significant, drug-related changes. The stability of the period-analytic descriptors following intravenous saline injections demonstrates the effectiveness of the attempt to reduce random, insignificant fluctuations. Even more notable is that the results of the drug experiments clearly demonstrate that sensitivity to significant drug-induced changes is retained.

The studies of the effects of chlorpromazine on the simian EEG were in good agreement with reports in the literature (Schalleck, Lewinson, and Thomas 1968; Pragay and Mirsky 1973; Fielding et al. 1973) and direct behavioral observation. The nature of the effects was striking. Since we had expected the 1.0 mg/kg and 10.0 mg/kg doses of chlorpromazine to cause some decrease in period counts for all brain areas and in all three period-analytic descriptors, it was somewhat surprising that the 1.0 mg/kg dose was nearly as effective as the 10.0 mg/kg dose. There were, of course, several parameters with very marked dose-response differences, such as intermediate period responses of the four brain areas and minor period responses of the frontal and occipital areas. Such differences notwithstanding, the profound effect of 1.0 mg/kg of chlorpromazine on the simian EEG deserves further consideration. The marked difference between the responses following saline and the responses following the 1.0 mg/kg dose of chlorpromazine suggests that an exploration of the chlorpromazine dose-response curve for doses from 0.001 mg/kg to 1.0 mg/kg would be a profitable research strategy. We are interested in finding the minimal effective dose of chlorpromazine in this laboratory system and in evaluating the effects of similar doses on the EEG of normal subjects and schizophrenic patients. Such studies could be important in providing adjuncts to therapy with this widely used antipsychotic agent.

Pentobarbital is one of the most commonly used barbiturates. Direct behavioral observation of animals has shown that low doses of pentobarbital are excitatory in nature, especially for thirty minutes following drug intake. Higher doses of this compound are hypnotic and induce surgical anesthesia at about 25.0 mg/kg. The major period responses to 20.0 mg/kg of pentobarbital clearly illustrate by means of the EEG the excitatory effect of low doses of pentobarbital. The EEG responses to high pentobarbital doses also correlate well with the observed behavioral effects, that is, hypnosis and decreased CNS arousal. We have done a limited group of studies (Gonzalez, Altshuler, and Burch 1973) examining the period-analytic responses to doses intermediate between 2.0 mg/kg and 20.0 mg/kg. These data, not presented here, suggest that the dose level at which pentobarbital begins to exert a depressant effect on the major period counts is between 6.0 and 8.0 mg/kg. It is curious that the different direction of change induced by the low and the high doses of pentobarbital is not reflected as profoundly in the intermediate and minor period summaries as it is in the major period. The 2.0 mg/kg dose altered intermediate and minor period counts slightly or not at all. The 20.0 mg/kg dose of this drug, on the other hand, profoundly decreased major, intermediate, and minor period counts. The excitatory effect of low doses of pentobarbital has been interpreted to be the result of differing levels of sensitivity to the drug of various portions of the brain. The excitatory effect of low doses of barbiturates is presumed to result from a greater sensitivity to barbiturates of cortical areas than deeper brain regions. Such greater cortical sensitivity to the drug is thought to result in decreased cortical inhibition of deeper brain regions and, consequently, increased reflexive motor activity. Our data did not demonstrate increases in intermediate and minor period counts, parameters which should represent to some extent the degree of asynchrony between the cortical and subcortical regions. It is conceivable that this finding casts some doubt on the interpretation of the differential effect of low and high doses of pentobarbital. This question, as well as a delineation of the major, intermediate, and minor period dose-response relationships of pentobarbital, will be the subject of future studies in our laboratory.

One of the most interesting hypotheses based on the EEG data from the *d*-amphetamine experiments is that the drug's primary locus of activity in the simian brain seemed to be in the occipital area. Although significant changes were observed in the other brain areas following this drug, the changes observed in the occipital area were by far the most dramatic.

An interesting contrast can be drawn between the occipital effects of cocaine and amphetamine. Substantial changes in all three period-analytic descriptors resulted from *d*-amphetamine, the changes in the major and intermediate periods being most profound. In contrast, the major period responses in the occipital area were markedly less pronounced than intermediate and minor period responses.

The EEG summary showed that the occipital area was the area most influenced by both cocaine and *d*-amphetamine. Such occipital specificity raised questions relating to the experimental protocol for each experiment. The protocol called for interspersed periods of photic stimulation (Table 2). We have recently examined the effect of the interspersed period of photic stimulation on the nonstimulated, spontaneous occipital EEG. The results of the experiments ruled out the possibility that the changes observed in spontaneous EEG were the result of the interspersed periods of photic stimulation.

Detailed analyses of the EEG during the periods of photic stimulation do suggest rather profound effects of both drugs on the ability of the occipital area to respond to photic stimulation in a fully integrated and synchronous manner. We are currently evaluating further the mechanism of the disruption of integrated occipital responses to photic stimulation. These studies will include explorations of the drug-induced changes on subcortical structures. We hypothesize that such explorations may provide some insight into the mechanism by which cocaine and d-amphetamine act in altering synchrony and modulatory control of the occipital area (Altshuler and Burch 1973).

Another major goal of this project was to evaluate this system of EEG analysis for its ability to distinguish between closely related compounds solely on the basis of the simian EEG. From the differences observed with the compounds employed in this study, it seems that this goal can be achieved.

The differences between cocaine and d-amphetamine are illustrative. These two compounds have traditionally represented a drug pair that was difficult to differentiate on the basis of EEG findings. Our data thus far suggest that each drug has a unique period-analytic profile. After expansion of the data base, it seems likely that computer recognition programs could be developed based on the period-analytic profiles of the two drugs in varying dosages.

Differentiation between chlorpromazine and pentobarbital on the basis of the EEG has not been as difficult as differentiation between cocaine and d-amphetamine. Several workers have reported characteristic EEG findings with each of the two drugs (Schalleck, Lewinson, and Thomas 1967, 1968; Doyle, Shimizu, and Himwich 1968; Killam and Gehrmann 1972; Fielding et al. 1973; Pragay and Mirsky 1973), but have not emphasized the same types of dose-related differences found in our study, especially using automated methods.

Our study uses period analysis, an established method for the automated analysis of the clinical EEG in a relatively unexplored application, pharmacological studies of the monkey. This new application may also represent a new dimension in our ability to recognize drug-induced changes in the EEG. We are evaluating the usefulness of this approach in studies of the mechanisms of specific drug effects on brain electrical activity; for example, studies of the mechanism of cocaine actions suggest a possible alteration in the central processing of visual sensory information following administration of the drug (Altshuler, Burch, and Dossett 1974).

Summary

These studies demonstrate that closely related pairs of drugs, cocaine versus *d*-amphetamine and chlorpromazine versus pentobarbital, may be distinguished from one another on the basis of the period-analytic descriptors of the EEG. The differences observed were in both magnitude and direction of change. In addition, different EEG characteristics in response to high or low doses of pentobarbital were clearly observed. These preliminary studies suggest that the period-analytic methodology should prove useful in future, more detailed studies of the mechanism of action of these and other centrally active drugs.

References

Altshuler, H.L., and Burch, N.R. 1973. The electroencephalographic effects of cocaine and *d*-amphetamine in the rhesus monkey as described by period analysis. *Proceedings of the Society for Neurosciences* 3:343.

Altshuler, H.L., Burch, N.R., and Dossett, R.G. 1974. The effects of cocaine and *d*-amphetamine on the spontaneous and photically-driven occipital electroencephalogram of the monkey. *Fed. Proc.* 33:293.

Burch, N.R. 1959. Automatic analysis of the electroencephalogram: A review and classification of systems. *Electroencephalogr. Clin. Neurophysiol.* 11:827.

Burch, N.R., Greiner, T.H., and Correll, E.G. 1955. Automatic analysis of electroencephalogram as an index of minimal changes in human consciousness. *Fed. Proc.* 14:23.

Burch, N.R., Nettleton, W.J., Sweeney, J., and Edwards, R.J. 1964. Period analysis of the electroencephalogram on a general purpose digital computer. *Ann. N.Y. Acad. Sci.* 115:827.

Burch, N.R., Whisenand, D., and Dossett, R. Period analysis of the electroencephalogram: Maturation and anoxia. In *Malnutrition and Brain Function*, Section III. Washington, D.C.: U.S. Govt. Printing Office (in press).

Doyle, C., Shimizu, A., and Himwich, H.E. 1968. Effects of chronic administration of some psychoactive drugs on EEG arousal in rabbit. *Int. J. Neuropharmacol.* 7:87.

Fielding, S., Cornfeldt, M., McGreevy, T., Outwater, B., and Pacifico, L. 1973. EEG correlates of behavioral toxicity of neuroleptic drugs. *Toxicol. Appl. Pharmacol.* 25:452.

Fink, M. 1969. EEG and human psychopharmacology. *Ann. Rev. Pharmacol.* 9:241.

Fink, M., and Itil, T. 1965. EEG analysis by digital computer. II: Relation of pentothal-induced changes to resting pattern. *Electroencephalogr. Clin. Neurophysiol.* 18:520.

Fink, M., Shapiro, D.M., Hickman, C., and Itil, T. 1968. Digital computer EEG analyses in psychopharmacology. In N.S. Kline and E. Laska (eds.), *Computers and Electrical Devices in Psychiatry*, p. 109. New York: Grune and Stratton.

Gonzalez, L.P., Altshuler, H.L., and Burch, N.R. 1973. Period analytic descriptors of the effects of psychotropic drugs in the subhuman primate. *Proceedings of the Society for Neurosciences* 3:226.

Killam, K.F., and Gehrmann, J.E. 1972. A comparison of EEG changes by drugs of social abuse. In E.I. Goldsmith and J. Moor-Jankowski (eds.), *Medical Primatology 1972*, part II. *Experimental Surgery, Transplantation, Immunology, Oral Medicine, and Neurophysiology and Experimental Psychology*, p. 260. Basel: S. Karger.

Pragay, E.B., and Mirsky, A.F. 1973. The nature and performance deficit under secobarbital and chlorpromazine in the monkey. *Psychopharmacologia* 28:73.

Schalleck, W., Lewinson, T., and Thomas, J. 1967. Power spectrum analysis of drug effects on electroencephalogram of the cat. *Int. J. Neuropharmacol.* 6:253.

Schalleck, W., Lewinson, T., and Thomas, J. 1968. Power spectrum analysis as a tool for statistical evaluation of drug effects on electrical activity of brain. *Int. J. Neuropharmacol.* 7:35.

Straw, R.N., and Sauer, R.A. 1973. Effect of selected centrally acting drugs on the electroencephalogram (EEG) of the monkey. *Fed. Proc.* 32:792.

information and mathematical quantification of brain state

Robert W. Thatcher, Ph.D.
E. Roy John, Ph.D.

Brain Research Laboratories
Department of Psychiatry
New York Medical College
New York, New York

"A certain Dr. Brown, on being rebuked because he had failed to acknowledge some previous work on the subject of his writings replied: 'I make no claim to originality for I have long since found that to consider oneself original one must read nothing at all. All I have done is to describe those methods which I have found to suit me best in practice.' "

This quote appropriately introduces a paper (Dawson 1954) that describes the use of the principle of signal averaging which was first proposed by Laplace in 1832 and successfully applied to the detection of atmospheric tides in 1847 (Regan 1972).

Our understanding of brain function has been greatly advanced by the application of "signal-to-noise" enhancement techniques. A major problem confronting today's users of these techniques, however, is the extraction of representative, reliable, and physiologically relevant signal averages and the precise and comprehensive evaluation of these averages. The problem is especially perplexing in behavioral experiments that involve electrophysiological recordings from chronically implanted electrodes over long periods of time, and in which enormous quantities of data are collected. In such experiments co-variation of component processes occurs over time and across anatomical structures. These patterns of co-variation provide insight into the operation of subsystems organized during various states of behavior (John 1967).

Several years ago John, Ruchkin, and Villegas (1963, 1964) showed that a large body of evoked potential (EP) data could be parsimoniously described by the set of regression equations obtained from a principal component factor analysis. It was possible, they reported, to reconstruct the evoked activity recorded from any brain region with a small number of mathematical descriptors common to all brain regions. Since that time factor analysis and other multivariate techniques have been applied to the study of such dynamic phenomena as habituation (Halas and Beardsley 1969), sleep-wakefulness cycles (Naitoh et al. 1971), audiometry (Suter 1969, 1970), attention (Donchin 1966), and thinking in human beings (Chapman 1973).

We now describe the application of a varimax rotation of principal component factor analysis to evaluate brain states and information storage and retrieval.

Although principal factor solutions account for the energy in the signal space most parsimoniously, the orientation of the axes is arbitrary and does not necessarily correspond to physiological processes; the orientation is selected to maximize the rate of reduction of residual variance for the total set of signals. In contrast, the varimax rotation orients axes in such a way as to maximize their contribution to some signals while minimizing their contribution to the remainder of the set.

In our studies with animal subjects, brain states were altered statically by administration of drugs, while dynamic changes in state were accomplished by electrical stimulation. In studies with human subjects, information storage and retrieval were investigated.

Factor Analysis Methods

Once electrophysiological data have been converted to a digital form, a number of methods exist for representing such data in a quantitative way. It is particularly important to seek mathematical methods that offer not only a precise description of the original activity, but also provide a way to extract from those complex details an economical representation of the fundamental processes that underlie electrophysiological phenomenology and the differences between those processes in different brain regions or in different brain states. We have made substantial progress toward these goals by using *factor analysis* of sets of average evoked potentials (AEP), and we will use those results to illustrate what such methods can accomplish. Since the focus of this paper is on concepts rather than on specific technical details, we will not describe our mathematical procedures. These are reported elsewhere as applications of this method to the analysis of changes during learning or the effects of various drugs (John, Ruchkin, and Villegas 1964; John et al. 1973). A general description of the method of factor analysis is essential, however.

Figure 1 depicts the factor analysis of a number of average evoked potentials, which appear in the top row. The first three factors are shown in the column at the left. The row of waves to the right of the first factor shows the contributions of this factor to each of the data wave shapes. Each of these is simply the factor multiplied by the appropriate weighting constant. The weighting constant may be negative, which has the effect of inverting the factor shape. The weighting constant is called the factor loading of the data wave shape and is, in fact, the correlation coefficient between the original data wave shape and the factor.

The next row, labeled first residuals, shows what is left after the contribution of the first factor has been subtracted from the original data wave shape. In the following rows, this process is repeated for the second and third factors, and the final residuals, which are unaccounted for by the three factors, are displayed at the bottom.

In this fashion, one can represent a great many diverse wave shapes as different combinations of only a few basic factors. Each data wave can be described by the set of its factor loadings, which makes possible a compression of the data.

If the final residual for a particular wave were zero, the sum of the squares of its factor loadings would equal one, and we could say that 100 percent of the energy of the wave was accounted for by the factors. As the residual becomes larger, the percentage of the energy accounted for by the factors becomes proportionately less.

The totality of evoked potentials that are describable by a given set of factors is called the *signal space* defined by those factors. The *dimensionality* of the signal space is the number of factors required to account for a predetermined percentage of the energy of the original set of wave shapes.

The most common method of factor analysis is called *principal component analysis* (Harmon 1960). Principal component analysis accounts for the energy in the set of signals in the most parsimonious way. Various rotations of this set of dimensions, or axes, that account for the energy in the space, or that *span* the space, can be defined just as the quadrants of a compass could be defined in various ways. We have found that *varimax* rotation (Kaiser 1958) yields orientations of axes that correspond best to physiological processes.

Whatever method is chosen to resolve the mathematical details, the general feature of the solution is that a set of evoked potentials, W_i, which represent the responses of different derivations to the same stimulus, or responses of the same derivation to different stimuli, can be described in terms of a common set of factors, or axes, as shown below:

$$W_1 = a_{11} F_1 (t) + a_{12} F_2 (t) + \ldots \ldots + a_1 K F_k (t)$$

$$W_2 = a_{21} F_1 (t) + a_{22} F_2 (t) + \ldots \ldots + a_2 K F_K (t)$$

$$W_N = a_{N1} F_1 (t) + a_{N2} F_2 (t) + \ldots \ldots + a_{NK} F_K (t)$$

Each wave W_i is described as an equation in which the amount of the process described by factor 1, $a_{i1} F_1 (t)$, is added to the amount of the process described by factor 2, $a_{i2} F_2 (t)$, and so on until a predetermined amount of the energy in the wave has been described with specified accuracy. Note that the sum of the squared coefficients for the terms in each equation must account for 100 percent of the variance. Thus each coefficient defines the percentage contributed by that factor to the whole process.

If the separate waves in the set are completely independent or individually determined, the number of dimensions K needed to describe a set of N waves will be equal to N. If the N waves are generated by the interaction of smaller numbers of underlying processes, K will be smaller than N. The important fact for electrophysiology is that the number of factors needed to account for a set of responses from different derivations is usually much smaller than the number of derivations. It has been shown that as the number of wave shapes recorded from electrodes chronically implanted in the cat increases, the number of dimensions necessary to span the signal space reaches an asymptote and stabilizes (John, Ruchkin, and Villegas 1964; John et al. 1972).

This method, then, meets the desired criterion of allowing the description of many different wave shapes with precision, in terms of a small number of common processes that are combined in differing amounts to account for the observed electrophysiological phenomena. Changes in state should either change the relative amount of these processes in particular regions of the brain or should cause new dimensions to appear. This method focuses particularly upon the subtle details of response wave shapes and replaces the eye of the expert by a pattern-recognition procedure.

FACTOR ANALYSIS OF EVOKED POTENTIALS

DATA WAVESHAPES

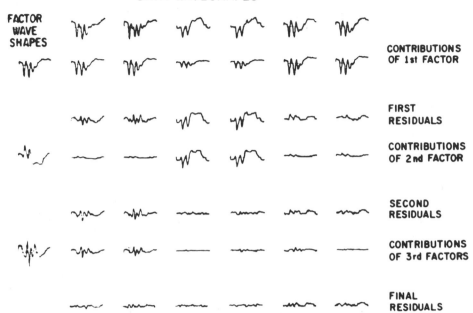

FACTOR
WAVE
SHAPES

CONTRIBUTIONS
OF 1st FACTOR

FIRST
RESIDUALS

CONTRIBUTIONS
OF 2nd FACTOR

SECOND
RESIDUALS

CONTRIBUTIONS
OF 3rd FACTORS

FINAL
RESIDUALS

Figure 1. This figure demonstrates how factors specific to wave shape are generated. The top line is a set of evoked potential averages to be described by the factor analysis. The computer scans the EPs and generates, through an iterative process, a waveform (factor 1) that accounts for the maximum variance of the body of data. The amount of energy in the raw data accounted for by the first factor is shown on line 2. Subtraction of the first factor from the original data results in the set of residual waveforms shown on line 3. This set of waveforms is evaluated by the computer and a second factor generated that accounts for the maximum variance of the residual data. Subtraction of the second factor from the wave shapes in line 3 yields a second residual (line 5). A third factor is then generated to optimally describe the second set of residuals, and this process is repeated until the requisite percentage of the total energy is accounted for by the factors. In this figure, 93 percent of the energy in the original evoked potentials on the first line was accounted for by three factors (John et al. 1973).

Application of Factor Analysis to the Classification of Drugs

Recently we reported the use of this method in evaluating the action of several different doses of each of four drugs on evoked potentials from arrays of electrodes chronically implanted into various brain structures in three cats (John et al. 1972, 1973). Drug administrations were at least one week apart.

Average evoked responses to two different stimuli were obtained from each of 12 derivations under each of 24 conditions (11 pre- and 13 post-injection sessions). The 576 wave shapes were arranged in a matrix of 24 columns (12 derivations x 2 stimuli) by 24 rows (11 control and 13 drug measures). Each column from this matrix, consisting of the 24 average evoked potentials recorded from a single derivation in response to one type of conditioned stimulus under 11 control and 13 postdrug conditions, was subjected to a separate factor analysis. We called the method *column analysis*. Figure 2 shows the raw data for a typical column analysis and the regression equations that described the data provided by the factor analysis.

The control wave shapes received most of their energy from factor 1, the post-chlorpromazine (CPZ) wave shapes from factor 2, the post-MJ (MJ is an experimental tranquilizer produced by Mead Johnson) wave shapes from factor 3, the post-phenobarbital (PHENO) wave shapes from factor 4, and the post-amphetamine (METH) wave shapes from factor 5. These results indicated that the set of control wave shapes co-existed in a space well described by factor 1. The various drugs added new dimensions to this space, defined by factors 2, 3, 4, and 5.

These new dimensions are shown in Figure 3, which depicts the vectors describing the state of three different cats provided by column analysis after three doses of chlorpromazine, three doses of MJ, three doses of phenobarbital, and two doses of amphetamine. Notice that each drug moves the state vector in a characteristic direction in this 2-3-5 factor hyperspace. Normally the signal vectors of the brain have no energy in this space at all. While some drugs act only in one dimension, merely increasing their loading in that direction as the dosage increases, other drugs change the dimension of their action at different dosages.

Epilepsy and Post-Tetanic Potentiation

In the next series of studies, the evoked potential was used as a non-contingent probe of neural excitability. The method involved using an irrelevant or noncontingent background flicker to produce responses in the brain. These responses interact with on-going processes, thus creating "interference" effects that are capable of disclosing subtle changes in background excitability (Hudspeth and Jones 1973). The noncontingent probe method has been used extensively in the past (Gershuni et al. 1960; Kitai 1965; Docampo, Suarez-Nonez, and Sierra 1967; Pampliglione 1967; Kamiya, Callaway, and Yeager 1969; Ciganek 1969; Sommer-Smith and Morocutti 1970).

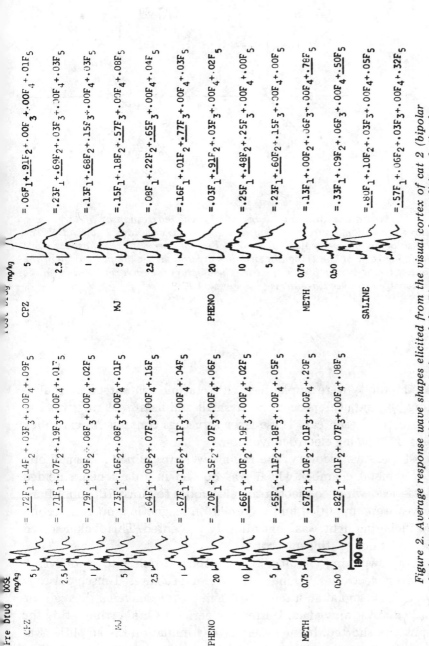

Figure 2. Average response wave shapes elicited from the visual cortex of cat 2 (bipolar derivation) in response to 200 presentations of the 5/sec approach conditioned stimulus (CS) during 11 control sessions (left) and 13 drug sessions (right). The regression equation to the right of each wave shape accounts for the energy of the wave shape as a linear combination of the varimax factors, with each coefficient defining the percentage of the total energy of the wave shape contributed by the corresponding factor analysis (John et al. 1972).

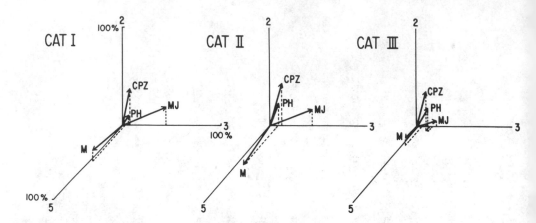

Figure 3. The effects of four different drugs on the evoked responses of three cats, described in three-dimensional subspace, representing varimax factors 2, 3, and 5. The length of each vector defines percentage of the total signal energy in the subspace while the component along each of the three dimensions corresponds to the percentage of the energy contributed to the vector by that factor. The diagram for each cat is based on the analysis of 576 average response waveforms (John et al. 1973).

Methods

Pigmented rabbits were implanted with chronic macrorecording electrodes. During the surgical procedure, a small stainless-steel ring was implanted in the base of each ear. These rings served as contacts for ear shock and as a means of inducing electroconvulsion.

After postoperative recovery, the rabbits were restrained in a small box and placed in a metal chamber which was housed in a darkened, shielded cage. Low-noise lead wires connected the electrodes to Grass 7P5 amplifiers. The brain waves were amplified and recorded on magnetic tape. A 2/second low-intensity flickering light was continuously presented. This flicker served as the source of the noncontingent probe.

A read-relay switching circuit allowed electrical pulses to be delivered through recording electrodes. To induce behavioral seizures, 1-msec pulses at a frequency of 55 Hz and at an intensity of 1 mA were delivered through the electrodes placed in the amygdala. During the period of brain stimulation the amplifier input was shorted. Immediately after stimulation the amplifier was reconnected to the leads from the amygdala. Amplifier blocking was seldom longer than 5 seconds.

Stimuli to arouse the animals were delivered through the ear electrodes with a second stimulator of 10-volt intensity. Electroconvulsion was produced by delivering high intensities of current (100-Hz, 1-msec pulses at 150 volts for 2 seconds) through the ear electrodes.

Results

Epileptiform Activity

Figure 4 shows averaged noncontingent visual flicker EPs (N=60) recorded during four different behavioral states. The top record is the spontaneous EEG recorded from the globus pallidus. The middle portion shows AEPs from the septum globus pallidus, visual cortex, and amygdala. The lower portion shows the vectogram descriptions of the EP wave shapes present in these four structures during the different behavioral states. Note that the EP wave shapes during the control and recovery periods, as reflected by the factor analysis, are basically identical except for the globus pallidus. That is, the globus pallidus is the only structure of the four that did not exhibit immediate recovery. The EP wave shapes generated during the amygdala seizure and during electroconvulsion due to ear shock differ significantly in every case. The electroconvulsive stimulus was delivered thirty minutes after amygdala seizure. The recovery period immediately followed electroconvulsion.

These results suggest that the noncontingent EP provides a probe of neural excitability and that the state of excitability during seizures produced by stimulation of the amygdala is distinctly different from the state present during seizures induced by electroconvulsion.

Table 1 shows the results of varimax factor analysis from the putamen during the two forms of seizure. Conditions 1 through 3 and 5 through 9 are for EPs when no seizures were present. Factor 3 contributes most (87 percent of the variance) to the averaged EP present during amygdala seizure while factor 1 contributes most (97 percent of the variance) to the average EP present during electroconvulsion. This table demonstrates that specific wave shapes correspond to particular states and that the varimax descriptors are stable over time.

Post-Tetanic Potentiation

Figure 5 demonstrates the use of varimax factor analysis to describe dynamic changes in wave shape following post-tetanic potentiation. Note the marked change in EP wave shape and amplitude produced by the arousing ear shock. In this example a 100 μA (55-Hz, 1-second duration) stimulus was delivered to the left amygdala only. These findings illustrate the now

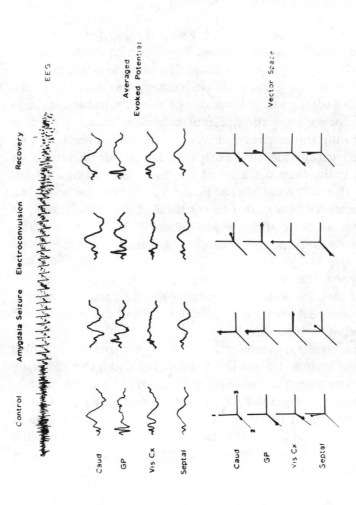

Figure 4. Represented are EEG, evoked potentials, and factor analytic descriptors of the evoked potentials during different neural states. The control period was taken two minutes before presentation of an amygdaloid stimulus that produced seizure. Electroconvulsion was produced minutes later by passage of current through ear rings. The recovery period represents recordings taken five minutes after the electroconvulsive seizure. The vectorgrams represent a three-dimensional factor description of the evoked potential wave shape. Factors 1, 2, and 3 represent the axes of the vectorgrams. It can be seen that evoked potentials recorded during the two seizure states have radically different shapes. Except for the globus pallidus, all structures exhibited recovery of the control wave shapes.

TABLE 1. Factor Loadings from Putamen
During Two Forms of Seizure

Condition	Factors		
	1	2	3
1	.03	.92	.04
2	.04	.93	.00
3	.01	.12	.87
4	.97	.03	.00
5	.07	.87	.02
6	.02	.91	.03
7	.05	.87	.04
8	.05	.89	.03
9	.04	.80	.08

well-replicated observation that post-tetanic potentiation in the amygdala produces EP waveform changes only in the first minute or two, whereas amplitude changes persist as long as 40 minutes following stimulation (Thatcher, in preparation). This method has also proved extremely useful in charting the excitability changes in widespread regions of the brain, which accompany the Goddard "kindling" phenomenon (Goddard 1967; Goddard, McIntyre, and Leech 1969).

These examples demonstrate the utility of factor analysis in parsimonious quantification of EP waveform changes that reflect dynamic brain states. This aspect of factor analysis is further exemplified in studies of information storage and retrieval in humans.

Information Retrieval in the Human

There are several advantages in using computers to present stimulus displays in electrophysiological experiments of human learning and memory. First, the duration, repetition frequency, intensity, and content of the display can be controlled precisely. Second, computer programs can require subject-computer interaction, which helps to control attention as well as to challenge the information-processing capacity of the subject. Third, considerable effort is saved by combining the data analysis and the instrumentation of the experiment.

These advantages led to the development of an experimental technique that uses computer displays to investigate information storage and retrieval in humans. The experiments are still in progress but several important find-

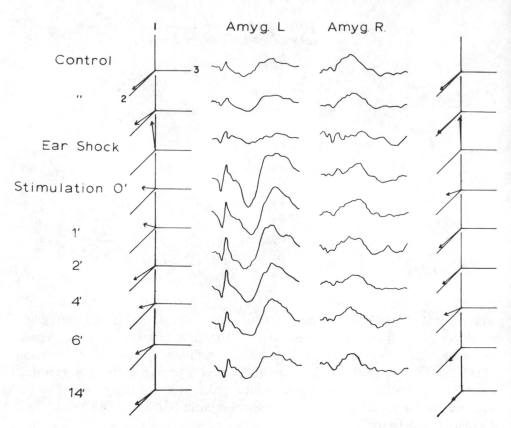

Figure 5. In this figure a kindling stimulus (100 μa p–p, 1-sec duration) was delivered to the left amygdaloid complex (Goddard, McIntyre, and Leech 1969). Averaged evoked potentials are from the ipsilateral and contralateral amygdalae. A large increase in amplitude of evoked potentials occurred in the left amygdala immediately following stimulation. There was some recovery of amplitude to control levels within 14 minutes. Only slight amplitude changes appeared in the right amygdala. Vectorgrams showing the factor structure of evoked potential wave shapes are on the left and right. Factors 1, 2, and 3 represent the three axes of the vectorgrams. Vectorgrams demonstrate that wave shape changes are short-lasting with a return to control shape in about two minutes.

ings have already been replicated and will be presented here. A more complete analysis of the findings is in preparation (Thatcher 1974).

Methods

Programs for a "delayed-matching from sample" paradigm were written for a PDP-12 computer and an accessory oscilloscope was used to present stimulus displays to human subjects. Brain waves from eight different areas were amplified, stored on magnetic tape, and subsequently analyzed.

Examples of 3 computer display programs are shown in Figure 6. In each case a series of blank displays (control displays) each lasting 20 msec are presented at a repetition rate of 1 per second. Following the presentation of the control displays, a blank filled with "information" is presented. The subject is instructed to remember the content of the information display. Following the information display, a variable series of 1 to 6 blank displays occurs and constitutes the "information-hold interval" (intertest interval—ITI). The last ITI display is followed by a test display that matches the information 50 percent of the time. Experiments A, B, and C represent experiments of increasing complexity.

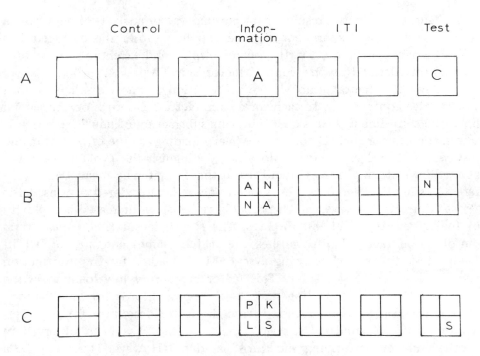

Figure 6. Examples of three computer display programs involved in delayed matching from sample experiments. In each case a series of blank displays are presented (control displays) followed by a blank filled with information (information display). The subject is instructed to remember the content of the information display. Following the information display, a variable series of blank displays occur and constitute the "information-hold" interval (intertest interval, ITI). The last ITI display is followed by a test display that matches the information display 50 percent of the time. The contents of the information and test displays are varied in a counterbalanced design. The subject is instructed to press a button in his left hand when it mismatches. Experiments A, B, and C represent experiments of increasing complexity.

The content of the information and test displays are varied in a counterbalanced design. The subject is instructed to press a lever to the left when
the test matches the information and to press the lever to the right when it
mismatches. In experiment A (Figure 6) three different test displays were
used. In experiment B four different information displays and eight different
test displays were used. Each subject was given 52 trials.

Data analysis involved computing the average EP for a given condition
across trials. These averages were then submitted to the varimax factor analysis.

Results

Figure 7 shows the results of the varimax factor analysis of data from a
subject performing experiment A. The top line shows the averaged EPs
(N=52) starting with the fourth control display and extending to the test.
Factor 1 is defined as the control factor since waves 4 through 9 load
heaviest on this factor although the information and test displays do not.
The relative contribution to each wave from factor 1 is shown on the second
line. The third line is the residual following subtraction of line 2 from line 1.
The second factor (line 4) contributes heavy loadings to the information and
test waves. However, factor 2 does not distinguish the evoked potentials
elicited by matching (same) stimuli from those elicited by mismatching (different) stimuli. Therefore, the second factor is considered a nonspecific
"post-information" wave, which probably reflects the increased complexity
of the information and test displays. The fourth factor (line 6), called an
"information factor," distinguishes the match (same) and mismatch (different) test displays by showing a shared high loading for the information
and the matching test display. This factor has a very low loading on the
mismatch EP. It is interesting that the factor descriptor for the "match"
wave is 180 degrees phase-reversed from the factor descriptor for the information wave. A similar 180-degree phase reversal has been observed in
another subject performing the same paradigm. However, this may be a
fortuitous finding and no significance can be attached to it as yet. One
purpose of Figure 7 is to demonstrate the ability of the varimax factor
analysis to describe a complex sequence of waveforms and at the same time
parcel out wave shapes specific to the different variables of the experiment.
All the major variables correlated with quantitatively distinct descriptors,
that is, control, content display, information, and match display, as well as
the ITI display (factor 4). The ITI factor (factor 4) may reflect processes
specific to the "information-holding" period.

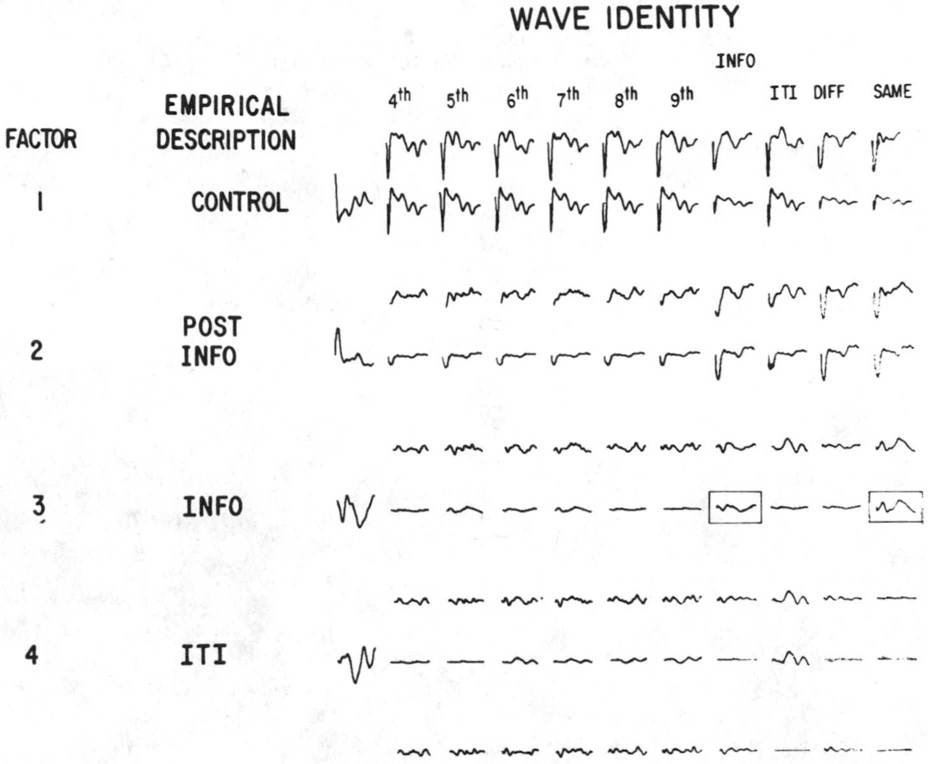

Figure 7. This figure shows the results of a varimax factor analysis from a subject performing experiment A (see Figure 6). The top row is averaged EPs (N=52 for all EPs
except same and different where N=26) starting with the fourth control display and
extending to the test. The four factors (accounting for 93 percent of the energy) are in
the first column of waves on the left. The empirical description of factors was determined
by the relative contribution of a factor to a specific variable of the exeriment. The
relative contribution of factor 1 to the top row of waves is represented by the waves in
row 2. The relative contribution of factor 2 to the residual waves in row 3 is represented
in row 4. This method of displaying the varimax factor analysis is described in Figure 1.
Note that the information factor (factor 3) loads heaviest on the EP produced by the
information display and on the EP elicited by the test stimulus that matches (same) the
information display. Note also a heavy loading by a factor (factor 4) specific to the ITI
display.

Figure 8 shows averaged EPs for three different information displays in
two subjects. The averaged response to the letter A in both subjects
differs from the waveforms produced by the letters B and C, indicating that
the wave shape of the EPs is specific to the information content of the
display. Additional support for information specificity is provided by factor
analyses of "sliding" EP averages. Each sliding average was made of five

TABLE 2. Evoked Potential Factor Loadings for
the Letters A, B, and C

Subject W.H.	A	1	2	3
		27	0	0
		83	0	0
		87	9	0
		89	10	0
		93	4	0
		86	1	5
		41	15	2
	B	25	50	6
		26	26	5
		1	86	3
		2	93	0
		4	95	0
		0	94	0
		0	83	5
	C	19	58	13
		19	56	19
		29	51	12
		23	32	40
		17	16	64
		48	6	13
Subject F.B.	A	77	17	0
		86	11	0
		88	11	0
		76	17	0
	B	21	75	0
		16	81	0
		15	83	0
		16	80	0
		16	81	0
		17	69	0
		19	56	0
		17	60	0
	C	24	53	21
		29	46	24
		27	55	16
		49	33	15
		66	23	8
		66	21	5
		59	30	1
		49	45	1
		39	50	4
		35	49	3

evoked potentials averaged in sequential order, that is, EPs 1, 2, 3, 4, 5, then
EPs 2, 3, 4, 5, 6, then EPs 3, 4, 5, 6, 7, etc. This moderate amount of
averaging was sufficient to create factor loadings specific to the information
content of the display. Table 2 shows that factor 1 loads heaviest for the
letter A, factor 2 for the letter B, and factor 3 loads heaviest for the letter C.

Figure 9 shows the results of a varimax factor analysis from a different
subject performing in an experiment corresponding to type B shown in
Figure 6. This subject displayed more variability, particularly in the control
space, than the subject in the previous example. However, the utility of the
varimax factor analysis is again demonstrated since, in spite of this variability, each of the relevant variables is described by unique factors. Note
that factor 5 (information factor) again distinguishes "same" from "dif-

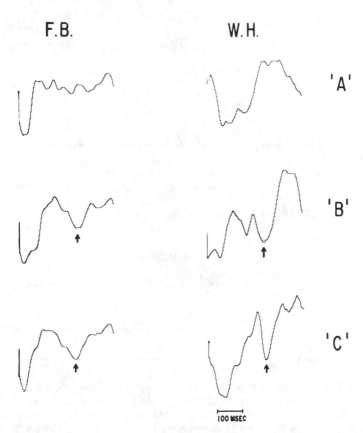

*Figure 8. This figure shows average EPs (Ns vary from 13 to 22) elicited by different
information displays (letters A, B, or C) for two subjects performing experiment type A
(see Figure 6). Note that the first 30 msec of the EPs are truncated in this figure as well as
in Figures 7 through 9.*

ferent" and contributes most to the averaged EP produced by the information display and the matching test display. The common factor loading indicates that the information and match-test waves share a common process. The mismatch test display yields an average EP that loads moderately well on the control factor (factor 2). Again it can be seen that unique waveforms are present for the first two ITI displays (factor 4).

Table 3 shows another example from a third subject of a common factor loading (factor 1) between the information EP and the match-test EP. Factor 2 is a control factor since it loads heaviest on the control and ITI displays. Factor 2 also loads on the mismatch EP. The consistent finding of a common factor loading between information and match suggests that the

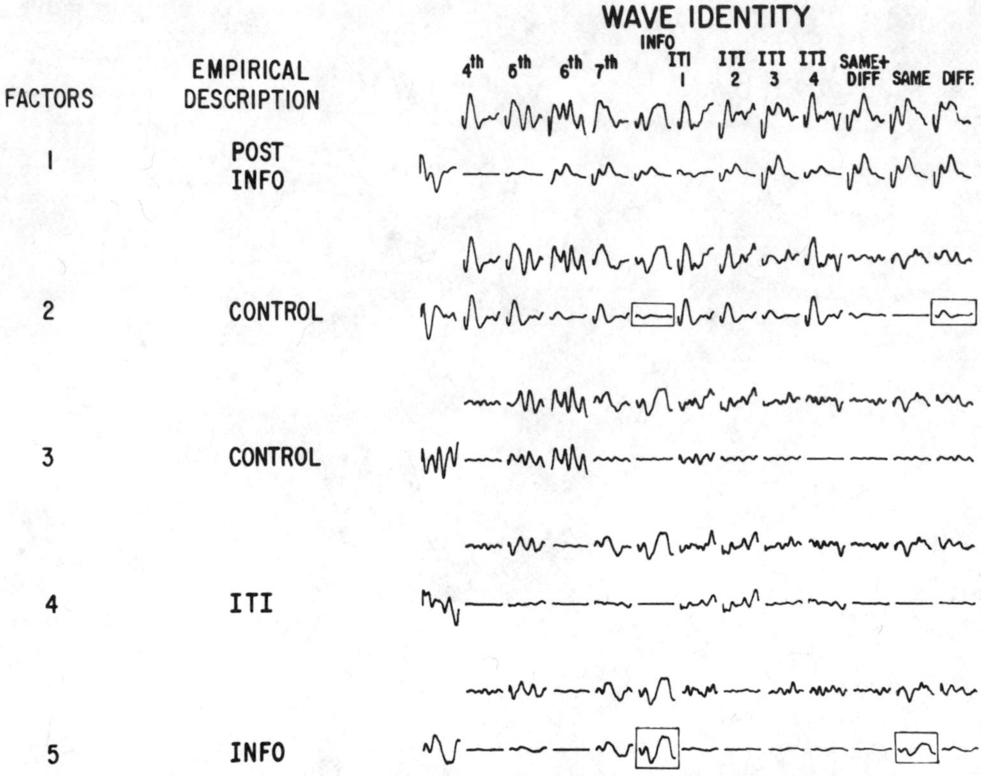

Figure 9. This figure shows the results of a varimax factor analysis from a subject performing experiment B (see Figure 6). The top row is averaged EPs (N=52 for all EPs except same and different where N=26) starting with the fourth control display and extending to the test. The five factors (accounting for 87 percent of the energy) are in the first column of waves on the left. The empirical description of factors was determined by the relative contribution of factors to specific variables of the experiment. This method of displaying the varimax factor analysis is described in Figures 1 and 7. (See text for interpretation of factors.)

presentation of the match-test stimulus results in the release or reproduction of some aspect of the information wave.

The content of the test display was identical for the match and for the mismatch condition. The only relevant difference within the design of the experiment was in the interaction of the present (test display) with the past (information display). Half of the time the identical test stimulus matched with the past and the other half of the time it did not. Figure 10 shows test waveforms from two subjects performing an experiment of type A. It can be seen that, when the test display was different from the previous information display, negative components at latencies of 250 to 350 msec appeared. These components were reliably absent when the test stimulus matched the information. It should be emphasized that differences between match and mismatch EPs may also occur at latencies of less than 100 msec (Thatcher 1974).

Summary

The question addressed by the various experiments described in this paper is whether the morphology of the evoked potential is a sensitive index of differences between brain states, and whether varimax factor analysis provides a precise and parsimonious method for quantitative distinctions between these states. Different brain states were induced in animals by administration of various drugs and by electrical stimuli delivered to the ear,

TABLE 3. Evoked Potential Factor Loadings for
Control, ITI, and Information Stimuli

Subject R.L.
Temporal L.

	Factors		
	1	2	3
Control	.22	.76	.00
Control	.33	.60	.06
Control	.18	.44	.38
Information	.85	.14	.00
ITI 1	.36	.60	.02
ITI 2	.24	.73	.02
ITI 3	.19	.77	.02
Match test	.74	.21	.03
Mismatch test	.49	.41	.08

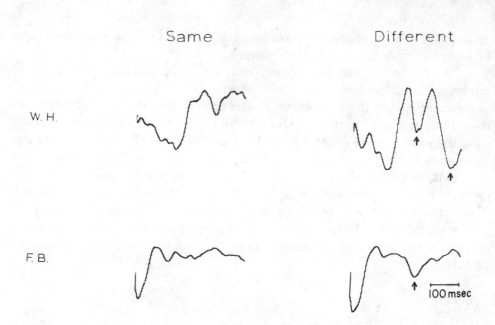

Figure 10. This figure shows the average EPs (Ns from 13 to 18) elicited by the match (same) and mismatch (different) test displays for two subjects. The subjects were performing an experiment of type A (see Figure 6).

causing arousal, and to the amygdala, causing convulsion. Different brain states were induced in human subjects by presentation of visual displays containing either no coded information or information concordant or discordant with a previous display. In each of these paradigms varimax factor analysis of the set of averaged evoked responses obtained under different brain states yielded a unique factor that accounted for most of the energy of the average responses characteristic of each state. The results show that the morphology of the AER reflects the differences between brain states under the various conditions explored, and that such changes in morphology are well detected by the method of varimax factor analysis. This method seems to fulfill the requirement we initially imposed; that is, varimax factor analysis provides a precise and parsimonious way to classify different brain states. We have applied this method in other studies and it has yielded excellent results in the detection of abnormal brain states caused by such neurological disorders as tumors and strokes. We believe that varimax factor analysis is of general utility in the evaluation and classification of the electrophysiological activity of the brain.

References

Chapman, R.M. 1973. Evoked potentials of the brain related to thinking. In F.J. McGuigan and R.A. Schoonover (eds.), *The Psychophysiology of Thinking*. New York: Academic Press.

Ciganek, L. 1969. Visually evoked potential correlates of attention and distraction in man. *Psychiatr. Clin.* 2:95.

Dawson, G.D. 1954. A summation technique for the detection of small evoked potentials. *Electroencephalogr. Clin. Neurophysiol.* 6:65.

Docampo, G., Suarez-Nonez, J.M.D., and Sierra, G. 1967. Reticular influences on the visual areas of the rabbit. *Brain Res.* 4:117.

Donchin, E. 1966. A multivariate approach to the analysis of averaged evoked potentials. *IEEE Trans. Biomed. Eng.* BME-13, p. 131.

Gershuni, G.V., Kozhevnikov, V.A., Maruseva, A.M., Avakyan, R.V., Radionova, E.A., Altman, J.A., and Soroko, V.I. 1960. Modifications in electrical responses of the auditory system in different states of the higher nervous activity. *Electroencephalogr. Clin. Neurophysiol.* 13:115.

Goddard, G.V. 1967. Development of epileptic seizures through brain stimulation at low intensities. *Nature* 214:1020.

Goddard, G.V., McIntyre, D.C., and Leech, C.K. 1969. A permanent change in brain function resulting from daily electrical stimulation. *Exp. Neurol.* 25:295.

Halas, E.S., and Beardsley, S.V. 1969. A factor analysis of neuronal responses during habituation in cats. *Psychol. Res.* 19:47.

Harmon, H.H. 1960. *Modern Factor Analysis*, Chicago: University of Chicago Press.

Hudspeth, W., and Jones, G.B. 1973. Stability of neural interference patterns. *First International Symposium on Biology and Holography*, New York, New York.

John, E.R. 1967. *Mechanisms of Memory*. New York: Academic Press.

John, E.R., Ruchkin, D.S., and Villegas, J. 1963. Signal analysis of evoked potentials recorded from cats during conditioning. *Science* 141:429.

John, E.R., Ruchkin, D.S., and Villegas, J. 1964. Experimental background: signal analysis and behavioral correlates of evoked potential configurations in cats. *Ann. N.Y. Acad. Sci.* 112:362.

John, E.R., Walker, P., Cawood, D., Rush, M., and Gehrmann, J. 1972. Mathematical identification of brain states applied to classification of drugs. *Int. Rev. Neurobiol.* 15:273.

John, E.R., Walker, P., Cawood, D., Rush, M., and Gehrmann, J. 1973. Factor analysis of evoked potentials. *Electroencephalogr. Clin. Neurophysiol.* 34:33.

Kaiser, H.F. 1958. The varimax criterion for analytic rotation in factor analysis. *Psychometrika* 23:187.

Kamiya, J., Callaway, E., and Yeager, C.L. 1969. Visual evoked responses in subjects trained to control alpha rhythms. *Psychophysiology* 5:683.

Kitai, S.T. 1965. Substitution of intracranial electrical stimulation for photic stimulation during extinction procedure. *Nature* 209:22.

Naitoh, P., Johnson, L.C., Lubin, A., and Wyborney, G. 1971. Brain wave "generating" processes during waking and sleeping. *Electroencephalogr. Clin. Neurophysiol.* 31:294.

Pampiglione, G. 1967. Some observations on the variability of evoked potentials. In W. Cobb and C. Morocutti (eds.), *The Evoked Potentials. Electroencephalogr. Clin. Neurophysiol.* suppl. 26.

Regan, D. 1972. *Evoked potentials in Psychology, Sensory Physiology and Clinical Medicine.* New York: Wiley-Interscience.

Sommer-Smith, S.A., and Morocutti, C. 1970. Cortical and subcortical evoked potentials during conditioning. *Electroencephalogr. Clin. Neurophysiol.* 29:383.

Suter, C. 1969. *Computer Analysis of Evoked Potential Correlates of the Critical Band.* Technical Report, Computer Science Center, University of Maryland, p. 68.

Suter, C. 1970. Principal component analysis of average evoked potentials. *Exp. Neurol.* 29:317.

Thatcher, R. 1974. A quantitative electrophysiological analysis of human memory. Symposium, Mechanisms of Memory, Eastern Psychological Assoc., Philadelphia, Pa.

biofeedback training of 40-hz eeg and behavior

Daniel E. Sheer, Ph.D.

Department of Psychology
University of Houston
Houston, Texas

The use of operant training techniques to control electrical brain activity is relatively recent, dating back some ten years to the beginning of the present series of publications (Mulholland 1968). As is generally true of new research, there is a focus on questions about the basic process itself—definitive training procedures, transfer and concomitant effects and, not the least of it, skepticism about the reliability of the phenomenon itself. The ever-accelerating literature reflected, in part, in a handbook (Barber et al. 1971a), in a recent bibliography (Butler and Stoyva 1973), and in a series of annual reviews (Barber et al. 1971b, Stoyva et al. 1972, Shapiro et al. 1973), has both clarified some issues and raised additional questions.

In spite of an amorphous surround of "mind control" distorting the question, it is now clear that patterns of electrical activity in the brain can be brought under operant control through response-reinforcement contingencies. This conditioning has been demonstrated in humans through a range of different EEG patterns: theta (Green, Green, and Walter 1972; Beatty et al. 1974), alpha (Brown 1970, Nowlis and Kamiya 1970, Mulholland and Peper 1971), a sensorimotor rhythm at 12 to 14 Hz (Sterman 1972), and beta (Beatty 1971). There is also some indication that asymmetrical control can be achieved with occipital alpha by differential feedback to homologous scalp areas of the two hemispheres (Peper 1971, 1972). Such localized control raises the possibility of more specific training, because the functional significance of laterality has also been demonstrated with EEG measures. Galin and Ornstein (1972) recorded from normal subjects during the performance of predominantly right (spatial) and left (verbal) hemisphere tasks. They found a significantly higher average spectral power (more alpha) in the right hemisphere, and thus more alpha blocking and beta in the left hemisphere, during performance of the verbal as compared with the spatial tasks.

Systematic information on optimal training procedures and conditions under which operant control will generalize beyond the training laboratory is simply not available. Among some relevant observations, Black (1971) has shown that peripheral skeletal muscle mediation is not an essential condition for operant control of CNS electrical activity. Hippocampal theta and non-theta waves can be conditioned in dogs whose skeletal musculature was paralyzed by gallamine. The possibility still remains, however, that hippocampal theta waves may be related to central circuits that control skeletal muscle activity because such drugs do not block central circuits. Indeed, rats who are free to move can be more quickly conditioned to theta than can immobile rats (Black 1972, and personal communication). This would imply a relationship between the circuitry for skeletal movement and hippocampal theta and/or demonstrate the importance of response state for conditioning theta.

At the human level the problem of mediative processing, particularly cognitive, becomes more difficult to dissect. Beatty (1972) compared alpha conditioning during one-hour training periods in one group of subjects who received feedback on EEG response-reinforcement contingencies, in another group who had only pretrial information on the behavioral state associated with the required alpha responses, in a third group who received both, and in a fourth group who received neither. Groups one, two, and three showed exactly the same magnitude and development of operant conditioning as compared with the fourth group, which showed no change. Prior information evidently produced the same effects as response-reinforcement contingencies, and a combination of these made no difference. Upon questioning, subjects in the "information only" group readily reported the typical correlates of alpha—relaxation, calmness, etc.—while the "feedback only" group gave a wide range of subjective reports. Apparently, in the absence of an external feedback system, the "information only" group of subjects cognitively monitored their own internal states to reinforce the required performance.

Subtle reinforcers can be established in human subjects, through cognitive processing, by the history of the subject, by instructional sets, and by momentary motivational states of the subject—to specify but a few conditions. Obviously it would be useful to have systematic data on cognitively mediated reinforcement and, when performance deteriorates for no apparent reason, on nonreinforcement as well. On the positive side, this cognitive processing at the human level may inevitably accompany neural response-reinforcement contingencies. It may thus provide a more effective method for achieving voluntary control, as compared with such other methods of control as reinforcement of overt behaviors, drugs, or direct stimulation (Black 1972).

It is difficult to demonstrate clear connections between changes in patterns of brain electricity and changes in concomitant behaviors, but there are encouraging signs. The first approach to the problem was subjective reports, in which alpha states were variously described as "pleasant feelings" (Brown 1970) and relaxing and "letting go" (Nowlis and Kamiya 1970). Mulholland and Peper (1971) associated alpha with passive observation of clearly visible targets and its attenuation with visual efferent control processes concerned with orienting and tracking. Galin (personal communication) recorded from symmetrical right and left central leads referred to the vertex while subjects were performing a mirror-tracking task that required visual spatial abilities. From computer analysis of the left-right ratios of EEG alpha he consistently found a comparative increase of alpha in the right (spatial) hemisphere in the 0.25-second period preceding the occurrence of an error.

An extensive series of studies by Sterman and his colleagues (Sterman, MacDonald, and Stone 1974) focused on a 12- to 14-Hz EEG rhythm recorded from sensorimotor cortex (SMR) in cats and man, which is associated with relaxation and inhibition of movement. The operant conditioning with cats showed that SMR-trained animals had enhanced EEG sleep-spindle activity, reduced motor disturbances during sleep, and increased resistance to seizures induced by convulsant doses of monomethyl hydrazine (Sterman 1972). Subsequently, seven human subjects—four epileptic and three normal—were trained for 6 to 18 months. After two to three months of regular and continuous training, the four epileptic patients began to show reductions in abnormal EEG signs and seizures, which were sustained throughout the training (Sterman, MacDonald, and Stone 1974).

Theta activity recorded from cortical leads has been associated with a subjective state somewhere between the relaxed wakefulness of alpha and the sleep state of delta (Green, Green, and Walter 1972). Subjective reports by persons trained in theta, include descriptions of hypnagogic-like imagery and reverie or wandering imagination which might be characterized as creative thought patterns. Beatty et al. (1974) investigated the effect of theta states associated with a very low level of arousal on a monotonous visual monitoring task requiring a high level of vigilance to maintain efficiency. They trained one group of subjects to augment occipital theta waves and another group to suppress them. Then both groups performed the continuous monitoring task in which contingent reinforcement was given for the group-appropriate response. The conditioned theta augmentation, also reinforced throughout the task, produced a significant deterioration in monitoring efficiency, while theta suppression produced a significant increase.

The substantial relationships shown in these studies between brain electricity and behavior are restricted entirely to inhibitory behavioral functions. The SMR rhythm is associated with relaxation and inhibition of movement. The alpha rhythm shows significant comparative increases in one hemisphere during a time when it is not maximally operative—the right hemisphere during verbal performance and the left during spatial performance. Again, the alpha shows significant comparative increases in the functional hemisphere—the right hemisphere during mirror-tracing performance—but only at the time when an error is made. The augmentation of occipital theta significantly depresses vigilant performance in a visual monitoring task, which shows improvement when the theta is suppressed.

For all these behaviors the following questions may well be asked. What are the patterns of brain electricity associated with facilitatory behavioral functions? What rhythm occurs in the sensorimotor cortex with facilitation of movement, and not inhibition? What waves show up in the right hemisphere during performance of spatial tasks, and in the left during verbal performance? What happens in the right hemisphere with mirror tracing during correct responding and not when an error is made? What brain electricity is in the occipital cortex when theta is suppressed with concomitant monitoring efficiency?

The first approximate answer is that the EEG is desynchronized at a very low amplitude with mixed fast frequencies. With the recording techniques and computer resolution now available, it is time that we took a much closer look at this low-amplitude, fast-frequency "desynchronized" EEG usually represented in charts as irregularly thickened black lines. The single designation, "desynchronized" or "arousal," for an EEG clearly refers to a number of different electrical patterns. In their study of conditioning in monkeys, Morrell and Jasper (1956) found that a generalized desynchronization was diffusely present in the cortex only during the first stage of sensory-sensory conditioning. When conditioning was established, a "stable, well-localized desynchronization" was limited to relevant cortical areas. Further, Morrell (1961) reported differences in units recorded from the brainstem reticular formation, hippocampus, and visual cortex during generalized cortical desynchronization as compared with the localized desynchronization in visual cortex.

The first stage of conditioning, diffuse cortical desynchronization, represents initial responding to novel stimuli within the complex matrix of irrelevant environmental stimuli. It is an oscillatory, unstable state of the organism, in which many different subassemblies of the intrinsic electrical activity are firing in different spatiotemporal patterns, that is, nonsynchronously. When connections become established, through spatiotemporal patterning of inputs, as in conditioned stimulus-unconditioned stimulus (CS-UCS) pairings, subassemblies of the electrical activity now fire in synchronous organizations restricted to the relevant circuitry. The desynchronized EEG is then no longer diffuse, but it still may appear as desynchronized without finer grained analysis because the synchronous subassemblies restricted to limited cortical areas are submerged within the total ongoing electrical activity. The limited subassemblies, defined by the relevant environmental inputs and the contingent reinforcement, are now firing at a synchronous frequency "optimal" for consolidation. We have proposed that a specific pattern of brain electricity, a narrow frequency band centered at 40 Hz, reflects this state of circumscribed cortical excitability or focused arousal (Sheer 1970, Sheer and Grandstaff 1970, Sheer 1972). The association of focused arousal-40 Hz represents an extension of the continuum from sleep-delta, through wakefulness-alpha, and diffuse arousal-beta.

Our focus on the 40-Hz EEG had its beginning in the large-amplitude, highly synchronous bursts recorded from the olfactory bulbs and other rhinencephalic structures of cats during sniffing, exploring, and orienting behaviors (Sheer, Grandstaff, and Benignus 1966). In quadruped animals, particularly, olfaction is an important distance receptor, and the associated motor feedback of sniffing is a highly adaptive orienting response for exploratory, feeding, and sexual behavior. This pronounced electrical rhythm occurs in rhinencephalic structures throughout the phylogenetic scale from catfish to man (Sheer and Grandstaff 1970).

At the neocortical level, where laminar structure is far more complex, the 40-Hz rhythm is at a much lower amplitude in a more complicated electrical background, but it can still be observed visually on the oscillograph from epidural leads at fast paper speeds. For systematic reliable data, however, computer analysis is clearly necessary. In a series of studies with the cat in a successive visual discrimination task (Sheer 1970, Sheer and Grandstaff 1970), consistent relationships were observed between 40 Hz and the acquisition phase of learning. In the 10-sec epoch of a 7/sec flickering light cue (S_D), a burst of 40 Hz occurred in visual and motor cortex about 0.5 sec before, and continuously for about 1.5 sec after, a correct bar-press response.

The few references to 40 Hz in the literature present a rather consistent picture. Galambos (1958), recording from the caudate nucleus and globus pallidus, observed 40 Hz when cats had learned that the last in a series of 11 clicks led to an unavoidable electric shock. Rowland (1958), recording from ectosylvian and lateral cortex and medial geniculate nucleus in cats, observed this activity during acquisition, when an auditory CS was paired with an electric-shock UCS. Killam and Killam (1967) also observed it in the lateral geniculate of cats when they were fully trained to discriminate a correct visual pattern from three presented. Pribram, Spinelli, and Kamback (1967) reported 40 Hz in the striate cortex of monkeys just after they made incorrect differential responses in a very difficult visual task. In the Russian literature, Dumenko (1961), recording from the auditory, somesthetic, and motor cortex of dogs, observed 40 Hz when limb responses were conditioned to tone as the CS and excitation of skin with induction current as the UCS. Sakhiulina (1961) observed it in the sensorimotor cortex of dogs when conditioned flexion of the contralateral leg was paired with different conditioned stimuli.

In recording from the scalp in humans, the meditation state provides a unique situation in which subjects are immobile and the recordings relatively free of muscle artifact. Das and Gastaut (1955), recording from occipital leads in seven trained yogis, reported high-amplitude levels of 40 Hz activity during the samadhi state, which is the final, most intense concentration stage in this form of meditation. Just recently Banquet (1973), studying 12 subjects practicing transcendental meditation with recording from left occipital and frontal leads, also observed 40 Hz during the third deep stage of meditation. Giannitrapani (1969), recording from scalp leads in middle- and high-IQ subjects, compared the EEG during mental multiplication activity and a resting condition. A 40-Hz rhythm occurred during the multiplication behavior just prior to the subjects' answering.

Considerable attention has been focused in recent years on a rather heterogeneous clinical grouping variously termed learning disability, minimal brain injury, and minimal brain dysfunction in children. One relatively clear subgrouping of such children can be characterized by no hard neurological signs, no primary sensory or motor defects, no apparent primary emotional disturbances, and low-normal to normal IQ. The main presenting problem is that these children cannot learn; they are either retarded in grade level or are in special classes. They are unable to assimilate new material and solve problems at the level of their chronological peers. Significant decrements were obtained specifically in the 40-Hz EEG band during problem-solving tasks in a carefully selected group of such children, as compared with matched children at normal grade level (Sheer and Hix 1971; Sheer 1974). One purpose of the present series of studies is to develop biofeedback training procedures for conditioning 40-Hz EEG in learning-disabled children.

Experimental Procedures and Controls

Reliable, consistent EEG recording of 40 Hz from the intact scalp is the first essential procedure to be accomplished, and it is by no means a simple task. This low-amplitude, fast-frequency part of the EEG spectrum, recorded from the human scalp, is of the order of 5 μ V. In addition, it completely overlaps with the muscle spectrum, which is broad and highly polyphasic, with generally a peak at 50 Hz (Chaffin 1969). Thus one must contend at the same time with a low signal level and muscle artifact at a much higher amplitude, both in the same frequency range. Over the past several years we have developed recording and analysis procedures that have been used both in the controlled laboratory situation and in such field situations as primary grade schools. The procedures have been control-tested with analog and digital computer analyses and implemented in portable hardware for on-line corrections and digital counts.

Our standard experimental procedure for operant conditioning of the 40-Hz EEG signal in both the field and laboratory situations is as follows: The subject is seated in a lounge chair in a slightly reclining position in front of a screen. His instructions are to turn on as many slides as possible in the conditioning period. The slides are colored, detailed, and cover a wide range of subjects with the interest level pegged for the particular group under investigation, adults or children. The slide-projector is automatically triggered through a stimulus control unit by pre-set criteria of the 40-Hz EEG signal, recorded from a specified set of bipolar leads.

The equipment and experimental set-up for biofeedback training in both the field and laboratory situations are shown in Figures 1A and 1B. In the former situation, the special electrode assembly consists of a Bionetics 10-mm porous silver chloride pellet (Kanter Associates, Santa Anna, Cal.) held in close reference (<¼") to a Texas Instruments TIS 58 Silent Field-Effect Transistor (FET) or Motorola equivalent configurated with a ZN 5089 NPN transistor to provide a current source for the FET and a 33K resistor to limit the current into the FET at 1 mA. This assembly is insulated with Insulex and encapsulated in a mold with No. 8751 epoxilite. The leads from the FET are a 50-ohm coaxial cable about four feet in length.

The effect of placing an FET at the immediate electrode site is to provide a low source impedance from the point of the FET of about 300 ohms which produces an excellent shunt to ground for all cable-induced or EMF noise detected along the length of the cable.

The electrode assemblies are applied to the scalp with adhesive rings, which are first attached to the rim of the epoxy mold and then fixed to the scalp. Standard electrode paste is applied between the pellet and the scalp with a syringe needle through holes in the rim of the mold. This electrode assembly fixes firmly to the scalp and can be easily removed by applying acetone.

The electrode leads go into a portable eight-channel differential AC

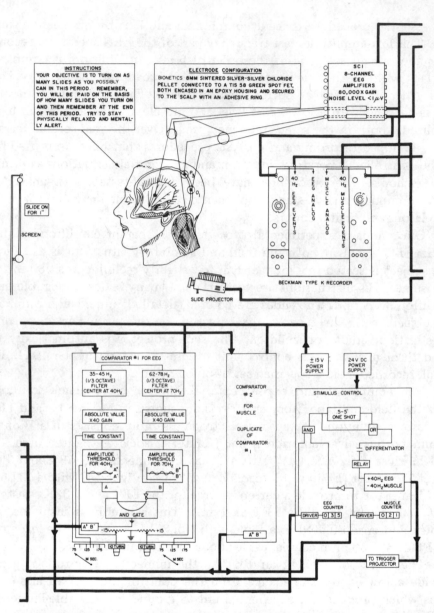

*Figures 1A and 1B.   Equipment and set-up for conditioning 40-Hz in the field situation.
The special electrode configuration changes the source impedance at the scalp to about
300 ohms in transmission over a 50-ohm cable to the first stage of amplification. This
configuration does not require shielding and attenuates movement artifact. The special
SCI amplifiers are high-gain, low-noise, with narrow-frequency windows. Their outputs
from the EEG and muscle leads go on to the two comparators and then to the paper and
FM tape recorders. At the same time they also activate the slide projector through the
stimulus control unit. In the laboratory situation, the recordings are made with standard
Grass electrodes and a 10-channel, Model 78 Grass polygraph with the same comparators
and feedback loop.*

amplifier assembly at 80,000 gain, with a narrow frequency window between 16 and 80 Hz and a common mode rejection above 100 db (Model MC 128E-4, SCI Systems, Houston, Texas). The power supply for this entire configuration is regulated at ± 15 volts and the internal noise level is of the order of 2 μV. The output from these amplifiers is monitored on-line with a two-channel Beckman Type-K Dynograph.

In the laboratory the recordings are made with standard Grass electrodes and a ten-channel Model 78 Grass polygraph. The Grass amplifiers are set at or close to maximum sensitivity; the high-pass filter cut-off is set at 10 Hz and the low-pass at 90 Hz, with the 60-Hz notch filter cut out. EEG records are monitored on-line on the Grass oscillograph by running the paper speed at 100 mm/sec during critical trial periods or for periodic samples during baseline conditions.

Electrode placements, in both laboratory and field situations, follow the standard Ten-Twenty System; in addition, a set of bipolar leads from the neck and temporal muscles are recorded from the side of the head on which the EEG signal is conditioned. Outputs from the Grass polygraph are stored on a seven-channel FM tape recorder for further computer processing.

Comparators. On-line, the EEG and muscle leads go into identical comparators or coincidence detection units, which are the hardware developed for feedback control of muscle artifact. A schematic drawing of these units is shown in Figures 2A and 2B. Each unit consists of two high Q, narrow-band twin-T analog filters (Model 3385, White Instrument Co., Austin, Texas) with rectified output compared against a DC level to develop a digital output. Both filters have a 23-percent band, one tuned at a center frequency of 40 Hz, the other at a center frequency of 70 Hz. The filter outputs are integrated with adjustable time constants and their threshold levels are set with amplitude comparators.

For the EEG leads an anion gate circuit allows the 40-Hz output to trigger a reinforcement only when it is not coincident with the 70-Hz output, which is used as an index of the polyphasic muscle. In addition, when a 40-Hz muscle signal from the muscle comparator coincides with a 40-Hz EEG signal, the slide projector will again not trigger.

When the output from the EEG comparator is neither coincident with the 70-Hz EEG signal nor with the 40-Hz muscle signal, it activates the stimulus control unit which triggers the slide projector. The outputs from the EEG and muscle comparators also go to digital counters, which keep a consecutive count of 40-Hz EEG bursts and 40-Hz muscle bursts for any specified time period.

The criteria of amplitude levels and burst durations are set by adjustable gain potentiometers and time constants for both the EEG and muscle comparators. The time constants are set at 75 msec, which represents three cycles of EEG at 40 Hz and five cycles of muscle bursts at 70 Hz. The amplitude levels are empirically determined for each subject at a preconditioning baseline session and are adjusted to allow for a low to moderate level of free operants. If there is any partial overlap of the three cycles of 40 Hz and the five cycles of 70 Hz from the same EEG leads, the slide is not triggered. This overlap can occur from a minimum of 20 msec before to 20 msec after the 40-Hz filter output because of the different time delays of the 40-Hz filter (54 msec) and the 70-Hz filter (31 msec), and a 40-msec one-shot time delay after the 70-Hz time constant circuit. These stringent criteria are probably an overcorrection for muscle artifact, resulting in a conservative estimate of the EEG signal.

Control procedures. The on-line control for muscle artifact with the comparators is essentially nonparametric contingency detection of the coincidence between EEG and muscle within the threshold limits specified. It is based on a correction for muscle using a parametric analysis of covariance, shown in Figure 3, developed with computer analysis on data obtained with matched groups of normal and learning-disabled children (Sheer and Hix 1971, Sheer 1974).

As can be noted in Figure 3, electrical activity in the range from 62 to 78 Hz with a center frequency at 70 Hz is specified as muscle (Σx^2) and, from the same leads, activity in the range from 36 to 44 Hz with a center at 40 Hz is specified as EEG (Σy^2). The corrected power function

$$\Sigma y^2 = \frac{(\Sigma xy)^2}{\Sigma x^2}$$

represents the variance or power of the EEG independent of muscle. We have carried out a number of independent control checks on this power equation to confirm its independence from muscle.

An analog-computer analysis procedure (Sheer 1970) was used to obtain these corrected spectral power functions for three 23-percent frequency bands, centered at 31.5, 40, and 50 Hz, on normal and learning-disabled children during control and problem-solving situations. Using the corrected power functions, there were significant increases in the 40-Hz power bands for the normal children during problem-solving situations but not in the bordering 31.5 and 50 Hz bands set up as controls (Sheer and Hix 1971, Sheer 1974). There is no reason why polyphasic muscle, with a relatively higher amplitude at 50 Hz, should show up differentially in the 40-Hz band but not in the 31.5- and 50-Hz bands.

Using a hybrid-computer analysis procedure with an IBM 360, high-resolution spectral-density functions were obtained with a Fast Fourier Transform program modified to provide covariance power functions. At the

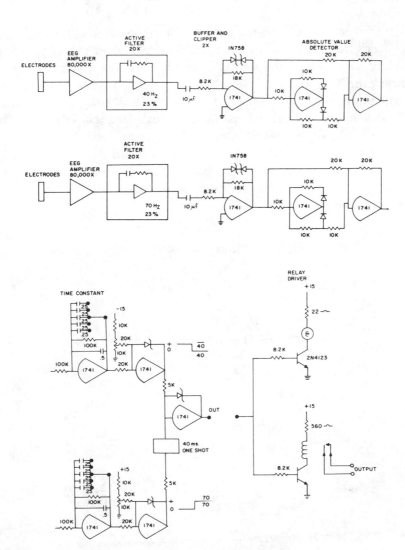

Figures 2A and 2B.   Schematic of the comparators used in the conditioning set-up to control for muscle artifact. The EEG leads to be conditioned go into one comparator and the muscle leads into another. Each comparator splits the input signal into a 40-Hz and a 70-Hz output with adjustable gain levels and burst durations, which are empirically determined for each subject. The EEG comparator will trigger the stimulus control unit; that is, count a 40-Hz burst and turn on the slide projector only when there is not a coincident 70-Hz burst. Also the muscle comparator and EEG comparator are connected so that when there is a 40-Hz muscle burst coincident with a 40-Hz EEG burst, the stimulus control will not trigger. The time constant or burst duration for both the EEG and muscle comparator is set at 75 msec, which represents three cycles of EEG at 40 Hz and about five cycles of muscle at 70 Hz. With a time delay in the 23% 40-Hz filter of 54 msec and in the 23% 70-Hz muscle filter of 31 msec, and a 40-msec one-shot after the time constant circuit, the 40-Hz EEG signal will not trigger the stimulus control unit if the 70-Hz muscle signal occurs from a minimum of 20 msec before to 20 msec after the 40-Hz filter output.

first stage of this analysis, during digitization of the analog signals, bursts of high-frequency components were automatically blanked out at pre-set levels by detecting the slope of the line of baseline crosses as the amplitude of the first derivative. The amplitude levels for blanking were empirically determined for each record and pre-set for automatically digitizing the analog EEG by balancing the maximal blanking of high-frequency bursts with the minimal effect on frequencies of interest. This procedure was the first step in the hybrid processing, primarily to keep the standard deviations of the EEG distributions within a homogeneous range for the subsequent covariance analyses. It is a gross correction, analagous to deleting obvious muscle bursts by visual inspection.

STATISTICAL   CONTROL OF MUSCLE

x = Observed   Muscle (70 H$_z$ Filter)

y = Observed EEG   (40 H$_z$ Filter)

y' = Predicted EEG from x

$y - y'$ = Difference between Observed and Predicted EEG
         ---- the EEG Independent of Muscle

$(y - y')^2$ = Power Function

$$y' = \beta x$$

$$y - y' = y - \beta x$$

$$(y - y')^2 = (y - \beta x)^2$$

where $\quad \beta = r \dfrac{\sigma_y}{\sigma_x}$; $r = \dfrac{\mathcal{E}xy}{\sqrt{\mathcal{E}x^2 \cdot \mathcal{E}y^2}}$; and $\dfrac{\sigma_y}{\sigma_x} = \dfrac{\sqrt{\mathcal{E}y^2}}{\sqrt{\mathcal{E}x^2}}$

then $\quad \beta = \dfrac{\mathcal{E}xy}{\sqrt{\mathcal{E}x^2 \cdot \cancel{\mathcal{E}y^2}}} \cdot \dfrac{\sqrt{\cancel{\mathcal{E}y^2}}}{\sqrt{\mathcal{E}x^2}} = \dfrac{\mathcal{E}xy}{\mathcal{E}x^2}$

therefore $\quad \mathcal{E}(y - y')^2 = \mathcal{E}y^2 - \dfrac{(\mathcal{E}xy)^2}{(\mathcal{E}x^2)^2} \cdot \dfrac{\cancel{\mathcal{E}x^2}}{1}$

$$= \mathcal{E}y^2 - \dfrac{(\mathcal{E}xy)^2}{\mathcal{E}x^2}$$

Figure 3. Corrected power function for the 40-Hz EEG signal is shown at bottom line. It is essentially a covariance analysis, in which the variance of the errors of estimate are determined for the 40-Hz frequency band when the spectral power functions are computer-analyzed.

A high-resolution print-out, shown in Figure 4, compares the corrected spectral-density function for an EEG signal with a spectral function for concurrent muscle. At one-half Hz resolution, it was possible to show clear differences in the spectral density distributions for EEG and muscle when the corrected power function was used for the EEG signal (Sheer 1973).

HIGH RESOLUTION POWER SPECTRA OF O_1-P_3 EEG AND LEFT TEMPORAL MUSCLE

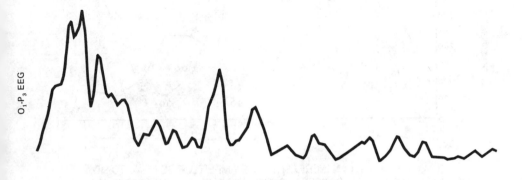

FREQUENCY (IN 58 Hz INTERVALS)

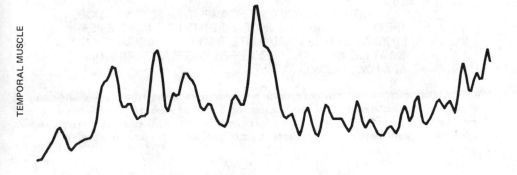

FREQUENCY (IN 58 Hz INTERVALS)

NOTE THE INCREASE IN THE 40 Hz BAND IN THE EEG WITH-OUT A COMPARABLE INCREASE IN THE TEMPORAL MUSCLE

NOTE THE INCREASE IN THE 50 Hz BAND IN BOTH THE EEG AND THE TEMPORAL MUSCLE

Figure 4. High-resolution spectral-density function print-out of concurrent EEG and muscle activity using the FFT digital-computer analysis. Ordinate is relative power; abscissa is the frequency spectrum in one-half Hz intervals.

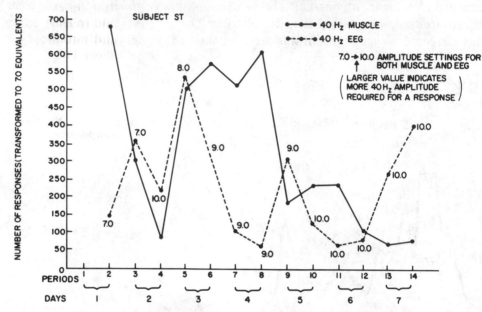

THE COMPARISON OF THE 40Hz MUSCLE AND EEG RESPONSES ACROSS DAYS (TWO PERIODS PER DAY) IN THE COURSE OF CONDITIONING WITH DIFFERENT AMPLITUDE SETTINGS.

WITH AN INCREASE IN THE AMPLITUDE SETTING TO 9.0, THE EEG RESPONSES DECLINE, BUT THE MUSCLE RESPONSES ARE MAINTAINED UNTIL THE EEG RESPONSES SHOW SOME CONDITIONING AT 9.0 WHEN THERE IS A SHARP DROP IN MUSCLE RESPONSES.

WITH AN INCREASE IN THE AMPLITUDE SETTING TO 10.0, THE EEG RESPONSES AGAIN DECLINE WITH THE MUSCLE RESPONSES HOLDING STEADY UNTIL THE EEG SHOWS CONDITIONING AT 10.0 WHILE THE MUSCLE RESPONSES ARE MAINTAINED AT A LOWER LEVEL.

Figure 5. Dissociation of EEG and muscle response during the course of conditioning in one subject. Ordinate represents the number of bursts at each of two 15-minute conditioning periods per day over seven days. It is clear that the EEG and muscle responses do not follow the same pattern with changes in amplitude settings and conditioning.

During the course of conditioning in biofeedback training sessions, learning curves for the EEG and muscle 40-Hz responses, obtained from the comparators, were compared. The EEG leads were a bipolar recording from O_1-P_3 and the muscle leads were a biopolar recording from the neck and temporal muscles on the same side. The responses were corrected 40-Hz bursts, 75 msec in duration, at the same amplitude threshold for both EEG and muscle. Figure 5 shows the learning curves for one subject when the amplitude thresholds were varied during the course of conditioning to emphasize the dissociation of EEG and muscle.

There were two 15-minute conditioning periods per day for seven successive days with the reinforcement contingent on the EEG responses only. At day 3, with an increase in the amplitude threshold from 8.0 to 9.0, there is a decline in EEG responses for three periods until the conditioning effect begins to show up as an increase in responses at the first period on day 5. The muscle responses follow a quite different pattern. Beginning at the second period on day 5, with an increase in amplitude threshold to 10.0, the EEG responses again show a decline for three periods until the conditioning increases the EEG responses for two periods on day 7. The muscle responses do not show the same decline with an amplitude increase to 10.0 on day 5, and actually show a decrease in responses on the two EEG conditioning periods of day 7. The differential pattern of these curves for EEG and muscle obtained with this subject typifies the consistent dissociation between EEG and muscle responses obtained during the course of conditioning with the on-line comparators.

Results

Conditioning and suppression. The data presented here are based on two groups of five adult subjects each who were trained to condition 40 Hz and one group of five who were trained to suppress 40 Hz. All subjects had one baseline session, during which the amplitude thresholds of both the EEG and muscle comparators were adjusted for each individual subject to allow a low to moderate level of EEG operants. They then received eight conditioning or suppression sessions with two 15-minute periods in each session. The subjects were instructed as follows: "The task is to learn to control your own brain waves. The best way to do this is to remain physically relaxed and mentally alert. You will know how well you are succeeding by how many slides you are able to turn on. The money you earn in these sessions will be based on the increased number of slides you turn on and remember, from session to session. After each session you will be asked to describe the slides you saw."

For the conditioning sessions the subjects were told that increases in a brain wave would turn on the slide projector. For the suppression sessions the subjects were told that decreases in a brain wave would keep a tone off, and that for each 30 seconds the tone remained off the slide projector would turn on.

In addition to the digital counts of 40-Hz EEG and muscle bursts, another comparator—set at the same burst duration and amplitude level but with a filter in the frequency range of 21 to 30 Hz—also counted beta bursts.

The EEG leads that were either conditioned or suppressed were O_1-P_3, the muscle leads were from the left neck and temporal muscles, and the beta responses were counted from the same O_1-P_3 leads.

The EEG from the O_1-P_3 leads, left neck and temporal muscle, and triangulated combinations of these were continuously monitored during the conditioning and suppression sessions. An EEG record from a 40-Hz conditioning session and another record from a beta conditioning session are shown in Figure 6. Beta conditioning at 21 to 30 Hz from the O_1-P_3 leads was carried out on additional subjects as control procedures.

In the 40-Hz conditioning session (Figure 6), the first-event pen indicates the occurrence of beta; the second pen, 40 Hz; and the third, muscle. For the 40 Hz on event pen 2 the 60-Hz marker only above the baseline indicates that the 40-Hz EEG is contingent with the 40-Hz muscle and thus not counted. It is only counted when the 60-Hz marker is above and below the line, indicating noncontingency with both 70-Hz EEG and 40-Hz muscle. In the beta conditioning sessions, the first event pen, now a 60-Hz marker, indicates the occurrence of beta; the second pen, muscle.

From the triangulation of these leads it is sometimes possible to infer a more specific locus for muscle bursts or for distinctive trains of the EEG. It is interesting to note that, with the paper speed at 100 mm/sec, it becomes clear that what is being conditioned as beta (21 to 30 Hz) is not "desynchronization" but quite synchronous bursts.

EEG records from the first and seventh suppression sessions are shown in Figure 7. The seventh session is distinctly different from the first, with the appearance of alpha and the absence of 40 Hz, beta, and muscle. Note also the spread of the high-amplitude alpha activity into the muscle leads, NM_L-TM_L. Apparently there can also be EEG artifact when recording muscle activity.

The conditioning data on the ten subjects and suppression data on five subjects are presented in Table 1. With session 1 as a baseline, the percentage changes on 40 Hz, beta, and muscle are shown for these two groups across sessions as a function of conditioning and suppression.

For the 40-Hz conditioning, Friedman signed-ranks analyses of variance with N = 10 were computed. On the 40-Hz EEG there was a significant difference across sessions at .01; on the beta there was a significant difference at .05; on the muscle the difference was not significant.

The same analyses with N = 5 were computed for the 40-Hz suppression. The only significant difference was on the 40 Hz at .05; beta and muscle were not significant.

On the 40-Hz conditioning all ten subjects showed a consistent trend toward conditioning. The group had a 160-percent increase in 40-Hz responses from session 1 to 8. On beta responses there was an increase of 65 percent. On muscle responses the session changes were more variable and the percentage change from session 1 to 8 of 16 percent was not significant.

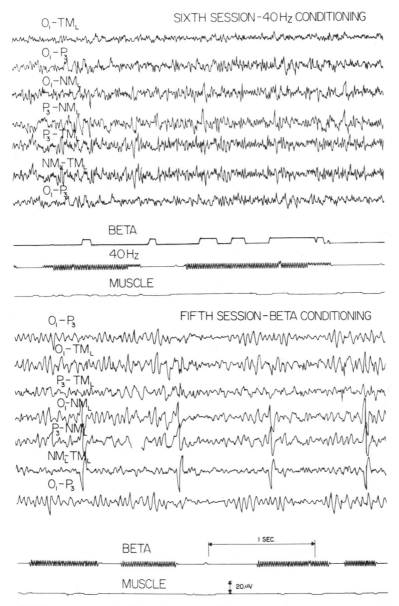

Figure 6. EEG records of 40 Hz and beta conditioning sessions, showing the bipolar leads recorded and three events in the top record and two events in the bottom record, indicating the occurrence of beta, 40 Hz, and muscle from the conditioned bipolar leads, O_1-P_3. NM_L = left neck muscle, TM_L = left temporal muscle. Note that with the paper speed at 100 mm/sec the conditioned beta (21 to 30 Hz) shows up as synchronous bursts instead of desynchronization.

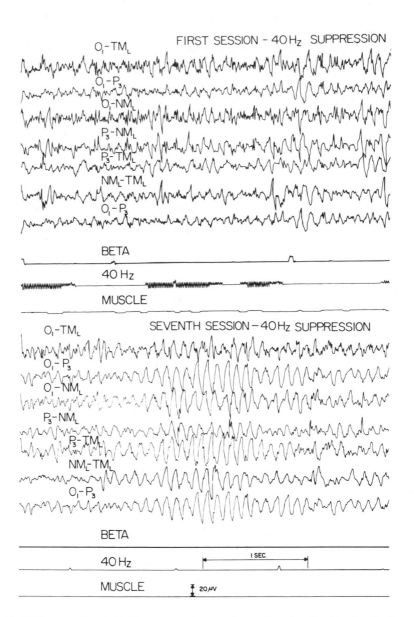

Figure 7. EEG records of 40-Hz suppression sessions, showing the bipolar leads recorded and three events, beta, 40 Hz, and muscle, from the suppressed bipolar leads, O_1-P_3. NM_L = left neck muscle and TM_L = left temporal muscle. Note the marked difference in the record during the seventh suppression session with the presence of alpha and an absence of beta, 40 Hz, and muscle.

TABLE 1.
Percentage Changes in 40 Hz, Beta, and Muscle Responses from Baseline During
the Course of 40-Hz Conditioning and Suppression
(Conditioning N=10; Suppression N=5)

40 Hz-Conditioning

% Changes from Session 1

	Session 1 Means	Session 2	Session 3	Session 4	Session 5	Session 6	Session 7	Session 8
40 Hz	186.4	+6%	+60%	+107%	+97%	+100%	+77%	+160% *
Beta	1017.6	-33%	+33%	+66%	+42%	+20%	+54%	+65% **
Muscle	3191.8	-2%	+.5%	+3%	+8%	+1%	+8%	+16%

40 Hz-Suppression

% Changes from Session 1

	Session 1 Means	Session 2	Session 3	Session 4	Session 5	Session 6	Session 7	Session 8
40 Hz	213.3	-23%	-2%	-3%	-22%	-64%	-75%	-79% **
Beta	1587.6	+10%	+11%	-3%	-14%	-19%	-15%	-18%
Muscle	3538.5	-21%	-34%	-17%	-20%	-17%	-23%	-15%

*significant at .01 level
**significant at .05 level

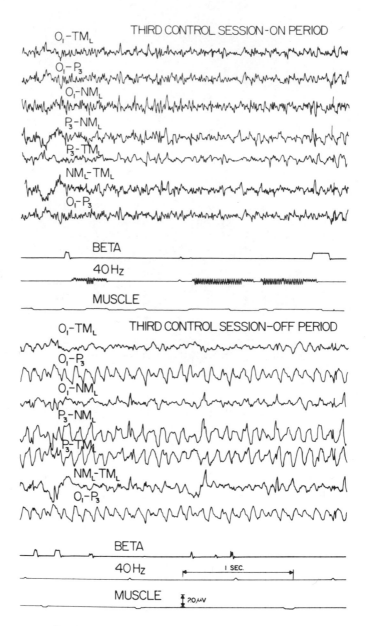

Figure 8. EEG records of alternate 2-minute control sessions in which subjects were required to turn 40 Hz "on" and "off" without reinforcement feedback. Note the absence of 40 Hz during the "off" period and marked presence of alpha with some beta and muscle in the O_1-P_3 lead. During the "on" period there is considerable 40 Hz and little beta.

On the 40-Hz suppression all five subjects showed a consistent trend toward suppression. For the group the percentage decrease was 79 percent on 40 Hz from session 1 to 8, 18 percent on beta, and 15 percent on muscle.

From these data it appears that a high degree of operant control of 40 Hz activity can be achieved by biofeedback training in both conditioning and suppression. With proper controls the conditioning of 40-Hz EEG can be dissociated from muscle activity. There is a significant but low degree of common variance between 40-Hz activity and beta (21 to 30 Hz). The distribution of correlations between 40 Hz and beta for the different sessions, combining conditioning and suppression, generally ranged from .35 to .45, which indicates about a 20 percent common variance. It is understandable that there should be a significant common variance—perhaps larger if error variance were reduced—because beta and 40 Hz represent different aspects or functioning of a common arousal process, diffuse and focused. At the same time it should be recognized that the different functions must have other parameters that are distinct and significant because there is a considerable variance which is not common.

Control testing. From one to three weeks after completion of the conditioning and suppression sessions, control-testing procedures were instituted to examine how much voluntary control the subjects had over the 40-Hz EEG. The test sessions were given once a week and consisted of one 8-minute-45-second warm-up period in which the same reinforcement feedback was provided as in the original conditioning and suppression. This was followed by ten consecutive 2-minute control periods consisting of alternate five "on" periods and five "off" periods, during which reinforcement was not given.

For the conditioning subjects the instructions for the "on" periods were to turn on the brain rhythm that had turned on the slides, and for the "off" periods to turn this brain rhythm off.

For the suppression subjects the instructions for the "on" periods were to turn on the brain rhythm (40 Hz) that kept the slides off. For the "off" periods they were told to turn on the brain rhythm (non-40 Hz) that turned on the slides.

EEG recordings from an "on" period and from the alternate "off" period during the third control session for one subject are shown in Figure 8. Differences between these two records are clearly evident. During the "on" period there is considerable 40 Hz present, little beta, and a good deal of 40-Hz muscle activity from the NM_L-TM_L leads. During the alternate "off" period the EEG picture had changed considerably. There is a complete absence of 40 Hz, about the same beta and less muscle, but now we see a straight run of alpha activity.

The EEG records during the sixth control session for the same subject are shown in Figure 9. Again the differences between alternate "on" and "off" periods are clear. During the "on" period the presence of 40-Hz EEG is strong, with some beta and 40-Hz muscle activity. During the "off" period there is now no 40-Hz EEG or beta, but about the same muscle. The pronounced run of polyphasic muscle activity in the NM_L-TM_L leads, primarily due to the neck muscle, does not appreciably affect the O_1-P_3 EEG leads.

The data on 40 Hz, beta, and muscle responses for one subject, carried through with control-testing sessions from the third to seventh postconditioning week, are shown in Table 2. There is consistent pronounced control over the 40 Hz activity without reinforcement feedback throughout this five-week period. On the 40-Hz EEG the mean for the "on" periods was 37.4 responses, with only two 2-minute periods at zero responses. The mean for the "off" periods was 0.48 responses with 17 out of 25 2-minute periods at zero responses. On beta the mean for the "on" periods was 151.04 responses and the mean for the "off" periods was 55.80 with no zero responses in either period. On muscle activity the mean for the "on" periods was 246.18 responses and the mean for the "off" periods was 180.56, with no zero responses in either period.

For the "on" periods a rank-order correlation (N = 25) between 40-Hz EEG and beta was .22; between 40 Hz EEG and muscle it was -.16; and between beta and muscle it was .34. For the "off" periods the 40-Hz EEG distribution had 19 zeros out of 25 scores and so correlations could not be computed.

On the eighth postconditioning week the subject was given the same control session with the same instructions, but he was also required to solve a series of problems during both the "on" and "off" periods. The subject was instructed, as in the previous five weeks, to turn on brain waves during the 2-minute "on" periods and to turn them off during the 2-minute "off" periods, but now he was also given three problems to solve during each period.

On the ninth postconditioning week the control session was repeated the same as before without problem-solving. The data for the eighth and ninth postconditioning weeks are shown in Table 3.

When the subject was required to solve the series of problems noted in Table 3, he could not turn off the 40 Hz activity as he had done for the previous five weeks and as he successfully did for the ninth postconditioning week without problem-solving. For the eighth postconditioning week the means for 40-Hz EEG were 41.2 responses for the "on" periods and 48.5 for the "off" periods. For the ninth postconditioning week they were 25.8 responses for the "on" periods and 0.4 for the "off" periods.

This experimental situation seems to be very sensitive to behavioral effects on the 40-Hz activity. This subject had achieved quite remarkable

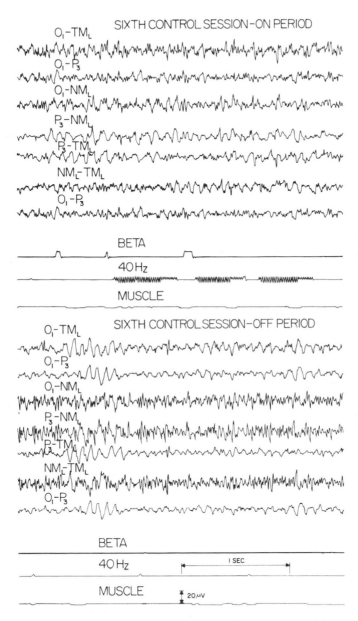

Figure 9. EEG records of alternate 2-minute control sessions in which subjects were required to turn 40 Hz "on" and "off" without reinforcement feedback. Note the absence of beta and 40 Hz during the "off" period and marked neck-muscle artifact which does not show up in the O_1-P_3 leads.

control over his EEG activity on the basis of conditioning and instructional set. He could not maintain this control when given what were apparently conflicting instructions to solve problems.

The voluntary control of 40 Hz activity has generality beyond this one subject. Data are presented in Table 4 for four additional postconditioning subjects and two postsuppression subjects who completed the control testing during the first postconditioning week.

Comparisons between the pairs of alternate "on" and "off" periods for the four postconditioning subjects show a definite trend for a higher level of 40-Hz responding during the "on" periods. However, they also clearly show the important effect of individual differences in motivation level when subjects attempt to maintain voluntary control over their own brain rhythms on the basis simply of instructional set. Subject 1 had a comparatively low level of 40-Hz but was able to maintain the distinction between alternate "on" and "off" periods except for the third pair, where he produced only one response for each period. Subject 4 maintained a consistently strong distinction throughout. Subjects 2 and 3 started out, for the first 3 alternate pairs, with very high levels of 40-Hz responses and clear distinctions between "on" and "off" periods, but they reversed on alternate pairs 4 and 5 and produced high levels of 40-Hz responses during the last "off" period in the session.

The two suppression subjects followed a consistent pattern. As instructed, they were able to suppress 40-Hz responses during all "off" periods as compared with their alternate "on" periods. The mean number of responses during the "off" periods was 0.6; for the "on" periods it was 4.2 responses. These can be compared with the means for the four conditioned subjects for whom the mean was 9.15 for the "off" periods and 33.25 for the "on" periods.

Concomitant behaviors. A number of different behavioral probes were tried in this training series to see what techniques might be effectively used for demonstrating relationships between 40 Hz change and behavior.

One series of measures focused on remembering the slides used as reinforcers. Detailed descriptions of these slides were obtained from subjects after each conditioning session. Quantitative and qualitative categorizations of this descriptive material as related to various measures of 40 Hz change failed to reveal any consistent trends.

Many different forms of self-reports—interviews, Q-sorts, adjective checklists, etc.—have been used with biofeedback training to try to establish connections with psychological variables. In the present series extensive structured and unstructured interviews were conducted with subjects after each conditioning session. From the voluminous material obtained almost any hypothesis could be partially substantiated, depending upon the classifications made and inferences drawn from these classifications.

TABLE 2.
Number of Responses of 40 Hz, Beta, and Muscle for Ten Consecutive
Control Periods of Alternate "On" and "Off"

		On	Off	On	Off	On	Off	On	Off	On	Off
Third post week	40 Hz	41	0	36	2	42	0	0	0	15	0
	Beta	213	24	175	50	111	24	16	33	117	46
	Muscle	273	201	259	217	350	168	216	134	279	182
Fourth post week	40 Hz	0	0	87	0	5	0	41	0	75	0
	Beta	13	7	137	11	33	15	54	7	139	15
	Muscle	290	163	107	109	271	182	109	115	85	208
Fifth post week	40 Hz	52	0	1	0	65	0	27	1	8	2
	Beta	268	155	209	170	167	174	195	203	207	202
	Muscle	273	156	240	216	274	164	169	113	251	270
Sixth post week	40 Hz	57	0	15	1	50	0	46	1	39	3
	Beta	186	11	83	41	219	17	167	39	204	23
	Muscle	240	277	194	195	326	106	286	278	332	258
Seventh post week	40 Hz	37	0	44	1	52	1	35	0	55	0
	Beta	156	32	185	29	172	26	210	17	140	24
	Muscle	307	211	285	135	233	144	287	176	223	136

Note: Subjects were instructed to turn on the brain rhythm that turned the slides on or to keep the rhythm off. Sessions were given once a week after 40-Hz conditioning. Data represent sessions from the third through the seventh post-conditioning weeks for one subject.

TABLE 3.
Number of Responses of 40 Hz, Beta, and Muscle for
Alternate "On" and "Off" Control Periods at Eighth and Ninth Postconditioning Weeks
for Same Subject Shown in Table 2.

	On	Off	On	Off	On	Off	On	Off	On	Off
Eighth post week 40 Hz	35	55	57	43	37	56	46	48	31	40
Beta	150	180	206	139	159	172	168	193	115	166
Muscle	287	226	210	158	293	184	278	276	281	240
Correct answers	2	1	3	1	3	2	1	2	0	1
Test items (N=3 in each period)	verbal analogies		verbal opposites		math. problems		math. problems		ravens matrices	
	On	Off	On	Off	On	Off	On	Off	On	Off
Ninth post week 40 Hz	4	1	27	0	32	1	19	0	47	0
Beta	74	36	102	17	140	30	122	17	158	19
Muscle	269	197	229	184	275	203	230	270	245	203

Note: At the eighth week the subject was also required to solve problems as shown, during both "on" and "off" periods. While solving problems he could not maintain suppression of 40 Hz during "off" periods. At the ninth week, under standard conditions, he again had control of the 40 Hz during "on" and "off" periods.

TABLE 4.
Number of 40-Hz Responses for Alternate "On" and "Off" Control Periods
at First Postconditioning Week for Four Additional 40-Hz-Conditioned
Subjects and Two 40-Hz-Suppressed Subjects

40-Hz Conditioning—First Post Week—40 Hz Bursts

Subjects	On	Off	On	Off	On	Off	On	Off	On	Off
1	13	1	1	0	1	1	4	0	2	1
2	35	13	66	11	86	6	6	15	5	31
3	56	2	72	15	61	5	2	9	20	61
4	30	1	26	2	30	1	22	4	27	4

40-Hz Suppression—First Post Week—40 Hz Bursts

Subjects	On	Off	On	Off	On	Off	On	Off	On	Off
1	0	6	3	4	1	2	1	1	1	2
2	0	4	0	10	0	2	0	5	0	6

Note: Instructions to suppressed subjects during "off" periods were to turn on brain rhythm (non-40 Hz) that kept slides on. During "on" periods they were instructed to turn on brain rhythm (40 Hz) that kept slides off.

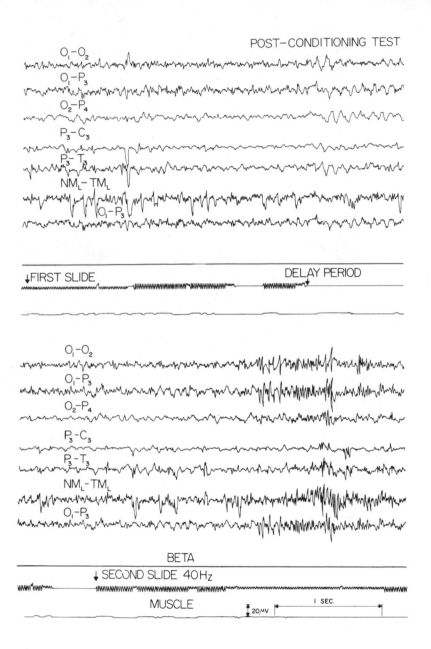

Figure 10. EEG record of a postconditioning test session in which subjects were required to solve problems presented as questions (first slide) and multiple choice answers (second slide). Note the marked occurrence of 40 Hz and the absence of beta with the presentation of the first slide and particularly at the beginning of the second slide in the O_1-P_3 leads. When a large muscle burst occurs with the verbal answer at the end of the second slide in the muscle leads as well as the O_1-P_3 leads, the 40-Hz bursts are not counted on the 40-Hz event pen because of comparator contingencies. Note also that the conditioning of the O_1-P_3 leads does not appear to carry over to the O_2-P_4 leads.

Based on the literature and our previous work on 40 Hz, we set up pre- and postconditioning test sessions on problem-solving tasks for five conditioned subjects. Each test session consisted of 5-minutes pre-baseline, two 10-minute sets of problems, a 10-minute interpolated activity, and 5 minutes post-baseline.

During each 10-minute problem-solving period five test items were presented. Each item consisted of a problem presented on a slide for 30 seconds, followed by a 15-second pause, and then another slide with multiple-choice answers on for 60 seconds. An EEG record of a postconditioning test trial is shown in Figure 10.

For the pre- and postconditioning test sessions, the electrode leads recorded include O_2-P_4, P_3-C_3, and P_3-T_3 to obtain some idea of what spread may have occurred from conditioning the O_1-P_3 leads. As can be seen in the figure, the marked occurrence of 40 Hz in the O_1-P_3 leads toward the end of the first slide and the beginning of the second slide does not generalize to the O_2-P_4 leads on the opposite side and also does not appear to spread in either the P_3-C_3 or P_3-T_3 direction. Of interest is the complete absence of beta even though there is considerable 40 Hz present during this problem-solving situation. Note also the high amplitude polyphasic muscle burst which represents the subject's verbal answer. It spreads into the O_1-P_3 leads, but the 40-Hz EEG event pen does not register any responses because of the comparator contingencies.

The data on 40-Hz responses and test performance, comparing pre- and postconditioning test sessions, are shown in Table 5. The pre- and post-baselines and memory for words were controls for the two problem-solving tasks, modified forms of the Minnesota Paper Form and Differential Aptitude Test. Mean number of 40 Hz responses before and after conditioning showed no significant differences on the baseline and "words" conditions. There were significant mean increases in 40-Hz responses on the two problem tasks, with all five subjects showing a rise during both problem-solving periods. On the test performance measure, that is, the number of correct responses on both sets of problems, there was a significant improvement by all five subjects after conditioning.

The data on behavioral correlates of the 40-Hz EEG appear promising. The results show that, with proper controls, this electrical activity can be conditioned and that some degree of voluntary control can be achieved, although with a good deal of individual variability. The important question still remains: can changes in this brain electrical activity bring along changes in behavior that have sufficient generality and stability to be significant? Systematic behavioral analysis, with a focus on generalization and transfer effects through a range of subject populations, is certainly required before firm conclusions can be drawn.

TABLE 5.
Data on Pre- and Postconditioning Test Sessions for Five
Subjects Conditioned on 40-Hz EEG

Mean number of 40-Hz bursts during baseline and test sessions before and after conditioning for five subjects

	Pre-Baseline	MPFB Problems	DAT Problems	Words	Post-Baseline
Before conditioning	21	37	41	77	58
After conditioning	23	141	158	121	22
Number subjects increasing	2	5	5	3	3

Mean number of correct responses in test sessions before and after conditioning for five subjects

	MPFB Problems	DAT Problems	Words
Before conditioning	2.6	1.6	11
After conditioning	4.0	4.4	16.6
Number subjects improving	5	5	3

Notes: Pre- and post-baseline: Five minutes of EEG recording during rest before and after test sessions. *MPFB problems:* Two equated sets of five items each from the Minnesota Paper Form Board Test, one set given before and another set after conditioning. For each item the problem was presented on a slide for 30 seconds, followed by a 15-second pause, and then followed by a multiple-choice answer slide which was on until the subject answered, or for 60 seconds if there was no answer. Score was the total number of correct answers. *DAT problems:* Two equated sets of five items each from the Differential Aptitude Test, one set given before and another set after conditioning. The procedure was the same as for the first group of problems. Score was the total number of correct answers. *Words:* Thirty words were presented on slides, one word per slide on for one second, with a 15-second pause between slides. Score was the number of words correctly remembered after the session.

Theory

The background for biofeedback training of 40 Hz has been reviewed in the introduction. Briefly, learning and problem-solving behavior must depend on short-term memory processing; and, in turn, memory traces in short-term store—dynamic organizations which are time-dependent, state-dependent, and context-dependent—must take the form of patterned electrical brain activity (Sheer 1970, Sheer 1972). The 40-Hz EEG reflects a state of localized cortical excitability or focused arousal, which is "optimal" for consolidation in short-term store.

There is a unique value in the EEG because it provides an index of the combined activity of masses of cells, and it is precisely this combination that is of major interest in the analysis of molar brain function. The effective use of EEG data lies in synthesizing the framework within which molecular analysis can be carried on, in the fashion that Sherrington reflex physiology provided the essential molar concepts on which the analysis of the electrical properties of the spinal motoneuron has been based. From our correlations between 40 Hz and problem-solving behavior, we can go on to a consideration of the mechanisms for this electrical activity.

The strongest, most pronounced 40 Hz occurs in rhinencephalic structures, particularly the olfactory bulb, through a range of species from catfish to man (Sheer and Grandstaff 1970). At the olfactory bulb the essential and sufficient stimulus is airflow; at the amygdala airflow is essential but a certain level of arousal is also necessary (Pagano 1966, Sheer, Grandstaff, and Benignus 1966); and at prepyriform cortex 40 Hz can be conditioned to neutral stimuli (Freeman 1963). All this is very interesting because in quadruped animals olfaction is a distance receptor, and sniffing—taking in stimuli—is an important orienting response.

In the olfactory bulb laminar structure is first encountered in a much simpler form than in neocortex and an analysis of mechanism should be easier to come by. The evidence is strong that the 40-Hz waves in the olfactory bulb are standing potentials derived from synaptic and postsynaptic events, with the synchrony attributable to successive trains of excitation and recurrent inhibition. The property of recurrent inhibition is essentially negative feedback which functionally contributes to the phasing of rhythmic discharges (Andersen, Eccles, and Loyning 1963; Granit 1963; Eccles 1965; Andersen and Andersen 1968).

Rall and Shepherd (1968) and Shepherd (1970) made an elegant detailed analysis of a dendrodendritic synaptic interaction as a mechanism for this rhythmic activity in the olfactory bulb. Air flow excites bipolar receptor cells in the olfactory mucosa, whose axons form the olfactory nerves synapsing within encapsulated glomeruli with dendrites of tufted and mitral cells.

Impulse discharge in mitral cells results in synaptic excitation of granule cells; these granule cells then deliver graded inhibition to mitral cells. This inhibition cuts off the source of synaptic excitatory input to the granule cells. As the granule-cell activity subsides, the amount of inhibition delivered to the mitral cells is reduced, which permits the mitral cells to respond again to excitatory input from the glomeruli. In this way a sustained excitatory input to the mitral cells would be converted into a rhythmic sequence of excitation followed by inhibition, locked in timing to a rhythmic activation of the granule-cell pool.

At the neocortex there exists a more complicated situation for which details on mechanism are lacking. Stefanis and Jasper (1964) and Jasper and Stefanis (1965) reported that the axon collaterals of cortical pyramidal cells in cats are facilitated at relatively high frequencies of repetitive excitation. The negative feedback of recurrent inhibition provides an automatic control of level of excitation—the greater the excitation, the more the feedback of inhibition.

The point is that the 40-Hz EEG reflects repetitive stimulation at a constant frequency for a limited time over a limited circuitry. The circuitry is defined behaviorally by the spatial-temporal patterning of sensory inputs, motor outputs, and reinforcement contingencies. It is "optimal" for consolidation because repetitive synchronous excitation of cells maximizes the efficiency of synaptic transmission over the limited circuitry.

Eccles (1964) has well documented this property of frequency potentiation by measuring the size of excitatory postsynaptic potentials that develop with repetitive activation at different frequencies. The duration of constant repetitive discharges is probably as significant in the transfer of information as is the intensity of neuronal firing or the number of cells involved. From quantitative studies in the spinal cord, Granit (1963) concluded that frequency of firing was the main code determining rate of continuous discharge in control of tonic motoneurons. At the human somatosensory cortex, Libet et al. (1967) have shown that subthreshold stimulus pulses could elicit conscious sensory experience only if they were delivered repetitively at 20 to 60 pulses per second.

A significant outcome of this feedback loop—wherein frequency potentiation sets up recurrent inhibition which sets up synchrony which sets up frequency potentiation—is the property of contrast. The negative feedback of recurrent inhibition particularly depresses those synapses that are weakly excited in the "surround" and so serves to further sharpen the focus of excitation. Behaviorally it is reflected, on the input side, in sharpening of attention to relevant stimuli and, on the output side, in decreasing extraneous responses and greater precision of relevant movements. The operation of contrast as a function of surround inhibition has been detailed for the somesthetic system (Mountcastle 1961), the visual system (Hubel and Wiesel 1962), and audition (Whitfield 1965).

There is evidence that this repetitive synchronous excitation of cortical cells is dependent upon cholinergic pathways approaching the pyramidal cells of *layer V*. These pathways provide the final stage in the ascending reticular activating system that arises from the tegmental and reticular nuclei of the brain stem (Shute and Lewis 1967). Direct stimulation of the mesencephalic reticular formation enhances the release of acetylcholine and is correlated with an EEG activation pattern (Celesia and Jasper 1966).

With the exception of its nicotinic action on Renshaw cells, acetylcholine's effect on neurons in the cortex is slow in onset and offset, not suitable for rapid "detonation" transmission, but functional in the modulation of the excitability of cortical input cells (Krnjevic 1969). In their early work Dempsey and his colleagues (Chatfield and Dempsey 1942, Morrison and Dempsey 1943) reported that repetitive excitation after single stimulation of a peripheral nerve was greatly increased after application of acetylcholine to the cortex of cats. This work has been extended by Krnjevic and Phillis (1963), who found that acetylcholine enhances rhythmic afterdischarges following sensory volleys, and by Spehlman (1971) who found that it facilitates the firing rate of cortical units activated by reticular stimulation.

Behaviorally, the importance of the reticular activating system in the consolidation process has been detailed by Block and his colleagues (Block 1970). They showed that direct reticular stimulation, when applied immediately after registration of information, considerably facilitates learning; the effect is less when the stimulation is delayed until 90 seconds after the learning trial. In addition, under certain conditions, posttrial reticular stimulation annuls the effect of fluothane anesthesia, which by itself prevents consolidation.

A series of studies has shown further that learning may be impaired by drugs that inhibit and facilitated by drugs that increase acetylcholine action. Atropine blocks the cortical postsynaptic effects of acetylcholine release and induces a slow-wave, high-voltage EEG pattern. Although behaviorally there is no concomitant appearance of drowsiness or sleep, atropine does affect learning. It depressed the performance of learned avoidance responses (Herz 1959) and auditory discrimination learning in rats (Michelson 1961), but, in both studies, only when administered during the early stages of training. Other impaired tasks include successive discrimination learning (Whitehouse 1964) and learned alternation and complex multiple-choice discrimination (Carlton 1963). On the other hand, physostigmine, which increases acetylcholine action, facilitated one-trial avoidance by rats when administered a few minutes before training trials (Bures, Bohdanecky, and Weiss 1962). It also improved the rats' learning of a Lashley III maze when administered 30 seconds after each daily trial (Stratton and Petrinovich 1963). Physostigmine impaired learning in both situations when given in larger doses, which recalls the U-shaped function between activation level and behavioral efficiency.

The network we have woven here is a long way from the correlation between 40-Hz EEG and problem-solving behavior, and its value is primarily heuristic. It makes connections between a number of related research areas in a context that should provide choice points for experimental testing.* The research strategy for such complex functions as memory processing would seem to require a two-step procedure as was followed here: first, to establish correlations between behavior and critical patterns of organized electricity; then, to focus attention on the physical and chemical mechanisms that are the basis for these organizations. The two steps seem required because, on the one hand, units and mechanisms in isolation are unlikely to be directly correlated with the complex behavior represented by memory traces; on the other hand, correlations between behavior and electrical organizations are only a first step toward an analysis of underlying mechanisms.

Summary

A specific pattern of brain electricity, a narrow frequency band centering at 40 Hz, reflects a state of circumscribed cortical excitability or focused arousal which is "optimal" for consolidation in short-term store. On-line control procedures have been developed to reliably record and digitally count this low-amplitude EEG activity independent of muscle artifact.

A high degree of operant control of the 40-Hz EEG can be achieved by biofeedback training in both conditioning and suppression. In control testing sessions following conditioning and suppression training, some degree of voluntary control has been demonstrated when subjects alternately turned the 40 Hz on and off only upon instructional sets. The generality and stability of relationships shown between the conditioned 40-Hz EEG and problem-solving behavior requires further systematic verification.

---

*Work in progress in our laboratory shows a significant spectral coherence, a lock-in at 40 Hz, between mesencephalic reticular and cortical visual and motor areas when the cat is beginning to meet learning criteria in a successive visual discrimination task.

Acknowledgments

Research reported here has been supported, during its equipment development phase, under NASA Grant No. NAS 9-1462. I would like to acknowledge the collaboration of Bruce Bird and Fred Newton, who assumed major responsibility for carrying out training experiments; Dr. Lyllian Hix for the hybrid computer programming; and David Ballard and William Ellis for technical assistance.

References

Andersen, P.O., and Andersen, S.A. 1968. *Physiological Basis of Alpha Rhythm*. New York: Appleton-Century-Crofts.

Andersen, P., Eccles, J.C., and Loyning, Y. 1963. Recurrent inhibition in the hippocampus with identification of the inhibitory cell and its synapses. *Nature* 198:540.

Banquet, J.P. 1973. Spectral analysis of the EEG in meditation. *Electroencephalogr. Clin. Neurophysiol.* 35:143.

Barber, T., DiCara, L.V., Kamiya, J., Miller, N.E., Shapiro, D., and Stoyva, J. (eds.) 1971a. *Biofeedback and Self-Control*. Chicago: Aldine-Atherton.

Barber, T., DiCara, L.V., Kamiya, J., Miller, N.E., Shapiro, D., and Stoyva, J. (eds.) 1971b. *Biofeedback and Self-Control 1970*. Chicago: Aldine-Atherton.

Beatty, J.T. 1971. Effects of initial alpha wave abundance and operant training procedures on occipital alpha and beta activity. *Psychonom. Sci.* 23:197.

Beatty, J.T. 1972. Similar effects of feedback signals and instructional information on EEG activity. *Physiol. and Behav.* 9:151.

Beatty, J. Greenberg, A., Derbler, W.P., and O'Hanlon, J.F. 1974. Operant control of occipital theta rhythm affects performance in a radar monitoring task. *Science* 183:871.

Black, A.H. 1971. The direct control of neural processes by reward and punishment. *Am. Sci.* 59:238.

Black, A.H. 1972. The operant conditioning of central nervous system electrical activity. In G.H. Bower (ed.), *The Psychology of Learning and Motivation: Advances in Research and Theory*, p. 47. New York: Academic Press.

Block, V. 1970. Facts and hypotheses concerning memory consolidation processes. *Brain Res.* 24:561.

Brown, B.B. 1970. Recognition of aspects of consciousness through association with EEG alpha activity represented by a light signal. *Psychophysiology* 6:442.

Bures, J., Bohdanecky, Z., and Weiss, T. 1962. Physostigmine induced hippocampal theta activity and learning in rats. *Psychopharmacologia* 3:254.

Butler, F., and Stoyva, J. 1973. *Biofeedback and Self-Regulation: A Bibliography*. Denver, Col.: Biofeedback Research Society.

Carlton, P.L. 1963. Cholinergic mechanisms in the control of behavior by the brain. *Psychol. Rev.* 70:19.

Chaffin, D.B. 1969. Surface electromyography frequency analysis as a diagnostic tool. *J. Occup. Med.* 11:109.

Chatfield, P.O., and Dempsey, E.W. 1942. Some effects of prostigmine and acetylcholine on cortical potentials. *Am. J. Physiol.* 135:633.

Celesia, G.G., and Jasper, H.H. 1966. Acetylcholine released from cerebral cortex in relation to state of activation. *Neurology* 16:1053.

Das, N.N., and Gastaut, H. 1955. Variations de l'activité electrique du cerveau, du coeur et des muscles squelcttiques au cours de la méditation et de l'extase yogique. *Electroencephalogr. Clin. Neurophysiol.* Suppl. 6:211.

Dumenko, V.N. 1961. Changes in the electroencephalogram of the dog during formation of a motor conditioned reflex stereotype. *Pavlov Journal of Higher Nervous Activity* 11:64.

Eccles, J.C. 1964. *The Physiology of Synapses.* New York: Springer-Verlag.

Eccles, J.C. 1965. The control of neuronal activity by postsynaptic inhibitory action. *23rd International Congress of Physiological Sciences*, p. 84. Amsterdam: Excerpta Medica Foundation.

Freeman, W.J. 1963. The electrical activity of a primary sensory cortex: Analysis of EEG waves. *Int. Rev. Neurobiol.* 5:53.

Galambos, R. 1958. Electrical correlates of conditioned learning. In M. Brazier (ed.), *The Central Nervous System and Behavior*, p. 375. New York: Josiah Macy, Jr. Foundation.

Galin, D., and Ornstein, R. 1972. Lateral specialization of cognitive mode: An EEG study. *Psychophysiology* 9:412.

Giannitrapani, D. 1969. EEG average frequency and intelligence. *Electroencephalogr. Clin. Neurophysiol.* 27:480.

Granit, R. 1963. Recurrent inhibition as a mechanism of control. In A. Moruzzi, A. Fessard, and H.H. Jasper (eds.), *Brain Mechanisms*, vol. I, *Progress in Brain Research*, p. 23. New York: Elsevier.

Green, E.E., Green, A., and Walter, E.D. 1972. Biofeedback for mind-body self-regulation: Healing and creativity. *Fields Within Fields . . . Within Fields* 25:131.

Herz, A. 1959. Effects of atropine on early stages of learning in the rat. *Arch. Exp. Pathol. Pharmacol.* 236:110.

Hubel, D.H. and Wiesel, T.N. 1962. Receptive fields, binocular interaction and functional architecture in the cat's visual cortex. *J. Physiol.* 160:106.

Jasper, H. and Stefanis, C. 1965. Intracellular oscillatory rhythms in pyramidal tract neurones in the cat. *Electroencephalogr. Clin. Neurophysiol.* 18:541.

Killam, K.F. and Killam, E.K. 1967. Rhinencephalic activity during acquisition and performance of conditional behavior and its modification by pharmacological agents. In W.R. Adey and T. Tokizane (eds.), *Progress in Brain Research*. vol. 27, *Structure and Function of the Limbic System*, p. 338. New York: Elsevier.

Krnjevic, K. 1969. Central cholinergic pathways. *Fed. Proc.* 28:113.

Krnjevic, K., and Phillis, J.W. 1963. Acetylcholine-sensitive cells in the cerebral cortex. *J. Physiol.* 166:296.

Libet, B., Alberts, W.W., Wright, E.W., Jr., and Feinstein, B. 1967. Responses of human somatosensory cortex to stimuli below threshold for conscious sensation. *Science* 158:1597.

Michelson, M.J. 1961. Effects of atropine on an auditory discrimination task in the rat. *Activatis Nervosa Superior* 3:140.

Morrell, F. 1961. Lasting changes in synaptic organization produced by continual neuronal bombardment. In J.F. Delefresnaye (ed.), *Brain Mechanisms and Learning*. p. 91. Oxford: Blackwell.

Morrell, F., and Jasper, H.H. 1956. Electrographic studies of the formation of temporary connections in the brain. *Electroencephalogr. Clin. Neurophsyiol.* 8:201.

Morrison, R.S., and Dempsey, E.W. 1943. Mechanisms of thalmocortical augmentation and repetition. *Am. J. Physiol.* 138:297.

Mountcastle, V.B. 1961. Duality of function in the somatic afferent system. In M.A. Brazier (ed.), *Brain and Behavior*, vol. 1, p. 67. Washington, D.C.: American Institute of Biological Sciences.

Mulholland, T. 1968. Feedback electroencephalography. *Activitas Nervosa Superior* 10:4.

Mulholland, T., and Peper, E. 1971. Occipital alpha and accommodative vergence, pursuit tracking and fast eye movements. *Psychophysiology* 8:556.

Nowlis, D.P. and Kamiya, J. 1970. The control of electroencephalographic alpha rhythm through auditory feedback and the associated mental activity. *Psychophysiology* 6:496.

Pagano, R.R. 1966. The effects of central stimulation and nasal airflow on induced activity of olfactory structures. *Electroencephalogr. Clin. Neurophysiol.* 21:269.

Peper, E. 1971. Comment on feedback training of parietal-occipital alpha asymmetry in normal and human subjects. *Kybernetik* 9:156.

Peper, E. 1972. Localized EEG alpha feedback training: A possible technique for mapping subjective, conscious, and behavioral experiences. *Kybernetik* 11:166.

Pribram, K.H., Spinelli, D.N., and Kamback, M.C. 1967. Electrocortical correlates of stimulus response and reinforcement. *Science* 157:94.

Rall, W., and Shepherd, G.M. 1968. Theoretical construction of field potentials and dendrodentritic synaptic interactions in the olfactory bulb. *J. Neurophysiol.* 6:884.

Rowland, V. 1958. Discussion under electroencephalographic studies of conditioned learning. In M. Brazier (ed.), *The Central Nervous System and Behavior*, p. 347. New York: Josiah Macy, Jr. Foundation.

Sakhiulina, G.T. 1961. EEG manifestations of tonic cortical activity accompanying conditioned reflexes. *Pavlov Journal of Higher Nervous Activity* 11:48.

Shapiro, D., Barber, T.X., DiCara, L.V., Kamiya, J., Miller, N.E., and Stoyva, J. (eds.) 1973. *Biofeedback and Self-Control 1972*. Chicago: Aldine-Atherton.

Sheer, D.E. 1970. Electrophysiological correlates of memory consolidation. In A. Ungar (ed.), *Molecular Mechanisms in Memory and Learning*, p. 177. New York: Plenum Press.

Sheer, D.E. 1972. Neurobiology of memory storage processes. *Winter Conference on Brain Research*, Vail, Colorado.

Sheer, D.E. 1973. Biofeedback training of 40 Hertz in animals and man. *Symposium on Learned Control of Brain Rhythms*, American Psychological Association, Montreal, Canada.

Sheer, D.E. 1974. Electroencephalographic studies in learning disabilities. In H. Eichenwald and A. Talbot (eds.), *The Learning Disabled Child*. Austin: University of Texas Press.

Sheer, D.E., and Grandstaff, N.W. 1970. Computer-analysis of electrical activity in the brain and its relation to behavior. In H.T. Wycis (ed.), *Current Research in Neurosciences*, vol. 10, *Topical Problems in Psychiatry and Neurology*, p. 160. New York:

Karger.

Sheer, D.E., Grandstaff, N.W., and Benignus, V.A. 1966. 40 c/sec electrical activity in the brain of the cat. *Symposium on Higher Nervous Activity*, Fourth World Congress on Psychiatry, Madrid, Spain.

Sheer, D.E., and Hix, L. 1971. Computer-analysis of 40 Hz EEG in normal and MBI children. *Society of Neurosciences Meeting*, Washington, D.C.

Shepherd, G.M. 1970. The olfactory bulb as a sample cortical system: Experimental analysis and function implications. In F.O. Schmidt (ed.), *The Neurosciences, Second Study Program*, p. 539. New York: Rockefeller Press.

Shute, C.C.D., and Lewis, P.R. 1967. The ascending cholinergic reticular system: Neocortical, olfactory and subcortical projections. *Brain* 90:497.

Spehlman, R. 1971. Acetylcholine and the synaptic transmission of non-specific impulses to the visual cortex. *Brain* 94:139.

Stefanis, C., and Jasper, H. 1964. Recurrent collateral inhibition in pyramidal tract neurons. *J. Neurophysiol.* 27:855.

Sterman, M.B. 1972. Studies of EEG biofeedback training in man and cats. *Highlights of 17th Annual Conference: VA Cooperative Studies in Mental Health and Behavioral Sciences*, Washington, D.C.: Veterans Administration.

Sterman, M.B., MacDonald, L.R., and Stone, R.K. 1974. Biofeedback training of the sensorimotor EEG rhythms in man: Effects on epilepsy. *Epilepsia* (in press).

Stoyva, J., Barber, T.X., DiCara, L.V., Kamiya, J., Miller, N.E., and Shapiro, D. (eds.) 1972. *Biofeedback and Self-Control 1971*. Chicago: Aldine-Atherton.

Stratton, L.O., and Petrinovich, L. 1963. Post-trial injections of an anti-cholinesterase drug and maze learning in two strains of rats. *Psychopharmacologia* 5:47.

Whitehouse, J. 1964. Effects of atropine on discrimination learning in the rat. *J. Comp. Physiol. Psychol.* 57:13.

Whitfield, J.C. 1965. "Edges" in auditory information processing. In *23rd International Congress of Physiological Sciences*, p. 245. Amsterdam: Excerpta Medica Foundation.

the influences of impressed electrical fields at eeg frequencies on brain and behavior

W.R. Adey, M.D.

Departments of Anatomy and Physiology
and Brain Research Institute
University of California
Los Angeles, California

In the search for functional correlates of information processing in brain tissue, early interest in the electroencephalogram proved disappointing. Although phenomena such as blocking of the alpha rhythm with eye closing and visual attention (Berger 1929, Adrian 1947) were quickly recognized, it has remained for much later studies with sophisticated computer analyses and pattern-recognition techniques to reveal EEG correlates of decision-making (Elazar and Adey 1967; Hanley, Walter, Rhodes, and Adey 1968), of psychological stress in hostile questioning (Berkhout, Walter, and Adey 1969), and of difficult perceptual tasks (Walter, Kado, Rhodes, and Adey 1967). Even though the latter studies have revealed EEG signatures for groups of subjects as well as for individuals, clear evidence has been lacking that would assign a causal role to the EEG in information processing. Indeed, it has been widely considered as a "noise" in cerebral tissue, having no direct physiological role, even though it could be correlated with specific behavioral states, including the brief epochs that accompany decision-making and perception, and even though these correlates might be reliable indicators of quite subtle differences, such as correct versus incorrect task performance at a later time (Hanley, Walter, Rhodes, and Adey 1968), or of opening versus closing of the hand in a phantasied motor performance (Nirenberg, Hanley, and Stear 1971).

How, then, may we proceed further to answer the question of a possible physiological role for the EEG in brain tissue? Do brain cells sense such field potentials as the EEG, and is their excitability in the genesis of propagated action potential modified thereby? What experimental paradigms and criteria should be used in testing for possible interactions between brain cells and extracellular fields? Very importantly, are there conditions in the anatomical and physiological organization of brain tissue that might make possible interactions with weak intrinsic or environmental electric fields in the aggregate behavior of a domain of elements, and thus preclude observation of these effects in so-called simpler systems?

There is a kinship with Heisenberg's uncertainty principle, not so much in the effects of measurement on the system being measured, but in the effects of experimental isolation of a tissue or its cellular elements in the hope that we may then better discern certain properties, which in fact may be miniscule properties of individual elements, but substantive in systems as a whole. In other words, complexity of cerebral tissue may be an inherent and essential quality.

Classical neuroanatomy and neurophysiology, and particularly synaptic neurophysiology, have drawn heavily on simple systems. Their exponents have often argued vociferously that spinal motoneurones, Aplysian ganglion cells, or cerebellar Purkinje cells are appropriate models in which to study the intrinsic processes unique to cerebral tissue in transaction, storage, and recall of information. The disappointing but inescapable conclusion that we are rapidly approaching an impasse in following cerebral models that consider only synaptic mechanisms and axonal connectivity should invite our attention to all the possible ways in which interactions may occur in cerebral tissue.

My colleagues and I have observed the effects of weak electric and electromagnetic fields on the behavior of man and animals, and we have correlated these observations with neurophysiological effects and brain chemistry. The most striking conclusion drawn from these observations is that mammalian central nervous functions can be modified by electrical gradients in cerebral tissue substantially less than those known to occur in postsynaptic excitation, and also substantially smaller than those presumed to occur with inward membrane currents at synaptic terminals in release of transmitter substances.

Neither these observations nor models of cerebral organization that arise from them are nihilistic to the impressive body of synaptic physiology. Rather, they invite consideration of hierarchies of excitatory organization in which synaptic mechanisms represent but one level.

Brain as a Tissue in Information Processing

No longer is information processing in brain tissue considered to involve only the nerve cells. In the past 25 years much new knowledge indicates strong physiological interactions between neurons and neuroglial cells. Concurrent electrical changes in neuronal and cortical "silent" cells, presumed to be neuroglia, have been noted in evoked potentials and seizure activity (Karahashi and Goldring 1966). Simultaneous and sometimes reciprocal changes in neurons and neuroglia have been physiologically induced in a variety of biochemical measures, including enzyme activity and protein synthesis (Hydén 1972). The inhibitory transmitter, gamma-aminobutyric acid (GABA) appears in cerebellar neuroglial cytoplasm but is difficult to detect in cerebellar neurons (Henn and Hamberger 1971). In the retina, glycine and GABA are taken up by neurons (Ehinger and Falck 1971) whereas glutamic acid, aspartic acid, and taurine are taken up by neuroglial cells (Ehinger 1973). By light microscopy, staining for calcium in hippocampal neuronal cytoplasm is low, but appreciable in neuroglia (Tarby and Adey 1968, Adey 1970). These few examples emphasize the sensitive interactions between these two cellular compartments.

Clearly, these interactions occur across the intervening intercellular space. Although only a small extracellular space can be detected in electron micrographs of cerebral tissue fixed with osmic acid, use of rapid freezing techniques by van Harreveld and his colleagues revealed a space of approximately 20 percent (van Harreveld, Crowell, and Malhotra 1965), a size confirmed in biochemical estimates (Reed, Woodbury, and Holtzer 1964). The space is occupied by highly hydrated macromolecular material forming a loose "fuzz" (Figure 1). Although polyanionic in character, it binds strongly to acidic solutions of phosphotungstic acid (Pease 1966, Rambourg and Leblond 1967). Despite its loose structure, this intercellular material appears to blend with other macromolecular material, glycoprotein in nature, forming the outer coats or "glycocalyces" of cell membranes (Bennett 1963). Weak electric currents, as used in impedance measurements in cerebral tissue, pass through the extracellular space as a preferred pathway, so that only a small portion of any extracellular current penetrates either neuronal or neuroglial membranes (Cole 1940). Extracellular fluid has a specific resistance of approximately 4 Ω cm, as compared with typical membrane resistances for neurons and neuroglial cells of the order of 5000 Ω cm^{-2} (Coombs, Curtis, and Eccles 1959; Nicholls and Kuffler 1964). Since impedance measurements therefore appear to primarily reflect conductance in the extracellular space, it is noteworthy that conductance changes in cortical and subcortical structures accompany a variety of learned responses, suggesting that the cell surfaces and intercellular macromolecular material may be one site of structural change in information storage and its retrieval (Adey, Kado, and Didio 1962; Adey et al. 1963 and 1966). As discussed below, this region of brain tissue may have other quite special functions in sensing and transducing weak chemical and electrical events at the membrane surface (Schmitt and Samson 1969, Adey 1973).

The hypothesis has been advanced elsewhere (Adey and Walter 1963, Adey 1972) that there may be an association between the characteristic phenomenon of overlapping dendritic fields in palisades of cells that characterize all vertebrate cerebral ganglia, and the concurrent development of a rhythmic electric wave process which may be fundamentally related to the ability of these tissues to undergo permanent changes in excitability as a

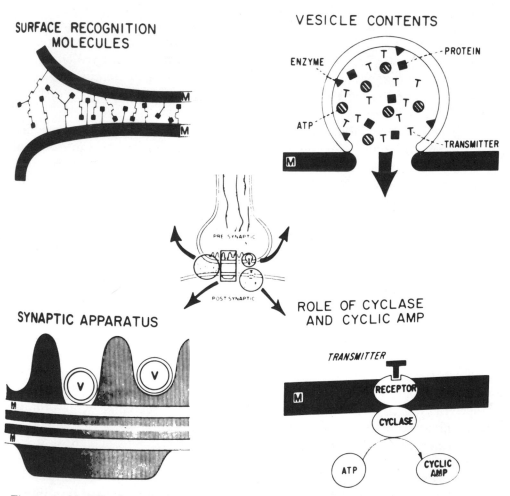

Figure 1. Models of presynaptic and postsynaptic membrane interfaces, with "surface recognition molecules" in the intercellular space. (From Schmitt and Samson 1969)

result of their prior participation in specified patterns of excitation. There is a noteworthy absence of dendritic overlap in such "nonlearning" structures as the spinal cord, and the slow components of spinal-cord electrical activity appear essentially irregular (Gasteiger 1959). Electron microscopy has confirmed that dendritic overlap in cerebral structures is indeed the basis of junctional contacts between dendritic branches of adjacent neurons (Rall et al. 1966) and that pre- and postsynaptic fine structures occur in these junctions (Pasik et al. 1973). This dendritic organization seems to constitute a specific arrangement in cerebral tissue, and it is discussed further below.

How May Information Be Processed in Brain Tissue?

Neurons in the central nervous system are activated synaptically by axon terminals bearing volleys of impulses that may arise in distant structures or from nearby regions. Fiber conduction and synaptic activation are clearly essential elements in brain function.

On the other hand, there are at least three other modes of information handling in cerebral neurons that deserve equivalent attention. They include dendrodendritic conduction, neuronal-neuroglial interactions across the intercellular space, and the sensing of weak stimuli that modify the immediate environment of the neuron. The last class would include sensitivity to weak electric (and perhaps magnetic) fields, and to minute amounts of chemical substances, including drugs, hormones, and neurohumors. Susceptibility of brain tissue to such drugs as LSD in body fluid concentrations of 10^{-9} (Adey, Bell, and Dennis 1962) are well known and generally accepted. Hormone concentrations that predictably modify brain function are even lower. It is therefore surprising that such scant consideration has been given to the possibility that brain tissue may be sensitive to field potentials in the environment of the neuron, including the intrinsic fields of the EEG. Our reluctance to proceed with studies that might reveal these sensitivities is understandable, however, as long as our viewpoint remains focused on classical synaptic pathways as the sole and sufficient mechanisms of cerebral neuronal interaction.

As a point of departure in our consideration of the possible functional role of cerebral field potentials, we may briefly review current knowledge on the genesis of the EEG. Intracellular records from cortical neurons have revealed waves with amplitudes up to 20 mV that resemble the EEG from the same region in their frequency characteristics (Creutzfeldt et al. 1964; Elul 1965, 1967a, 1972; Fujita and Sato 1964). Components of evoked field potentials have also been correlated with membrane potential deflections in intracellular records (Elul and Adey 1965; Creutzfeldt, Watanabe, and Lux 1966; Purpura, Shofer, and Musgrave 1964). Elul

(1967a) has investigated relationships between these neuronal waves and the EEG, concluding that in normal cerebral tissue the neuronal wave is only coherent with the gross EEG at chance levels. Moreover, the EEG appears to be the summed contribution of waves from many neuronal generators, with volume conduction through the extracellular medium. Thus, about 100 microvolts of signal would be contributed to the volume conductor by a neuronal wave 10 millivolts in amplitude in intracellular records. Elul (1962) has shown that the EEG maintains this general amplitude with recording dipoles progressively reduced to cellular dimensions.

How, then, could such a weak extracellular field influence neuronal excitability? A typical depolarization of at least several millivolts is necessary with a membrane potential of 50 mV in order to initiate a propagated spike discharge. Nevertheless, comparably small field gradients significantly alter firing thresholds in spinal motoneurones (Nelson 1966). Clearly, a mechanism of "membrane amplification" could be hypothesized that would account for sensing these effects. As a working model, let us consider some of the possible sequences of events in activation of a domain of cortical neurons.

We may assume that neuronal spikes would be generated in the axon hillock of the neuronal soma and pass by short axons or axon collaterals to adjacent neurons in the same "domain," here considered to be a group of several hundred cells (Anninos et al. 1970). In a similar fashion, interdendritic connections would provide paths for the spread of slower neuronal wave activity generated in the dendrites and which might sweep longitudinally toward the soma (Green et al. 1960). Jointly these processes would generate an EEG in the enclosing extracellular space. A system of macromolecular sensors on the membrane surface might transduce components of the extracellular field by altered ion binding and an associated conformation change. This altered membrane surface would then trigger a transmembrane amplification in ionic movements, thus modifying the initial events mediated by neuronal slow waves and concurrent membrane potential changes induced by synaptic activation. Parenthetically, it is not yet clear whether intracellular waves in cerebral neurons arise from postsynaptic potentials or relate to membrane oscillations of a different kind, perhaps in partially depolarized dendrites.

We may summarize this working model:

Slow waves (dendrites)	Activation of neuronal
Spike generation (soma)	domain
Membrane amplification	
Membrane macromolecular	
sensors	Genesis of EEG

Clearly, such a model is hierarchically organized. Molecular events at the membrane surface would influence the excitability of a particular neuron. In turn, this neuron would influence others in its domain through conduction processes. Joint activity of other neurons would produce a volume-conducted field through the domain. In turn, this field would again modify the environment at each neuronal surface. It is noteworthy that this field is an "enchanted loom" when recorded at cellular dimensions, showing great differences and complexities in adjoining tripolar records along different electrical axes (Elul 1962).

To be useful, such a model must be necessary and sufficient to explain phenomena not adequately accounted for by other schemes. The following observations of central nervous interactions with weak electric and electromagnetic fields invite serious consideration of this type of model, since they occur at energy levels far below those seen in classical synaptic activation. In turn, these observed field effects will lead to a more detailed consideration of membrane surface phenomena that might be involved.

Effect of Low-Level, Low-Frequency Electric Fields
on EEG and Behavior

Relatively little research has been conducted on the effects of weak environmental electric fields on behavior or brain electrical patterns in man or animals. Wever (1968) exposed human subjects to 10-Hz fields with an electric gradient of 2.5 volts/meter. Their patterns of circadian rhythms were measured from sleep-wake cycles and from peaks and troughs in diurnal temperature cycles. After 7 to 10 days of control measurements, the fields were activated for an approximately equal period. During field exposure, the circadian rhythms were shortened by 1 to 2 hours in many subjects. About the same time, studies in our laboratory by Hamer (1968) and elsewhere by König and Ankermüller (1960) showed changes in human reaction times with low-level fields between 5 and 15 Hz.

Pilot studies in our laboratory suggested that subjective estimates of the passage of time in man are influenced by these fields. A more detailed study was therefore undertaken of time estimation in the presence of weak electric fields in the pigtail macaque monkey (Gavalas et al. 1970). Scheduling of reinforcements for a simple lever-press can alter an animal's rate of response, or the timing of that response, or both. Our monkeys were therefore trained to press a lever in a fixed-interval schedule of reinforcement. The animal was gradually conditioned to wait 5 sec between presses, and to press within a 2.5-sec reward-enable interval. If the animal pressed within the specified time interval, he was rewarded with apple juice. Bar presses that were too early or too late were not rewarded, and the timer was then recycled to the start of another 5-sec interval. Trained animals performed with an accuracy of 70 to 80 percent, and performance was relatively stable from day to day.

In this initial study EEG recording electrodes were placed in structures in which it was intuitively anticipated that changes in EEG records might be induced by the fields. They included the hippocampus, the amygdala, the nucleus centrum medianum, and the visual cortex.

Three trained animals were exposed to the fields for 4 hours each day. The fields were applied to two large metal plates 50 cm square and 40 cm apart, so that the animal's head was completely within the field. Field amplitude was 2.8 volts peak-to-peak (p-p). Each monkey was tested in two experiments of 20 exposures to 7-Hz fields and two comparable control experiments without fields. Two of the three monkeys were also tested twice with 10-Hz fields and in two control series without the fields. Daily tests for 4 hours with fields on were randomly interspersed with 4-hour daily control runs without fields.

Behavioral effects of low-frequency fields. Consistent differences in interresponse time distributions were observed in the 7-Hz experiments, but the 10-Hz field failed to produce reliable changes in behavior. For one animal the mean interresponse time (IRT) was unchanged by the 10-Hz field in the first experiment of 20 tests, and the responses were slightly faster (but not significantly so) in the replication. In another animal IRTs were faster in the first 10-Hz experiment and slower in the second.

With 7-Hz fields, however, quite large and consistent shifts in IRTs were observed in all three animals (Figure 2). Animal Z showed a shortening of the 5-sec estimate by 0.5 sec in both first and second experiments. These differences were highly significant statistically ($p = 0.001$ or better). In animal J, the mean IRT shifted significantly in the direction of faster responses in the first experiment, but the difference was not replicated in the second experiment. Animal A, like animal Z, showed a statistically significant shift to faster responses in both experiments. The proportion of correct responses did not shift significantly with fields on for monkeys J and Z, but monkey A, which had a large number of very long IRTs in the fields-off condition, showed gains of 16 percent correct and 21 percent correct when the fields were on.

In summary, five of the six experiments showed a shift to significantly faster interresponse times in the 7-Hz fields compared with performance in the absence of fields. All these mean differences were 0.4 sec or greater. Shifts in model values also occurred in all five experiments and were all 0.2 sec or greater. As shown in Figure 2, the total output of responses and the variability of those responses differed considerably from monkey to monkey. Nevertheless, the trend to shorten IRTs in the presence of the fields was remarkably consistent, and the size of the shift was relatively large.

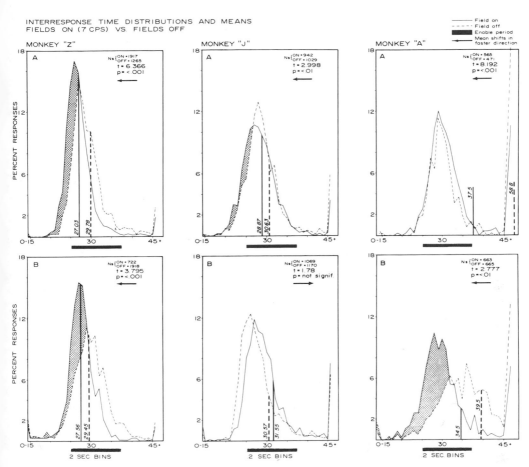

Figure 2. Behavioral data showing shifts in interresponse time under 7-Hz fields. The abscissa shows time between responses in 0.2-sec bins; the ordinate shows percentage of total responses at each interval. Note that only bins 15 to 45 are plotted; bins 0 to 144 were used in calculation of means and standard deviations. (From Gavalas, Walter, Hamer, and Adey 1970)

These initial findings have been confirmed and extended in further experiments with five monkeys. We have tested the effects of fields at 7, 10, 45, 60, and 75 Hz, at gradients ranging from 10 to 100 volts/meter. These later studies have indicated that higher voltage gradients decrease variability in IRTs, and that a threshold for altered IRTs may be in the range of 1 to 10 volts/meter. Moreover, effects at higher frequencies, including 60 Hz, were first seen with fields of 60 to 100 volts/meter, as a decreased variability in IRTs. Since questions of antenna effects with implanted electrodes that might produce a focal field enhancement within the tissue have been widely raised, it is noteworthy that these thresholds and frequency differentials show close similarity between unimplanted and implanted subjects (Tables 1 and 2). Thus it seems clear that the field is sensed directly by the organism without intercurrent effects attributable to an implanted electrode system.

TABLE 1. Unimplanted Monkey

ANIMAL C HIGH VOLTAGE (56 V/m)

Rank-Order Weighted Mean Interresponse Times
(last bin excluded)

Entire Experiment			Hour 1			Hour 2			Hour 3		
Hz	V/m	x̄IRT	Hz	V/m	x̄IRT	Hz	V/m	x̄IRT	Hz	V/m	x̄IRT
7	56	5.347	7	56	5.440	7	56	5.697	75	56	5.659
75	56	5.576	75	56	5.498	75	56	5.922	60	56	5.784
60	56	5.756	60	56	5.698	0	0	5.976	7	56	5.819
0	0	5.960	0	0	5.883	60	56	5.987	0	0	6.121

TABLE 2. Unimplanted Monkey

ANIMAL C HIGH VOLTAGE (56 V/m)

Rank-Order Weighted Standard Deviations
(last bin excluded)

Entire Experiment			Hour 1			Hour 2			Hour 3		
Hz	V/m	x̄IRT	Hz	V/m	x̄IRT	Hz	V/m	x̄IRT	Hz	V/m	x̄IRT
75	56	0.796	75	56	0.714	0	0	0.872	75	56	0.814
60	56	0.897	7	56	0.821	7	56	0.929	60	56	0.858
7	56	0.913	60	56	0.826	75	56	1.050	0	0	0.943
0	0	1.016	0	0	1.027	60	56	1.081	7	56	1.039

Electrophysiological effects of low-frequency fields. EEG records during field exposure were not markedly changed by the fields. Spectral density plots revealed small peaks in power in some brain structures at the field frequency, for epochs of predominantly incorrect responses near the end of the four-hour run. The effect of the imposed field on EEG power was further tested by a special statistical test to which we have applied the term *peak quotient* (Gavalas et al. 1970). This test considers the relationship of the EEG spectral plot to a logarithmic distribution over the frequency range of 4 to 20 Hz, since the spectral curve of the EEG in this frequency range closely approximates an exponential shape in many brain structures in the absence of fields. Activity contributed by this field would then be a peak above the line containing those points not at the field frequency or its harmonics. Peak quotients for these peaks were compared by t-tests for EEG epochs in fields-on vs. fields-off conditions, for the three monkeys J, Z, and

A, and for each brain structure (Table 3). In animal J, significant differences were observed in the left and right hippocampi, and in the right amygdala for both 7- and 10-Hz fields. Animal A was tested only with 7-Hz fields and showed differences significant at the 0.01 probability level in both hippocampi and in the left nucleus centrum medianum. Its EEG records while sitting quietly prior to training were also evaluated. Again, differences for peak quotients for 7-Hz fields-on vs. fields-off records were observed in four of six structures tested: right nucleus centrum medianum, left amygdala, and both hippocampi.

TABLE 3. EEG Peak Quotients—Fields On vs. Fields Off
Probability of Observed Differences (t-tests)

Performing DRL task. 80-second segments near end of the 4-hour runs. Combined data from two experimental-control runs.		7 Hz on vs. off	10 Hz on vs. off
Monkey J	left hippocampus	$p = .048$	$p = .025$
	right hippocampus	$p = .001$	$p = .011$
	right amygdala	$p = .003$	$p = .001$

(Other structures observed: left midbrain reticular formation, left visual cortex, right motor cortex, right visual cortex)

Monkey Z	right hippocampus	$p = .006$	$p = .020$
	left centre median	$p = .001$	$p = .001$

(Other structures observed: auditory cortex, right visual cortex, right amygdala, left hippocampus)

Monkey A	right hippocampus	$p = .001$	
	left hippocampus	$p = .001$	no run
	left centre median	$p = .059$	

(Other structure observed: left amygdala)

Nonperforming: sitting quietly		7 Hz on vs. off
Monkey A	right hippocampus	$p = .001$
	left hippocampus	$p = .036$
	right centre median	$p = .045$
	left amygdala	$p = .003$

(Other structures observed: left centre median, right amygdala)

Source: Gavalas, Walter, Hamer, and Adey 1970.

EEG records were also evaluated by coherence calculations and by discriminant analyses methods. Coherence measures between the 7-Hz signal generator were always higher for the fields-on condition than for fields-off in responsive brain structures, but coherence patterns between responsive brain structures were not consistent. Although EEG changes at nonfield frequencies could not be detected by visual inspection, discriminant analysis of spectral parameters revealed strong driving at harmonics of the field frequency, with increased intensity and increased coherence. These harmonic responses, which exceeded the harmonic content of the field waveform, are compatible with biological transduction (Van der Tweel and Verdyn Lunel 1965, Walter and Adey 1966), although an artifactual transduction is not precluded. After excluding all bands containing harmonics of the field frequency, discriminant analyses still showed a clear separation of EEGs from fields-on and fields-off conditions, principally in the raised total EEG power in the presence of fields, even in nonharmonic frequency bands.

In summary, all three monkeys in this low-frequency field study showed altered EEG power at 6 to 8 Hz in the hippocampus and less consistently in the amygdala and nucleus centrum medianum with 7-Hz fields. The field amplitude was 7 volts p-p/meter. The component of this field induced in the head of the monkey and flowing to ground was measured by Dr. J. Miller and his colleagues at the Illinois Institute of Technology at 0.8 nanoamp. No precise measurement of the intracerebral electric gradient produced by the field has so far been technically feasible.

If, however, we assume a specific impedance for brain tissue at those frequencies of the order of 300 Ω cm (Ranck 1963), then the electric gradient would be about 0.02 μV/cm in a brain with a conducting cross-section of about 10 cm^2 and a maximum linear dimension of 7 cm in the axis of a field of 10 volts/meter. Our experiments suggest that this intensity may be close to threshold for discernible behavioral and electrophysiological effects. That such a weak field should be an effective stimulus is baffling in terms of classical synaptic excitation. Depolarization of the postsynaptic membrane in generation of an action potential transiently abolishes a gradient of about 1 kV/cm, some 10 orders of magnitude larger than these weak fields; nor would such a weak field be expected to elicit significant release of transmitter substances from within the membranes of presynaptic terminals. Clearly, it is this disparity between observed effects of these fields on the central nervous system as a whole and the unlikely possiblity of their direct action on synaptic transmitter mechanisms that invites fresh consideration of more subtle membrane sensitivites.

Effects of Low-Level Modulated, Very High-Frequency (VHF) Fields on Specific Brain Rhythms in Cats

Our search for more definite evidence that the membrane surface might transduce weak extracellular fields as a step in excitation led us to the use of

VHF electromagnetic fields, amplitude-modulated at EEG frequencies. Our general hypothesis related to the heavy fixed-charge distribution on polyanionic macromolecular material characteristic of these surfaces. These surface glycoproteins form sheets with a strong asymmetry in charge distribution with respect to extracellular fluid and to deeper layers of the membrane. Such a phase partition would be expected to demodulate the envelope of a high-frequency carrier wave, much in the fashion of a semiconductor, although remaining unresponsive to the carrier frequency itself. If this hypothesis were correct, it would be anticipated that the presence of low-frequency modulation on the carrier wave would be a prerequisite for central nervous effects, and that differential effects at specific brain sites would be dependent on particular modulating frequencies. Our findings support this hypothesis.

We have studied the effects of 147-MHz fields, amplitude-modulated over the frequency range of 0 to 30 Hz, with an intensity of 1.0 mW cm^{-2} or less (Bawin, Gavalas-Medici, and Adey 1973). At this weak field level, no significant heating of the cat's head occurs (Mumford 1970). The fields were applied between two aluminum plates that flared from a narrow apex at which the feedline was attached. These triangular plates were about one-half wavelength long at the field frequency and 4100 cm^2 in area. To further ensure a uniform field distribution between the plates, the unbalanced coaxial transmission line from the VHF generator was coupled to the two plates by a half-wave coaxial "balun," so that identical voltages were applied to the two plates with a 180° phase shift. Modulation depth could be varied from 0 to 90 percent, and was typically maintained at 80 percent. The cat's body was held in a hammock, and it was free to sit or lie, but lateral movement of the head was prevented by a painless retaining device. Twelve adult female cats were used, and bipolar electrodes were implanted in the caudate nucleus, amygdala, nucleus ventralis anterior thalamic, nucleus centrum medianum, midbrain reticular formation, and presylvian cortex. Eye movements were also monitored.

Effects of VHF fields on conditioned EEG patterns. The first experiment was based on the following hypothesis. Different brain structures produce "bursts" of EEG rhythms that can be used as EEG "signatures" for that particular brain region. Moreover, these signatures can be elicited as conditional responses to behavioral training (Fox and Rudell 1968; Sterman, Wyrwicka, and Clemente 1969; Delgado et al. 1970; Sterman, Howe, and Macdonald 1970; Fox and Ahn 1971). If the cats were trained to produce a particular burst in the presence of a VHF field modulated at the same frequency as the burst, then effects of the field might be detected during either acquisition or extinction of the learned response, or both.

The EEG patterns to be reinforced were arbitrarily selected from any one of the implanted sites. The selected rhythms were narrow in band width (±2 Hz from the dominant frequency) and had a mean duration of 0.5 sec, with a probability ($p \geqq 0.25$) that at least one burst would be present in any 2.5-sec interval. The training paradigm consisted of a series of 100 flashes at 30-sec intervals, followed 2.5 sec later by electrical stimulation of the frontal eye field. This stimulation acted as an aversive unconditional stimulus (Us) and appeared unpleasant, although behaviorally it produced only ocular movements. The operant response was defined as the occurrence of the selected patterns during the 2.5-sec epochs following the flash (Cs). The criterion for conditioning was arbitrarily chosen as a doubling of operant response rates seen with flash presentations in preconditioning trials. Further details of training and extinction procedures are given elsewhere (Bawin, Gavalas-Medici, and Adey 1973).

All five animals in this series were first conditioned and extinguished in the absence of VHF fields. Learning and extinction curves were practically identical for all animals (Figure 3). Less than seven sessions were required for the animals to double their operant levels. The animals were then overtrained three or four days, during which performances remained at 70 to 80 percent. Extinction profiles were very sharp in each case. Performances dropped rapidly to baseline levels in less than six days (third extinction session). The most clearly visible rhythms were found in the visual cortex, the hippocampus, and the nucleus centrum medianum. The fully developed responses showed increased amplitude and sharply defined peak frequencies, for example 16, 6, and 3 Hz in the visual cortex, 4.5 to 3 Hz in the hippo-

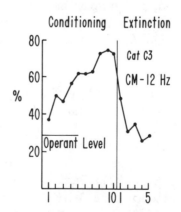

Figure 3. Performances of a cat (C3) in conditioning and extinction of a 14-Hz rhythm in nucleus centrum medianum, without VHF fields. Data normalized over total number of Cs presentations within session. (From Bawin, Gavalas-Medici, and Adey 1973)

campus, and 13 to 16 Hz in the centrum medianum.

As a preliminary to VHF field exposure, these five cats were then retrained. Two served as controls and were overtrained and extinguished in the absence of fields. The other three were irradiated with the VHF fields, amplitude modulated at 3, 4.5, and 14 Hz respectively, during overtraining and extinction.

The two control cats maintained regular levels of performance during the training sessions but never exceeded their previous achievement. They did not perform at all for long periods, because of sleep or inattention. The extinction in the absence of fields was again very rapid. Performance dropped to 40 percent during the first session.

By contrast, the irradiated animals remained quiet but fully awake during the six overtraining sessions. Their performance finally reached levels equal or superior to the highest scores in the first conditioning. These high performance levels persisted for 25 to 40 days into the extinction schedule (Figure 4). Drowsiness, slow-wave sleep, and rapid-eye-movement (REM) epochs then appeared at the end of testing periods until approximately day 55, when the animals ceased performing and again became alert and restless.

Spectral analysis revealed a concentration of power around the imposed

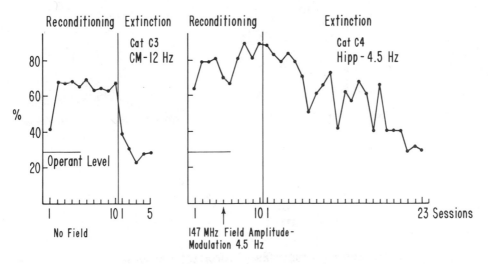

Figure 4. Comparison of performance in two cats during reconditioning and extinction; cat C3 (centrum medianum, 14 Hz—no field) and cat C4 (hippocampus, 4.5 Hz—VHF field amplitude-modulated at 4.5 Hz). Data normalized over the total number of Cs presentations within session. The arrow indicates the first day of exposure to the fields. (From Bawin, Gavalas-Medici, and Adey 1973)

modulation frequency. However, daily controls with the fields amplitude-modulated at different frequencies for short epochs and also with brief field-off conditions failed to produce any changes or any artifactual patterns in these highly stable responses. No change was ever elicited in the EEG records by application of fields in the absence of the conditioning procedure. Figure 5 compares the autospectra of the hippocampal EEG in one animal accompanying correct and incorrect responses during irradiation with fields modulated at 4.5 Hz (the peak frequency of the response) on day 5 of reconditioning. The peak shifted away from the imposed frequency when the animal was not performing. The hippocampal responses shifted to 2 to 3 Hz as the performances returned to operant levels during extinction trials.

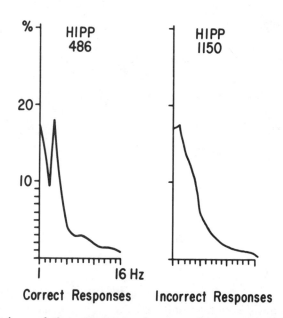

Figure 5. Comparison of the autospectra (average of 20 epochs of 2.5 sec each) of the hippocampal patterns (cat C4) in cases of correct and incorrect responses during exposures to VHF fields amplitude-modulated at 4.5 Hz Reconditioning day 5. (From Bawin, Gavalas-Medici, and Adey 1973)

Effects of VHF Fields on Spontaneous Transient EEG Rhythms

Two animals were used in this complementary study. Two different patterns occurring in two different brain locations were selected for each animal in preliminary testing sessions. Two mutually exclusive rhythms in one cat (14 Hz in nucleus centrum medianum and 10 Hz in presylvian gyrus) and two concurrent patterns (13 Hz in caudate nucleus and 4 Hz in centrum medianum) were selected for manipulation in the VHF fields. The output of filters tuned to these frequencies was then used to trigger the VHF fields, amplitude-modulated at various frequencies, for 20 sec (Figure 6). The occurrence of a second or third burst during the fields-on epochs recycled the chain of events, so that every occurrence was similarly reinforced. In this way the specificity of the modulation frequency could be tested.

The experimental results clearly indicated that the fields were acting as reinforcers, increasing the rate of occurrence of the spontaneous rhythms only when modulated at frequencies close to the biologically dominant frequency of the selected intrinsic EEG rhythmic episodes. As seen in Figure 7, imposition of fields modulated at a frequency (3 Hz) different from the triggering one (10 Hz, sessions 7 and 8) dramatically decreased the 10-Hz

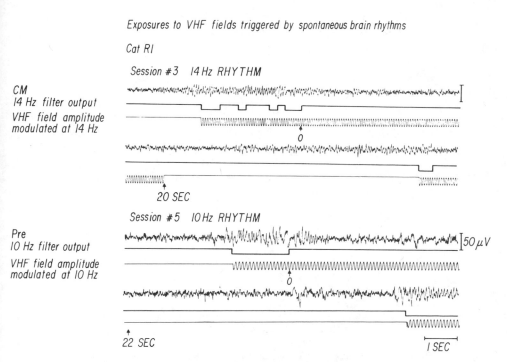

Exposures to VHF fields triggered by spontaneous brain rhythms

Cat RI

Session #3   14 Hz RHYTHM

CM
14 Hz filter output
VHF field amplitude
modulated at 14 Hz

20 SEC

Session #5   10 Hz RHYTHM

Pre
10 Hz filter output
VHF field amplitude
modulated at 10 Hz

22 SEC   1 SEC

Figure 6. Selected EEG patterns and mechanisms of reinforcement. Cat R2. Sessions 3 and 5. (From Bawin, Gavalas-Medici, and Adey 1973)

rhythm in the presylvian gyrus and increased the nonreinforced pattern (14 Hz, centrum medianum). These results provide strong evidence that the modulation was indeed responsible for both enhanced and decreased rhythms seen in the preceding sessions.

In summary, we may hypothesize that the fields acted as contingent reinforcers in both series of experiments. If antenna effects on the electrode leads, despite their shielding up to the head, had induced even small potentials at the tip of the electrodes, spectral analysis would be expected to reveal voltages so induced and rectified at the electrode-tissue contact. Such effects would be expected to appear uniformly at all electrodes and to be present, unchanged, throughout the fields exposure. The EEG changes reported here were anatomically localized, highly specific in terms of frequency, and associated with transient patterns. It therefore seems unlikely that the tissue effects are attributable to direct injection of field voltage via the electrodes.

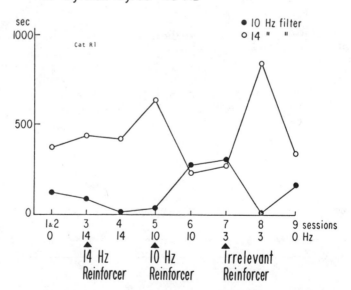

Figure 7. Selected reinforcement of intrinsic EEG rhythmic episodes by VHF fields. Cat R1. Experimental conditions: no field (0), VHF fields amplitude-modulated at 14 Hz, 10 Hz, and 3 Hz. (From Bawin, Gavalas-Medici, and Adey 1973)

Macromolecular Effects in Membrane Excitation; the "Greater Membrane"
and the Sensing of Weak Fields

It was pointed out above that the neuronal membrane surface is characterized by outer coats of fragile, highly hydrated macromolecular material that appears to be glycoprotein in nature and polyanionic, with numerous negative fixed charge sites. The presence of these fixed charges may be detected by electrokinetic effects in membrane fragments and in metabolically poisoned cells, as well as in cultured neurons and in isolated fresh neurons (Elul 1966, 1967b).

The presence of this surface glycocalyx (Bennett 1963) greatly extends the effective membrane thickness, perhaps to as much as 2000Å, in what has been described as the "greater membrane" (Schmitt and Samson 1969). In this greater membrane model, a sensing role has been proposed for the material of the glycocalyx, with specialized receptor sites for hormones and neurohumoral substances effective in minute amounts, as well as in the binding of transmitter substances. The effectiveness of substances in minute amounts at the membrane surface may involve conformation changes in macromolecules at the binding site. Thereafter, as a transmembrane effect, molecular "switches," such as prostaglandins, may trigger a transmembrane response in the presence of calcium ions (Ramwell and Shaw 1970), with activation of powerful metabolic enzymes, such as adenyl cyclase, and conversion of ATP to cyclic AMP in energy-releasing mechanisms (Sutherland and Robison 1966). Clearly this sequence of events in chemical sensing involves major "membrane amplification" between the initial surface binding and the release of metabolic energy.

Does a comparable mechanism of membrane amplification underlie central nervous sensing of weak electric fields? It is possible that the broad surface sheet of macromolecular material with its numerous fixed negative charges may function as a sensor of these fields. These negative charges bind cations as a "counter-ion" layer at their surface. Katchalsky (1964) noted that divalent cations are more powerfully bound than are the monovalent with the exception of hydrogen ions, and that calcium is much more powerfully bound to macromolecular polyelectrolytes than to other divalent ions, including magnesium. Bass and Moore (1968) have proposed that calcium ions are displaced from macromolecular binding sites by hydrogen ions. The ensuing local alkalosis would entail only a restricted movement of calcium ions to adjacent binding sites, and not their freeing in a major diffusion flow. Our data support the possibility that the binding of calcium to membrane surface polyanions may be in the class of "cooperative" processes, with a weak trigger at one point initiating macromolecular conformation changes over considerable distances, and perhaps triggering metabolic energy release through transmembrane signals. Schwartz and co-workers (Schwartz 1967 and 1970; Schwartz, Klose, and Balthasar 1970; Schwartz and Balthasar 1970) have proposed a cooperative model of this type for linear biopolymers, such as poly *l*-glutamic acid, in the binding of acridine dyes. They envisaged the development of cooperativity by assuming that immediately neighboring segments of the polymer are more likely to be found in like charge states than unlike ones. If this occurs on the membrane surface, decremental dendritic conduction could be based on a "virtual" wave of altered calcium binding, traveling longitudinally on dendritic structures, leaving modified states of binding sites on the macromolecular sheet behind the advancing wave, but involving only small displacement of calcium ions to adjacent sites. Movement of calcium ions grossly through cerebral tissue at rates around 0.3 μM/sec (Adey 1971; van Harreveld, Dafny, and Khattab 1971) would support this hypothesis, but it leaves open the question of small, focal displacements of calcium to adjacent binding sites.

The role of calcium in the release of calcium and GABA from cat cerebral cortex. To test the effects of modified calcium levels in cerebral tissue, we have equilibrated cat cerebral cortex with $^{45}Ca^{2+}$ and ^{3}H-GABA in the absence of general anesthesia (Kaczmarek and Adey 1973, 1974a). A small increase in unlabeled Ca^{2+} in the solution bathing the cortex elicited a large release of labeled $^{45}Ca^{2+}$ and labeled GABA (Figure 8). Moreover, the effect of a 1-mM increment in Ca^{2+} concentration was only slightly less than that of a 20-mM increment. Mg^{2+} failed to produce increases comparable to added Ca^{2+}. Thus, calcium triggers its own release and the release of GABA. A possible mechanism may be the displacement of $^{45}Ca^{2+}$ bound to polyanionic sites on the membrane surface. To be consistent with the observed $^{45}Ca^{2+}$ efflux and net Ca^{2+} and net Ca^{2+} binding, this mechanism may take the form:

$$Ca^{2+} + {}^{45}Ca\text{-}M^{n-} \rightarrow Ca\underline{{}^{45}Ca}\text{-}M^{(n-2)-}$$

$$Ca\underline{{}^{45}Ca}\text{-}M^{(n-2)-} \rightarrow {}^{45}Ca^{2+} + Ca\text{-}M^{n-}$$

where M represents a membrane anionic species. The efflux of Ca ion from the membrane would then be proportional to a higher power of the bound Ca ion concentration.

Effects of weak electric gradients on calcium ion and GABA fluxes in cortex. This sharp nonlinearity in the release of bound calcium by a small increase in extracellular calcium suggested the possibility of triggering calcium release with a weak electric gradient. We therefore tested the effects of electrical stimulation of cat cortex with gradients in the range of 20 to 60 mV/cm on the efflux of ^{3}H-GABA and ^{45}Ca^{2+} from the cortical surface in the cat (Kaczmarek and Adey 1974b).

To produce a nonfocal electric field through the brain, we used electrodes of agar in lucite cylinders 2.5 cm high and 1.0 cm in diameter. Three stainless steel screws made contact with the agar at the top of the cylinder. The potential gradient generated by the stimulus was measured progressively from the cortical surface to the ventral diencephalon with a bipolar electrode (1-mm tip separation) and shown to be reasonably uniform throughout. The stimulus was a 200/sec pulse train (pulse duration 1.0 msec).

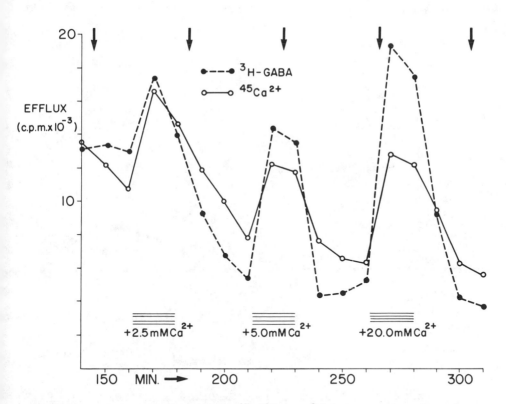

Figure 8. The simultaneous efflux of ^{45}Ca^{2+} and ^{3}H-GABA from cat cortex in an experiment in which aminooxyacetic acid (AOAA), 5 mg/kg body weight, had been administered before incubation with ^{3}H-GABA. The superfusion medium contained 2.16 mM Ca^{2+} before the Ca^{2+} concentration was increased by the amount indicated. Time after the start of superfusion is shown on the abscissa and the arrows indicate gallamine triethiodide administration. (From Kaczmarek and Adey 1973)

There was an increased efflux of both $^{45}Ca^{2+}$ and ^{3}H-GABA with gradients of 20 to 50 mV/cm (Figure 9). The increases in efflux were smaller than those noted above with small increments in the calcium concentration of the medium or with seizure activity (Kaczmarek and Adey 1973), but they were clearly reproducible. The mean results of six experiments with a gradient of 50 mV/cm were a 1.29 ± 0.06-fold increase for $^{45}Ca^{2+}$ and 1.21 ± 0.04 for ^{3}H-GABA, but these may reflect much larger changes in the rate of binding and release in the tissue.

If these weak fields acted through classical processes of transmitter release, important questions may be raised. If a typical synaptic terminal is 0.5 μ in diameter, the extracellular gradient imposed by these fields is, at most, 2.5μV across the terminal. It is unclear how such a weak stimulus may affect the transmembrane potential of 50 mV sufficiently to influence transmitter release. The gradients in these experiments are more than four orders of magnitude less. Similar considerations apply to effects of the fields

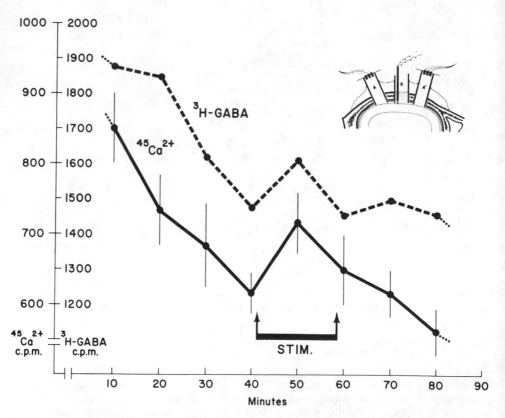

Figure 9. Effects of low-level electrical stimulation with cortical electrical gradient of 50 mV/cm, 200 pulses/sec, 1.0-msec duration, on efflux of $^{45}Ca^{2+}$ and ^{3}H-GABA. (From Kaczmarek and Adey 1974b)

of postsynaptic excitability.

An equally important question raised by these results is the extent to which the field generated by the activity of one cortical neuron may influence a nearby cell. For the spinal motoneurone, the extracellular gradients generated by the neurons are greater than 50 mV/cm and do alter neuronal excitability (Nelson 1966). In these experiments we induced seizures by topical glutamate or by intravenous thiosemicarbazide. EEG gradients as high as 37.5 mV/cm were observed across a 1.0-mm dipole. Elul (1962) observed considerably higher extracellular EEG gradients in the absence of seizures using bipolar microelectrodes with a tip separation of 30 μM. Thus, the applied fields in these experiments are in the range of naturally occurring gradients and support the hypothesis that cortical neurons are sensitive to the natural electric field gradients that surround them.

Preliminary findings of altered calcium efflux in the isolated chick brain with modulated VHF fields. The positive findings of calcium release with weak electrical stimulation have led to the testing on the freshly isolated chicken brain of the effects of the modulated VHF fields used in the experiments described above. These studies by Dr. Suzanne Bawin and Dr. Leonard Kaczmarek are continuing, but the results so far appear to warrant inclusion here.

The heads of one-week-old chickens were removed by decapitation and the whole cerebrum dissected from the cranium. The cerebrum was then placed in a $^{45}Ca^{2+}$ Ringer solution for 30 min and the efflux of calcium subsequently observed in a 90-min period, with and without VHF field exposure. Results of 180 experiments to date are shown in Figure 10. The unmodulated VHF field produced very little increase in $^{45}Ca^{2+}$ efflux by comparison with nonirradiated control brains. However, a sharp increase in efflux occurred with fields modulated at frequencies between 11 and 16 Hz. Moreover, the results were identical in brains first killed with 10^{-4} M potassium cyanide prior to equilibration with $^{45}Ca^{2+}$.

These findings strikingly confirm the sensitivity of cerebral tissue to the low-frequency modulation components of the VHF field, with a frequency specificity in the low-frequency range. Previous studies in this laboratory (Elul 1967b) have shown the persistence of membrane fixed surface charges after cyanide poisoning of cultured neurons, so that it seems reasonable to assume that the binding of calcium and its subsequent efflux relates to persisting properties of membrane surface polyanions.

Conclusion

In the unique structural and functional organization of cerebral tissue,

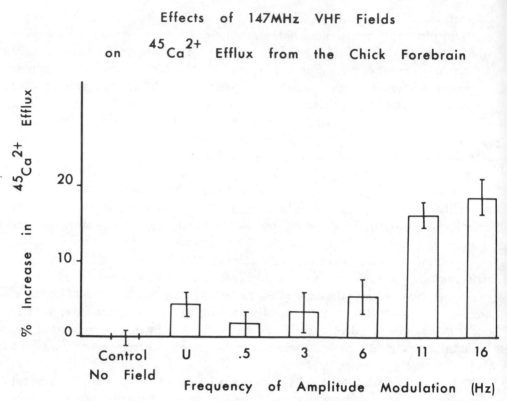

Figure 10. Increase in release of $^{45}Ca^{2+}$ by VHF fields, amplitude-modulated at indicated frequencies, from isolated chicken brains. Means calculated from 180 experiments.

critical experiments that define beyond reasonable doubt some essential aspects of information transaction, or its storage or recall, are difficult to design and usually even more difficult to perform. In this mansion of many rooms, or perhaps more aptly, in this city of many houses, it is easy to be preoccupied with one pattern of organization to the exclusion of others, and to believe that this or that particular level of patterned organization is the one that is essential and sufficient for our understanding of brain mechanisms. In the studies presented here, my colleagues and I have invited attention to the hierarchical organization that assuredly underlies structuring and functioning of the brain, and to emphasize that these indeed appear to be interacting hierarchies in the intimacy of cerebral tissue. In particular, we emphasize the apparent role of intrinsic cerebral electric fields as functional elements in neuronal excitability and in interactions between groups of neurons.

Acknowledgment

Studies reported from this laboratory were supported by NSF Grant GB-27740, Air Force Contract F44620-70-C-0017, and ONR Contract N00014-69-A-200-4037.

References

Adey, W.R. 1970. Cerebral structure and information storage. *Progress Physiol. Psychol.* 3:188.

Adey, W.R. 1971. Evidence for cerebral membrane effects of calcium, derived from direct-current gradient, impedance, and intracellular records. *Exp. Neurol.* 30:78.

Adey, W.R. 1972. Organization of brain tissue: Is the brain a noisy processor? *Internat. J. Neurosci.* 3:271.

Adey, W.R. 1973. Continuity-discontinuity problems: mixed systems. In *Dynamic Patterns of Brain Cell Assemblies*. Massachusetts Institute of Technology, *Neurosciences Research Program Bulletin* (in press).

Adey, W.R., Bell, F.R., and Dennis, B.J. 1962. Effects of LSD, psilocybin and psilocin on temporal lobe EEG patterns and learned behavior in the cat. *Neurology (Minneap.)* 12:591.

Adey, W.R., Kado, R.T., and Didio, J. 1962. Impedance measurements in brain tissue of animals using microvolt signals. *Exp. Neurol.* 5:47.

Adey, W.R., Kado, R.T., Didio, J., and Schindler, W.J. 1963. Impedance changes in cerebral tissue accompanying a learned discriminative performance in the cat. *Exp. Neurol.* 7:259.

Adey, W.R., Kado, R.T., McIlwain, J.T., and Walter, D.O. 1966. The role of neuronal elements in regional cerebral impedance changes in altering, orienting and discriminative responses. *Exp. Neurol.* 15:490.

Adey, W.R., and Walter, D.O. 1963. Application of phase detection and averaging techniques in computer analysis of EEG records in the cat. *Exp. Neurol.* 7:186.

Adrian, E.D. 1947. *The Physical Basis of Perception*. New York: Cambridge University Press.

Anninos, P.A., Beek, P., Csermely, T.J., Harth, E.M., and Pertile, G. 1970. Dynamics of neural structures. *J. Theor. Biol.* 26:121.

Bass, L., and Moore, W.J. 1968. A model of nervous excitation based on the Wien dissociation effect. In A. Richard, and C.M. Davidson (eds.), *Structural Chemistry and Molecular Biology*, pp. 356-368. San Francisco: Freeman.

Bawin, S.M., Gavalas-Medici, R.J., and Adey, W.R. 1973. Effects of modulated very high frequency fields on specific brain rhythms in cats. *Brain Res.* 58:365.

Bennett, H.S. 1963. Morphological aspects of extracellular polysaccharides. *J. Histochem. Cytochem.* 11:14.

Berger, H. 1929. Über das Elektroenkephalogramm des Menschen. *Archiv. Psychiat.* 87:527.

Berkhout, J., Walter, D.O., and Adey, W.R. 1969. Alterations of the human electroencephalogram induced by stressful verbal activity. *Electroencephalogr. Clin. Neurophysiol.* 27:457.

Cole, K.S. 1940. Permeability and impermeability of cell membranes for ions. *Cold Spring Harbor Symp. Quant. Biol.* 4:110.

Coombs., J.S., Curtis, D.R., and Eccles, J.C. 1959. The electric constants of the motoneurons membrane. *J. Physiol. Lond.* 145:505.

Creutzfeldt, O.D., Furster, J.M., Lux, H.D., and Nacimiento, A. 1964. Experimentaler Nachweis von Beziehungen zwischen EEG-wellen und Activitat corticaler Nervenzellen. *Naturwiss* 51:166.

Creutzfeldt, O.D., Watanabe, S., and Lux, H.D. 1966. Relations between EEG phenomena and potentials of single cortical cells. II. Spontaneous and convulsoid activity. *Electroencephelogr. Clin. Neurophysiol.* 20:19.

Delgado, J.M.R., Johnson, V.S., Wallace, J.D. and Bradley, R.J. 1970. Operant conditioning of amygdala spindling in the free chimpanzee. *Brain Res.* 22:347.

Ehinger, B. 1973. Glial uptake of taurine in the rabbit retina. *Brain Res.* 60:512.

Ehinger, B., and Falck, B. 1971. Autoradiography of some suspected neurotransmitter substances: GABA, glycine, aspartic acid, glutamic acid, histamine, dopamine, and L-DOPA. *Brain Res.* 33:157.

Elazar, Z., and Adey, W.R. 1967. Electroencephalographic correlates of learning in subcortical and cortical structures. *Electroencephalogr. Clin. Neurophysiol.* 23:306.

Elul, R. 1962. Dipoles of spontaneous activity in the cerebral cortex. *Exp. Neurol.* 6:285.

Elul, R. 1965. Specific site of generation of brain waves. *Physiologist* 7:125 (abstract).

Elul, R. 1966. Use of non-uniform electric fields for evaluation of the potential difference between two phases. *Transactions of the Faraday Society*, London 62:3484.

Elul, R. 1967a. Statistical mechanisms in generation of the EEG. In L.J. Fogel and F.W. George (eds.), *Progress in Biomedical Engineering*, p. 131. Washington, D.C.: Spartan Books.

Elul, R. 1967b. Fixed charge in the cell membrane. *J. Physiol. Lond.* 189:351.

Elul, R. 1972. The genesis of the EEG. *Internat. Rev. Neurobiol.* 15:228.

Elul, R., and Adey, W.R. 1965. The intracellular correlate of gross evoked responses. *Proceedings 23rd International Congress of Physiological Sciences*, Tokyo. Abstract 1034, p. 434.

Fox, S.S., and Ahn, H. 1971. Identification of functional bioelectric configurations in spontaneous activity of the brain. *Proceedings First Annual Meeting Society for Neuroscience*, Washington, D.C., p. 81.

Fox, S.S., and Rudell, A.P. 1968. Operant controlled neural event: Formal and systematic approach to coding of behavior in brain. *Science* 162:1299.

Fujita, Y., and Sato, T. 1964. Intracellular records from hippocampal pyramidal cells in rabbit during theta rhythm activity. *J. Neurophysiol.* 27:1011.

Gasteiger, E.L. 1959. The electrogram in deafferented spinal cord. *Proceedings 21st International Congress of Physiological Sciences*, Buenos Aires, p. 105.

Gavalas, R.J., Walter, D.O., Hamer, J., and Adey, W.R. 1970. Effect of low-level, low-frequency electric fields on EEG and behavior in *Macaca nemestrina*. *Brain Res.* 18:491.

Green, T.D., Maxwell, D.S., Schindler, W.J., and Stumpf, C. 1960. Rabbit EEG "theta" rhythm; its anatomical source and relation to activity in single neurons. *J. Neurophysiol.* 23:403.

Hamer, J. 1968. Effects of low-level, low frequency electric fields on human reaction time. *Communications in Behavioral Biology* 2, part 2A.

Hanley, J., Walter, D.O., Rhodes, J.M., and Adey, W.R. 1968. Chimpanzee performance data; computer analysis of electroencephalograms. *Nature* 229:879.

Henn, F.A., and Hamberger, A. 1971. Glial cell function: Uptake of transmitter substances. *Proc. Natl. Acad. Sci. USA* 68:2686.

Hyden, H. 1972. Macromolecules and behaviour. In G.B. Ansell and P.B. Bradley (eds.), *The Arthur Thomson Lectures*, University of Birmingham, England. London: Macmillan, 75 pp.

Kaczmarek, L.K., and Adey, W.R. 1973. The efflux of $^{45}Ca^{2+}$ and ^{3}H-gamma-aminobutyric acid from cat cerebral cortex. *Brain Res.* 63:331.

Kaczmarek, L.K., and Adey, W.R. 1974a. Some chemical and electrophysiological effects of glutamate in cerebral cortex. *J. Neurobiol.* (in press).

Kaczmarek, L.K., and Adey, W.R. 1974b. Weak electric gradients change ionic and transmitter fluxes in cortex. *Brain Res.* 66:537.

Karahashi, Y., and Goldring, S. 1966. Intracellular potentials from "idle" cells in cerebral cortex of cat. *Electroencephalogr. Clin. Neurophysiol.* 20:600.

Katchalsky, A. 1964. Polyelectrolytes and their biological interaction. In *Connective Tissue: Intercellular Macromolecules*, p. 9. New York Heart Association. Boston: Little, Brown.

König, H., and Ankermüller, F. 1960. Über den Einfluss besonders niederfrequenter elektrischer Vorgänge in der Atmosphäre auf den Menschen. *Naturwiss* 21:486.

Mumford, W.W. 1970. Heat stress due to RF radiation. In S.F. Cleary (ed.), *Proceedings Second Annual Triservice Conference on Biological Effects of Microwave Energy*, p. 21. Rockville, Maryland: Bureau of Radiological Health. Document BRH/DBE 70-2, PB 193898.

Nelson, P.G. 1966. Interaction between spinal motoneurons of the cat. *J. Neurophysiol.* 29:275.

Nicholls, J.G., and Kuffler, S.W. 1964. Extracellular space as a pathway for exchange between blood and neurons in the central nervous system of the leach: ionic composition of glial cells and neurons. *J. Neurophysiol.* 27:645.

Nirenberg, L.M., Hanley, J., and Stear, E.B. 1971. A new approach to prosthetic control: EEG motor signal tracking with an adaptively designed phase-locked loop. Institute of Electrical and Electronics Engineers. *Transactions in Biomedical Engineering* 18:389.

Pasik, P., Pasik, T., Hamori, J., and Szentagothai, J. 1973. Interneurons in monkey lateral geniculate nucleus: Participation in "triadic" and "non-triadic" synapses. *Proceedings 3rd Annual Meeting Society for Neuroscience*, San Diego, California, p. 298 (abstract), Washington, D.C.

Pease, D.C. 1966. Polysaccharides associated with the exterior surface of epithelial cells: Kidney, intestine, brain. *J. Ultrastruc. Res.* 15:555.

Purpura, D.P., Shofer, R.J., and Musgrave, F.S. 1964. Cortical intracellular potentials during augmenting and recruiting responses. II. Patterns of synaptic activities in pyramidal and non-pyramidal tract neurons. *J. Neurophysiol.* 27:133.

Rall, W., Shepard, G.M., Reese, T.S., and Brightman, M.W. 1966. Dendrodendritic synaptic pathway for inhibition in the olfactory bulb. *Exp. Neurol.* 14:44.

Rambourg, A., and Leblond, C.P. 1967. Electron microscope observations on the carbohydrate-rich cell coat present at the surface of cells in the rat. *J. Cell. Biol.* 32:153.

Ramwell, P.W., and Shaw, J.E. 1970. Biological significance of the prostaglandins. *Recent Prog. Horm. Res.* 26:139.

Ranck, J.B. 1963. Specific impedance of rabbit cerebral cortex. *Exp. Neurol.* 7:144.

Reed, D.J., Woodbury, D.M., and Holtzer, R.L. 1964. Brain edema, electrolytes and skeletal muscle. *Arch. Neurol.* 10:604.

Schmitt, F.O., and Samson, F.E. (eds.) 1969. Brain-cell microenvironment. Massachusetts Institute of Technology, *Neurosciences Research Program Bulletin* 7:277.

Schwartz, G. 1967. A basic approach to a general theory for cooperative intramolecular conformation changes of linear biopolymers. *Biopolymers* 5:321.

Schwartz, G. 1970. Cooperative binding to linear biopolymers. 1. Fundamental static and dynamic properties. *Eur. J. Biochem.* 12:442.

Schwartz, G., Klose, S., and Balthasar, W. 1970. Cooperative binding to linear biopolymers. 2. Thermodynamic analysis of the proflavine-poly (*l*-glutamic acid) system. *Eur. J. Biochem.* 12:454.

Schwartz, G., and Balthasar, W. 1970. Cooperative binding to linear biopolymers. 3. Thermodynamic and kinetic analysis of the acridine-poly (*l*-glutamic acid) system. *Eur. J. Biochem.* 12:461.

Sterman, M.B., Howe, R.C., and MacDonald, L.R. 1970. Facilitation of spindlebursts sleep by conditioning of electroencephalographic activity while awake. *Science* 167:1146.

Sterman, M.B., Wyrwicka, W., and Clemente, C.D. 1969. EEG correlates of behavioral inhibition. *Cond. Reflex* 4:124.

Sutherland, E.W., and Robison, G.A. 1966. The role of 3, 5-adenosine monophosphate in responses to catecholamines and other hormones. *Pharmacol. Rev.* 18:145.

Tarby, T.J., and Adey, W.R. 1968. Cytological chemical identification of calcium in brain tissue. *Anat. Rec.* 157:331 (abstract).

van Harreveld, A., Crowell, J., and Malhotra, S. 1965. A study of extracellular space in central nervous tissue by freeze substitution. *J. Cell. Biol.* 25:117.

van Harreveld, A., Dafny, N., and Khattab, F.I. 1971. Effects of calcium on the electrical resistance and extracellular space of cerebral cortex. *Exp. Neurol.* 31:358.

Van der Tweel, L.H., and Verdyn Lunel, H.F.E. 1965. Human visual responses to sinusoidally modulated light. *Electroencephalogr. Clin. Neurophysiol.* 18:587.

Walter, D.O., and Adey, W.R. 1966. Linear and non-linear mechanisms of brain wave generation. *Ann. New York Acad. Sci.* 128:772.

Walter, D.O., Kado, R.T., Rhodes, J.M., and Adey, W.R. 1967. Electroencephalographic baselines in astronaut candidates estimated by computation and pattern-recognition techniques. *Aerospace Med.* 33:371.

Wever, R. 1968. Einfluss schwacher elektromagnetischer Felder auf die circadiane Periodik des Menschen. *Naturwiss* 1:29.

afferent input: a critical factor in the ontogenesis of brain electrical activity [1]

Peter Kellaway, Ph.D.

Baylor College of Medicine, The Methodist Hospital,
Blue Bird Clinic Research Unit, Houston, Texas

The existence of critical periods in the ontogenesis of behavior, such as that associated with imprinting (Sluckin 1972), has been well-documented in recent years in morphologic, cytochemical, and electrophysiologic studies of the developing nervous system. Behavioral scientists have suggested that ontogenetic criticality can be understood if growth and behavioral differentiations are based on organizing processes and if organization can be modified only when active processes of organization are in progress (Scott 1962).

On the basis of the evidence, there appear to be three critical periods of behavioral development: the period of infantile stimulation, the period of learning, and the period of formation of basic social relationships (Scott 1962). The course of each successive stage must be significantly influenced by the characteristics of the antecedent epoch. The period of infantile stimulation, or, in neurophysiological terms, of critical afferent input, must indeed set the stage in terms of the neural substrate for the operational processes involved in the subsequent development of behavior. The extent to which the substrate at a given point in time demonstrates plasticity will determine the possibility for reorganization.

The mammalian brain exhibits for some time after birth a continuation

[1]Partially supported by the Blue Bird Research Foundation, The Playtex Foundation (1955), and The Cannafax Fund of The Methodist Hospital.

of histogenesis, neuronal and glial mitosis, cell migration, and growth differentiation of axonal and dendritic processes. The continued maturational evolution is currently conceived as an orderly sequence of interactions between the genome and the milieu, similar to that which characterizes embryonic development (Detwiler 1936). It would appear that the subsequent emergence and differentiation of behavior depend not only upon the genetic substrate but upon environmental variations, notably, the character, quality, and quantity of afferent input to the central nervous system.

The incompleteness of neuronal and glial differentiation for an undetermined period following birth is presumably the basis of a plasticity that permits a degree of modification by afferent input of neural circuitry (connectivity), protein synthesis, and electrical activity. The extent to which growth differentiation, or maturation, which are regulated primarily by the genome in terms of rate and form, may be modified by "normal" and "abnormal" afferent factors has yet to be determined. The length of time postnatally that CNS maturational processes may be modified by extrinsic environmental factors is also not yet known. Recent evidence (Dews and Wiesel 1970) indicates that the sensitive period during which a given neural system or "behavioral organ" is subject to significant modification may be a circumscribed time epoch within a more general early period in which neural circuitry may be influenced by the life history of the organism.

That the formulation of specific interneuronal connections can be modified by functional influences is a concept that has almost completely escaped the notice of modern clinical neurology, and it is only gradually finding its way via behavioral neurobiology (Mason, Davenport, and Menzel 1968; Jacobson 1970; Horn, Rose, and Bateson 1973) into clinical psychiatry (Freedman 1971; Harlow, Harlow, and Suomi 1971). The idea is not, however, a new one. It is implicit in the writings of Ramon y Cajal (1959) and explicit in early experimental studies of von Gudden (1869) and Berger (1900) on the visual system of infant animals.

It is probable that the latter investigators chose the visual system for study because it, of all afferent systems, best lends itself to this type of investigation. Because partial to total interference with visual input may be easily effected, and because visual function may be precisely assessed physiologically and behaviorally, it is in this system that the role played by afferent input in the development and maintenance of nervous system structure and function has been most actively investigated.

The wealth of new and exciting experimental data in this area, and my own observations of human subjects who have suffered aberrations of visual input in early life as a consequence of disease, are the bases for my selecting the visual system as a model for discussion of the role of afferent input as an ontogenetically important determinant of brain function as expressed in its electrical activity.

The Visual System as a Model

Since von Gudden's (1869) first eyelid-suturing experiments in the late nineteenth century, there has been evidence that animals reared in the absence of adequate visual stimulation subsequently display functional and structural aberrations of their visual systems. All mammalian species that have been reared in total darkness or in diffuse light appear to be behaviorally blind when first exposed to a normal visual environment. Subsequently, this blindness gradually recedes, but in some instances the visual defect is permanent. Concomitant with the defective vision are various histological, cytochemical, and neurophysiological disturbances of the neurons in the visual system.

The extent and permanency of these changes have been shown to depend on several critical variables; of these, the most important is the *age*, or stage of neural development, at which deprivation is instituted. Other critical factors are the *duration* and the *nature* of the deprivation. Dews and Wiesel (1970), using eyelid suturing as a means of excluding patterned-light stimulation, demonstrated that deprivation is only effective if it occurs within a certain critical period and that this period has a lower as well as an upper age limit. In the kitten, the period of maximal susceptibility is between the fourth and twelfth weeks after birth. The vulnerability is greatest at the beginning of this period. At this time, toward the end of the third postnatal week, a few days of visual occlusion have the same drastic consequences that only two weeks later will require weeks of occlusion to effect. The *character* of the deprivation is also an important variable. Paradoxically, monocular deprivation has been shown by Wiesel and Hubel (1963b, 1965a, and 1965b), Kupfer and Palmer (1964), and Ganz, Fitch, and Satterberg (1968) to have a more profound effect than binocular deprivation. There are also significant qualitative and quantitative effects morphologically, cytochemically, and behaviorally when the alteration of the afferent input is a consequence of visual deprivation as contrasted with afferent denervation. Thus, Kupfer and Palmer (1964), studying the histology and cytochemistry of neurons in the lateral geniculate in kittens, have compared the findings following unilateral afferent denervation produced by enucleation and unilateral visual deprivation produced by lid closure. Enucleation at five weeks resulted in a rapid and severe transneuronal atrophy in the neurons in the appropriate geniculate laminae, and there was a concomitant decrease in enzyme[2] activity in the atrophied laminae, as compared with the adjacent normal laminae. On the other hand, visual deprivation at five weeks resulted

[2]TPN-diaphorase, DPN-diaphorase, cholinesterase, dihydrogenases of 6-phosphogluconate, succinate, and lactate-DPN.

only in decreased size of geniculate neurons in those laminae receiving input from the closed eye. These small neurons had an appearance that is normal for neurons of a five-week-old kitten. Cytochemical studies indicated no difference in enzyme activity between the smaller neurons and adjacent neurons of normal size. Since the normal geniculate neuron increases in cross section or area about 50 to 60 percent from birth to 15 weeks of age, it would appear that visual deprivation arrests normal growth of the neuron but does not significantly alter its metabolic activity.

Another clearly documented fact from animal studies is that the rate and severity of transneuronal atrophy vary with the species, being more rapid and severe in monkeys (Matthews, Cowan, and Powell 1960; Glees 1961; Matthews 1964) than in the cat or rabbit (Cook, Walker, and Barr 1951). Thus, there is an ontogenetic and phylogenetic parallel in terms of susceptibility.

Human Studies

Animal studies carried out in the last ten years provide the basis for interpretation of clinical observations that the author and his associates made twenty years ago. These observations demonstrate an effect of significant alterations of afferent input at a critical stage of development on the electrical activity of the human brain.

In 1951, we had begun a systematic analysis of electroencephalographic patterns and their ontogenetic evolution in premature and term infants. Gibbs and Gibbs (1952) had reported that premature infants were prone to develop foci of spike discharge in the occipital area. We had not observed this phenomenon in our own longitudinal EEG studies of infants born prematurely. The reason for this disparity of findings soon became clear when, in 1952, colleagues in ophthalmology and pediatrics, who were studying the characteristics and natural history of retrolental fibroplasia, suggested that as the retina is an extension of the brain, studies should be made using the EEG to determine if the agent responsible for the changes in the eye might also produce brain damage. It soon became evident that the occipital spikes observed by the Gibbs in premature infants were not an association of prematurity *per se* but an association with coexistent retrolental fibroplasia (Kellaway, Bloxsom, and MacGregor 1955), a revelation that came simultaneously to Gibbs, Fois, and Gibbs (1955). This association has since been confirmed by Cohen, Boshes, and Snider (1961).

Retrolental Fibroplasia (RLF)

We noted in our first 15 patients that not all of the infants and children showed occipital spike foci and that it was in the younger patients that the spikes were not present (Kellaway, Bloxsom, and MacGregor 1955). In the entire group of 71 RLF patients that we have now studied, the earliest occurrence of occipital spike foci was at 10 months, in an infant we were following prospectively. The time of detection of the occipital spike focus or foci in 21 patients studied is prospectively shown in Figure 1. The other 50 cases (Figure 2) were identified and recruited for the study after they were one year of age or more. Thus, the time at which the spike focus was first demonstrated does not necessarily reflect the true time of the initial emergence of this electrical abnormality. It would appear, from findings in the infants who were studied prospectively, that the spike focus takes a certain period to develop after retinal damage has occurred. No other serial studies have been reported, but Gibbs and Gibbs (1952) illustrated a case in which an occipital spike focus was present as early as 7 months.

On the basis of our initial data, it appeared that foci were more likely to appear if both eyes were severely involved than if one eye was partially

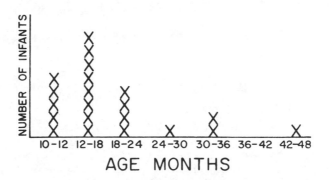

Figure 1. Time of first detection of occipital spike foci in 21 infants with RLF studied prospectively. EEGs were recorded every two months for the first year, every four months during the second year, and every six months thereafter. After the spikes were first detected, repeat studies were made at yearly intervals.

sighted (Kellaway, Bloxsom, and MacGregor 1955). This suggestion has not been borne out in our subsequent studies, in which all RLF children followed serially have developed unilateral or independent bilateral occipital spike or spike and slow wave foci. An example of occipital spike foci associated with RLF is illustrated in Figure 3.

The spike discharge did not, in our series, evolve from a slow wave focus, but the spikes were low in voltage when they first appeared and gradually increased in amplitude and incidence with time. In about 80 percent of the infants, the spike focus initially could be demonstrated only during sleep. The amount of spike activity, the character of the activity (single or multiple spikes), the time course of the spikes, and the occurrence of spike and wave complexes varied considerably among individual patients, and these variables were not statistically related to the severity of bilateral

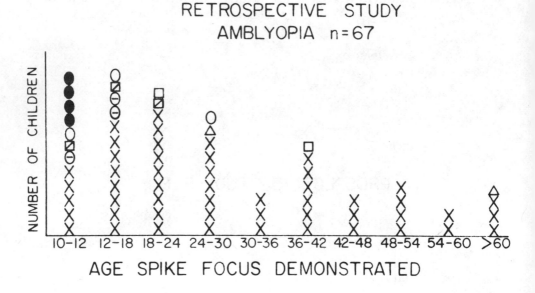

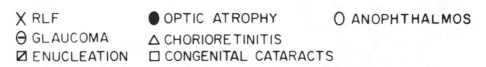

Figure 2. *Age at which an EEG showing occipital foci was first made in a series of infants and young children with various types of amblyopia. In some of these, the study was prospective in that the initial study was made within a few days or weeks after birth or after the blindness had occurred. However, in most cases, the study was retrospective in that the first EEG was made at any time between 10 months and 6 years. The 50 cases of RLF who were not part of the group studied close to the time of birth are included in this figure.*

involvement or to age, although there appeared to be a trend toward the occurrence of single spikes of slower time course with increasing age (Figure 4). Similar observations have been reported by Gibbs, Fois, and Gibbs (1955).

The clinical observations of Campbell in 1951, extended and elucidated by experimental studies carried out between 1952 and 1953, established that RLF was a direct consequence of the damaging influence of high pO_2 levels on the developing retinal capillaries—an iatrogenic disease related to the conviction of many pediatricians at that time that high concentrations of atmospheric oxygen were essential to the well-being of the premature infant. Although the fundus has a normal appearance in the premature infant, the development of the retinal vasculature is incomplete. High atmospheric pO_2 was shown by several groups of workers (Gyllensten and Hellstrom 1952; Patz, Hoeck, and DeLaCruz 1952; Ashton, Ward, and Serpel 1953) to distort the maturational development of the retinal vessels, resulting, when exposure was prolonged, in detachment of the retina, complete disorganization of the vitreous with fibrovascular scar tissue, and incorporation of the newly formed tissue and the retina into a retrolental mass (Owens and Owens

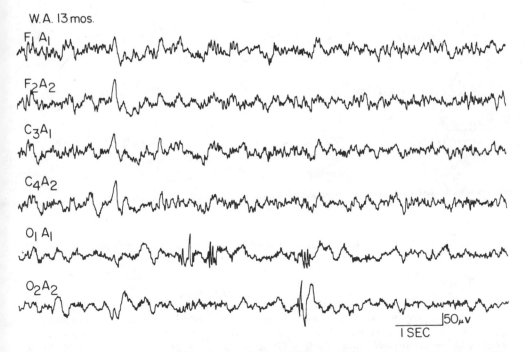

Figure 3. Infant W.A. independent spike foci in left and right occipital regions at age 13 months. Premature, birth weight, 2 lbs., 2 oz. When foci first appear, the spikes have a rapid time course and after occur in brief bursts of 2 to 5 spikes as illustrated in this section of the sleep record. The foci were not evident awake.

1949). Some regression of the structural changes is possible in the early stage of this process, but all of the children whom we studied had a gross reduction in visual acuity in both eyes. This ranged from total blindness in 75 percent to partial sight in one or both eyes in 10 percent; perception of light in one eye was present in the remaining 15 percent.

It appeared to us that if, indeed, the causative agent of RLF was acting directly upon the brain, the consistent occurrence of the spike foci in the occipital region was a unique phenomenon. Why the predilection for the occipital cortex, or, alternatively, for subcortical nuclei projecting to this area? Could it not be that the damage to the peripheral sensory organ in some manner secondarily induced a functional abnormality in the primary

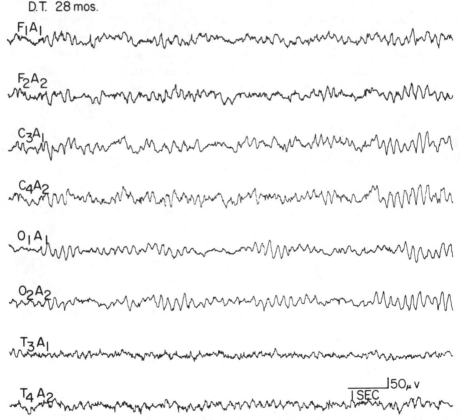

Figures 4 and 5. *D.T. Enucleation for retinoblastoma: Right eye at age 3 months and left eye at 5½ months. Homolateral ear to scalp recording at age 20 months shows awake (Figure 4) an occipital rhythm of 6 to 7 cfs per sec with no spike activity. Occipital alpha rhythm may persist in children who are initially sighted but become blind in infancy. During sleep (Figure 5), quite active foci of spike and slow wave discharges are present in the right and left occipital regions independently. The focus on the right side shows more and higher voltage spikes and slow wave complexes. Note rapid time course of the spikes.*

projection areas of the cortex?

In order to find an answer to this question, we initiated a study of children with other optic diseases that produced either (1) deafferentiation or (2) deprivation of patterned vision in one or both eyes.

Congenital Glaucoma

Four infants were followed. Occipital foci were demonstrated in three infants, at 11 months, 16 months, and 17 months of age, respectively. One infant, studied at 8 months and again at 36 months, did not show spike foci.

Enucleation for Retinoblastoma or Injury

Five patients were followed serially. One infant had bilateral enucleation: the right eye at 3 months and the left eye at 5½ months and developed a right occipital spike focus at 11 months (Figures 4 and 5). This infant's

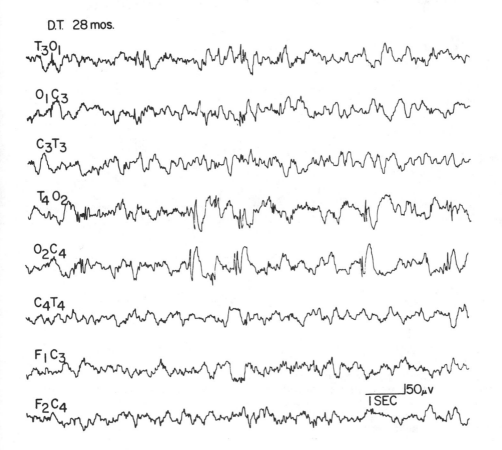

D.T. 28 mos.

older sibling, who had a bilateral enucleation at 23 months, was followed for one year but did not develop a spike focus. Two other infants with bilateral enucleation at 2 and 5 months developed occipital spike foci at 20 and 14 months, respectively.

A fifth patient suffered a penetrating injury to the right eye with subsequent enucleation at 4 years. This child was studied at ages 4 years 6 months, 6 years, and 7 years 2 months. No electroencephalographic abnormality was demonstrated.

Optic Atrophy

Four cases were followed; all demonstrated foci when first seen, two at 10 months and two at 12 months (Figure 6). In one case treated with ACTH,

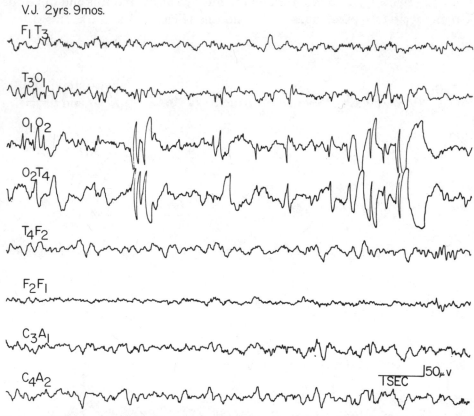

Figure 6. V.J. Congenital optic atrophy of unknown etiology. Spike focus in right occipital region present when first studied at age 10 months. In this sample, from a recording made at age 33 months, the right focus is very active with very high voltage spike and spike and slow wave complexes. Only occasional lower voltage spikes arise independently in the left occipital region.

the focus first demonstrated at 12 months, was absent at 18 months and again at 24 months.

The etiology of the optic atrophy in one infant was believed to be congenital syphillis. The etiology was not determined in the other three.

Chorioretinitis

Two cases were studied. Occipital spike foci were present in both, when first studied at the age of 26 months and 63 months, respectively (Figure 7).

Anophthalmos

Four infants with anophthalmos were studied one or more times. In three, occipital spike foci were present when they were first studied, at 12,

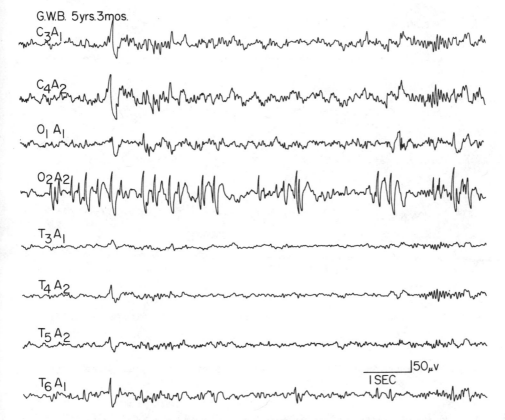

Figure 7. G.W.B. Acute uveitus and chorioretinitis at age of 3 months. Noted to have detached retina of the left and left optic atrophy. Spike discharges were seen in the left and right occipital regions in the first EEG made at age 63 months. The focus on the right side was extremely active with very high voltage spikes and spike and wave complexes.

13, and 29 months, respectively (Figures 8, 9 and 10). The fourth infant did not show foci when studied at 6, 12, and 18 months; he died at 19 months.

Congenital Cataracts

Eight patients were studied serially. Of these, five with congenital rubella were followed from the neonatal period to age 4 years. None of these showed occipital spikes.

In three cases of congenital cataracts of undetermined cause, occipital spike foci were demonstrated at 11 months (Figure 11), 21 months and 37 months, no previous EEG studies having been made.

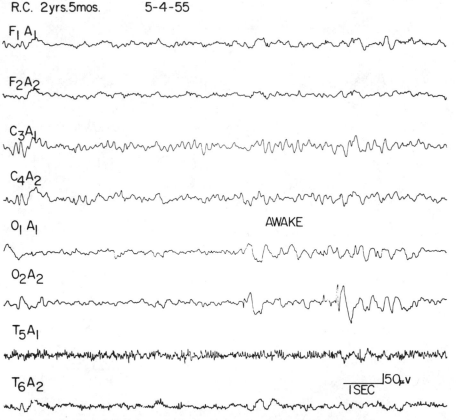

Figure 8. R.C. Anophthalmos. Note absence of sustained occipital alpha rhythm with a well sustained central alpha. Occasional random spike and slow wave discharges occur in the right occipital region.

Strabismus

The 34 children in this group were aged 3 to 7 years when first studied. Two or more electroencephalograms, including sleep recordings, were made in all cases, but systematic longitudinal studies were not attempted (Figures 12 and 13).

Eighteen children had esotropia, twelve had exotropia, and four had an alternating strabismus. Twenty-two children were amblyopic and, of these, thirteen showed occipital spike foci. Twelve children were not amblyopic, and none of these had occipital spike foci.

The RLF, glaucoma, optic atrophy, chorioretinitis, and enucleation findings indicate that early deafferentation in man results in neuronal changes in the visual system that are of a type which is prone to generate EEG spikes. The presence of similar spikes in the children with congenital cataracts suggests that deprivation of pattern vision from birth results in

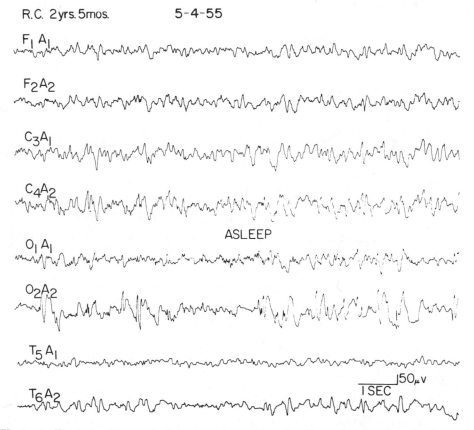

Figure 9. Illustrates the marked increase in spike and spike and slow wave discharges in the right occipital region that occurred during sleep.

similar neural changes.[3]

The findings in the children with strabismus indicate that asymmetry of binocular input to the geniculostriate system may also lead to neuronal changes that are prone to generate spikes. In this regard, it is of interest that von Noorden (1973b) has demonstrated morphologic changes inthe geniculate of infant monkeys rendered esotropic that are similar to those produced in this animal when one eye is occluded during infancy. Stillerman, Gibbs, and Perlstein (1952), who first reported an association between occipital spikes and strabismus, considered the spikes to be a sign of a primary central nervous system abnormality which had a causal relationship to the strabismus. The finding that occipital spike foci occur in children with anophthalmia is of special interest in that it suggests that the necessary neural substrate in the geniculostriate system is laid down in fetal life in the absence

[3]Profound disturbances in space perception and visual behavior have been thoroughly documented in human subjects following surgical removal of cataracts dating from early life (von Senden 1960).

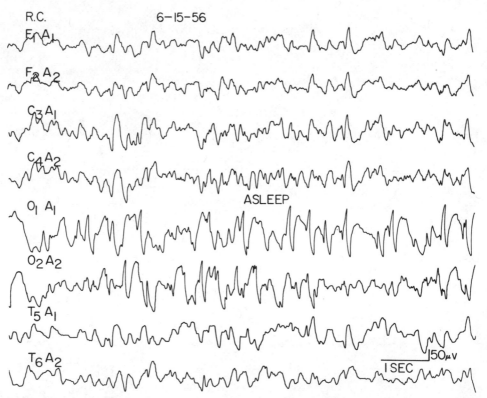

Figure 10. Shows the marked increase in spike activity that was present a year later. The spikes have a slower time course and are present bilaterally; the focus of the left side now being the more active of the two.

of afferent connections with the peripheral sense organ.

The Pathophysiological Significance of the EEG Spike

Goldensohn, Zablow, and Stein (1970) have demonstrated that an EEG spike recorded at the scalp is the consequence of the synchronization of multiple cortical sources of similar but highly circumscribed discharges which individually are not manifest in scalp recordings. Each of these circumscribed electrocortical spikes is the product of synchronized single-cell discharges of a finite neuronal aggregate. This synchronization of unit activity involves significant modification of individual cell behavior and of intraneuronal function within the cortical feltwork in which the localized spike activity is generated. Thus, the EEG spike is not merely an epiphenomenon but a manifestation of a complex neuronal process which may interfere with

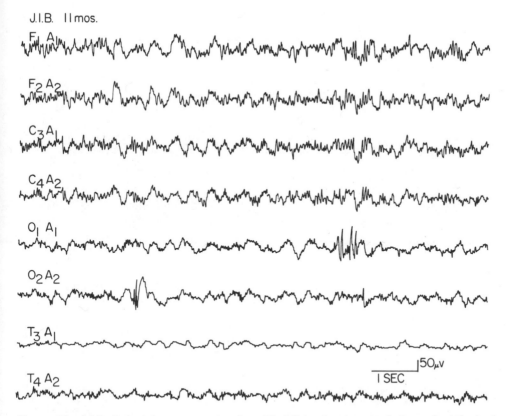

J.I.B. 11 mos.

Figure 11. J.I.B. Infant born prematurely with bilateral cataracts. Independent foci of spike discharge in the left and right occipital region awake and asleep. This sample is of Stage II sleep.

the ability of the involved and perhaps contiguous neurons to process information (Goldensohn and Purpura 1963).

Animal studies (Schmidt, Thomas, and Ward 1959; Ajmone Marsan 1961; Ward 1969) have demonstrated that EEG spikes are associated with bursts of action potentials in individual cortical units, and Ward and Schmidt (1961) and Rayport (1968) have shown that this is true of human spike foci. Intracellular recordings have demonstrated that these bursts of action potentials are produced by slow depolarizations of large magnitude, termed paroxysmal depolarization shifts, or PDSs (Prince 1968; Dichter and Spencer 1969; Matsumoto, Ayala, and Gumnit 1969).

The PDS is apparently an extraordinarily large synaptic potential, reflecting the response of the neuron to intense synaptic activation (Prince 1968; Matsumoto, Ayala, and Gumnit 1969). If this is true, some mechanism for producing this intense synchronization of synaptic drives must be pres-

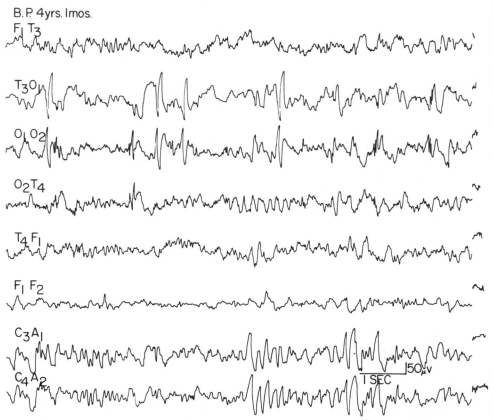

Figure 12. B.P. Right esotiopia from birth. Unsuccessful surgical correction attempt at age one year. Left occipital sharp and slow wave complexes and spikes in the left occipital. Occasional low voltage spikes in the right occipital independently.

ent. In the calcarine cortex, even in the adult, most synapses are of intrinsic origin, and less than 10 percent are derived from the cells of the lateral geniculate nucleus (Cragg 1971; Gary and Powell 1971). One possible mechanism for the intensification of synchronization might be a proliferation of loops of axodendritic excitation, as has been described in chronically denervated cortex of the kitten (Purpura and Housepian 1961).

Mechanism of Generation of the Occipital Spike

The mechanism underlying the generation of focal occipital spike activity in deafferentation, visual deprivation, and asymmetry of binocular afferent input (strabismus) can now be inferred on the basis of recent experimental data. In 1964, we (Smith and Kellaway 1964a) suggested that the fundamental mechanism responsible for cortical spike generation in the

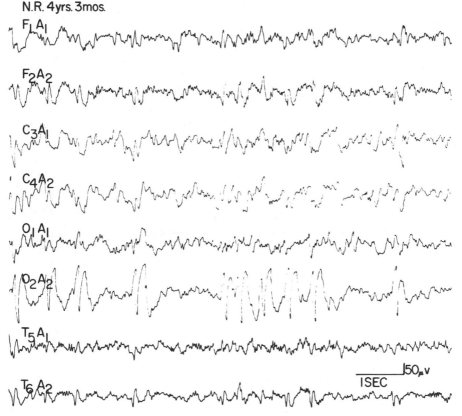

Figure 13. N.R. Exotropia left eye first noticed at age three weeks. High voltage, sharp and slow wave complexes in the right occipital, occasionally evident in the left.

presence of retinal destruction, visual deprivation, or asymmetry of visual input may be identical. The experimental evidence supports this hypothesis.

It is clear that functional and morphologic changes, similar to but not as profound as those consequent to deafferentation, may be induced by early visual deprivation. However, as the receptive fields of geniculate neurons are largely determined by their retinal input, it is, as we have previously suggested (Smith and Kellaway 1964a), probably more germane in terms of the generation of occipital spikes to consider the output from these cells as measured by the characteristics of the activity of neurons in the visual cortex. Wiesel and Hubel (1965b) found that kittens deprived either monocularly or binocularly by lid suturing during the first three months of life show profound visual deficits which demonstrate little recovery when the deprived eye or eyes have been open for as long as one year after the deprivation period. Such animals show some unusual properties of single units, such as to suggest that a "significant derangement" of the innate cortical connections had occurred (Wiesel and Hubel 1963a). Hyden (1943), twenty years earlier, had shown that the functional state of nerve cells in various brain regions depends upon the activity level of their inputs. More recent evidence indicates that qualitative differences between afferent input patterns from the two eyes may exert a more powerful influence on the organization and functional responses of cortical neurons in the developing brain than does binocular deprivation. The development of normal binocular connections apparently requires synchronous and coherent inputs from the two eyes during the critical period (Barlow, Blakemore, and Pettigrew 1967; Nikara, Bishop, and Pettigrew 1968). In the normal adult animal, each visual cortical neuron receives excitatory input from each eye and, if the neuron is to respond appropriately, the two retinal images must lie in an exact spatial relationship with one another (Pettigrew, Nikara, and Bishop 1968; Bishop, Henry, and Smith 1971). The specific relationship varies between neurons, but the optimal relationship is sharply demarcated (Rose and Blakemore 1974). The fact that the establishment of binocular connections is dependent on a dynamic and synchronous interaction of the patterns of input from each eye has been demonstrated by Hubel and Wiesel (1965), who showed that alternate occlusion of each eye, day by day, produces a progressive shift in eye dominance until only monocularly excitable neurons are present in the cortex. The results of monocular deprivation have been interpreted (Dews and Wiesel 1970) as evidence that geniculate cell axons from adjacent laminae compete with one another during development for synaptic surfaces of binocular cortical neurons, and that the reduced growth in the lateral geniculate nucleus is a consequence of the unbalanced axonal development of the binocular portion of the geniculocortical projections. (The deprived cells are conceived as being at a disadvantage in the competition.)

Guillery and Stelzner (1970) and Guillery (1972) have studied cell size in the lateral geniculate of the kitten following early monocular deprivation with concomitant destruction of a patch of temporal retina in the nonoccluded eye. They were able to demonstrate that cell growth in a visually deprived geniculate lamina is influenced by the conditions of the cells in an adjacent lamina. Deprived cells lying opposite an atrophic segment produced by local retinal destruction grow more than cells which lie opposite a normally innervated segment.

Spatial alignment also appears to be an important aspect for development of normal binocular connections. Surgically-induced strabismus within the critical period of development produces a population of exclusively monocular neurons in the cortex (Hubel and Wiesel 1965), and small vertical misalignments (circa 10-degrees), produced with the use of prisms, have similar consequences (Shlaer 1971). Similarly, von Noorden and Dowling (1970) have been able to produce amblyopia in two monkeys as a consequence of surgically-induced esotropia at the ages of 1 and 7 months, respectively. Baker, Grigg, and von Noorden (1974) studied single-cell activity in the visual cortices of these two animals. In one monkey, which, in the deviated eye, had light perception only, 2 out of 47 neurons could be influenced through the deviated eye. Both of these neurons were binocularly driven and were located close to each other in one penetration through the posterior lunate bank. Fifty-five percent of the neurons sampled could not be driven by visual stimulation of either eye. The second monkey, whose acuity in the deviated eye improved with time to 20/360, had more neurons driven from the deviated eye (39 of 68). Only three of these neurons were binocularly responsive, and these were highly dominated by the deviated eye. Although in esotropia the deviated eye is not deprived of light or pattern stimulation, the net morphologic effect and degree of visual impairment are similar to those seen in the monkey with monocular deprivation due to lid closure in the sensitive period (von Noorden 1973b). The only common denominator of the two conditions is the dissimilarity of input from the two eyes.

This evidence supports our original suggestion (Smith and Kellaway 1964a), based on the EEG evidence, that the basic mechanism underlying the development of occipital spikes in strabismus with unilateral argambly-opia is similar to that associated with visual deprivation or retinal destruction. The structural/functional characteristics of the neural substrate of the spike foci in these three conditions have not been precisely defined, but they appear to be based on a rearrangement of cortical connections common to each.

We suggested originally that the occipital spikes seen clinically following deafferentation arise in the striate cortex as a consequence of a denervation sensitization effect similar to that which occurs in effector organs. This phenomenon is apparently based on a supersensitivity of the denervated end-organ to transmitter substances (Sharpless 1969) and is common to various types of excitable tissue (Cannon and Rosenblueth 1949). A slowly developing increase in excitability to the point of spontaneous epileptiform discharge is a characteristic feature of neuronally isolated cortex (Echlin 1959). This phenomenon has been variously attributed to a chemical sensitizing effect similar to that seen in denervated muscle or to a proliferation of recurrent axon collaterals (Purpura 1964).

The phenomenon of axodendritic proliferation has been described only in denervated (undercut) cerebral cortex in neonatal kittens. The hyperexcitability and spontaneous focal discharges that occur in such isolated-cortex preparations are associated with precocious development of intracortical axon collaterals of elements whose main-stem axons are interrupted in the process of undercutting. An extraordinary development of axon collaterals in the involved neuron results in conversion of large, type I neurons into type II cells, with axons ramifying entirely in the cortex. The spontaneous spike activity arising in undercut, immature cortex is believed by Purpura (1964) to reside in a hyperexcitability initiated by recurrent axon collaterals that effect synaptic relations with adjacent pyramidal neurons via the cell body as well as with basilar dendrites and proximal portions of apical dendrites. As Purpura conceives it, the major developmental alterations underlying the hyperexcitability are related to reorganization of subsurface synaptic pathways, leading to an overall increase in net excitatory synaptic drives on pyramidal neurons. The existence of such changes following transneuronal degeneration or attenuation of visual input in the cortex of immature animals is yet to be demonstrated. Globus and Scheibel (1967) and Valverde (1968) have found that after enucleation in rabbits and mice, there is a statistically significant loss of dendritic spines on the apical dendrites of certain pyramidal cells in the striate cortex. The loss of spines is generally confined to a specific segment of the dendritic tree that is assumed to be the site of termination of the geniculate cortical fibers; but even in this segment, an appreciable number of normal spines persist (Valverde and Esteban 1968). In mice raised in darkness, Valverde (1967) has also demonstrated a statistically significant diminution of the mean number of dendritic spines per segment in the apical shafts of layer V pyramidal cells of the visual cortex. The number of dendritic spines in the visual cortex has been shown to be significantly altered in visually deprived rabbits, and Coleman and Riesen (1968) have shown that stellate cells of layer IV in the visual cortex of cats reared in the dark have shorter and fewer dendrites than those of normal animals.

The extraordinary sensitivity of the primate brain to deafferentation or deprivation may render it unique in the capacity to develop occipital spiking. Kellaway, Druckman, and Moore (unpublished) were unable to induce occipital spiking in the rabbit or kitten by surgical enucleation in newborn animals. Recordings made from chronically implanted cortical electrodes for periods up to eight months after enucleation at three to twenty days after birth failed to reveal any evidence of abnormal electrical activity in striate cortex.

Baxter (1966) was unable to find any difference in the spontaneous electrical activity of the visual cortex in dark-reared as compared to light-reared kittens. However, recent studies of the effects of acute deafferentation on spontaneous single-unit activity in adult cat visual cortex have reported a strong tendency toward rhythmic synchronous firing of neighboring visual cortical neurons, accompanied by characteristic bursts of 6 to 8 per second waves in the EEG (Kasamatsu and Adey 1974a, 1974b). The same authors also reported that visual cortical units following enucleation showed long-lasting spike trains with short to moderate interspike intervals.

In the monkey occipital cortical spike activity has been seen following deafferentation (Doty 1970). Sakakura and Doty (1969) report that after bilateral enucleation in the squirrel monkey, "the EEG of striate cortex becomes flat (!), punctuated by sporadic spikes." This effect occurred acutely and in adult animals and was interpreted by the authors to indicate that "some aspect of normal retinal activity must exert continual control over the . . . excitability of the striate cortex." The significance of these findings in the squirrel monkey in relation to the late-developing spike foci seen in man following enucleation is not clear, and elucidation must await serial electrical studies of deafferentation in infant primates.

It is possible only to speculate on the precise mechanism of generation of spikes in visual cortex in children as a delayed consequence of deafferentation, form deprivation, or disparity of binocular input in infancy. The one factor that the animal work indicates is common to all three situations is a change in cortical connectivity. The dynamics of spike generation might involve, therefore, a decrease in inhibitory input or an increase in synchronized excitatory synaptic drives or a combination of both of these.

The primary sensory receiving areas of the cortex in the human infant have less dendritic arborization and fewer interconnections between cells than all other regions of the cortex, except the so-called association areas (Conel 1939, 1941, and 1947). The number of neurons and the density of their interconnections increase over a period of at least two years after birth. Clearly, the conditions in the cortex of the human infant are such as to favor, in the absence of appropriate afferent input, proliferation of recurrent axon collaterals and a net increase in excitatory synaptic activity.

Whatever the fundamental mechanism of spike generation may finally prove to be, the demonstration that spike foci may arise in a primary projection area of the cortex as a consequence of altered afferent input during a critical period of ontogenesis has important implications for developmental neurology and for clinical electroencephalography.

Spike foci are the most common of all the specific, abnormal, electrical phenomena encountered in the EEGs of children, and in a high percentage of cases it is not possible to identify retrospectively the etiologic agent responsible for the focus. For example, in a retrospective study, Smith and Kellaway (1964b) were able to determine a cause in less than 40 percent of 200 children with rolandic spike foci, and even in those in whom a possible etiology was identified, the evidence in most cases was circumstantial rather than conclusive. This has proved true of all foci, regardless of location (Kellaway, unpublished data). It would appear, therefore, that most electrographic foci in children are a consequence of etiological factors yet to be identified.

Another factor of apparent importance which emerged from this study of children with focal EEG abnormalities was the large percentage who had onset of central nervous system problems very early in life. More children with spike foci had onset of symptoms in the first six months of life than in any one-year epoch thereafter, and three times as many developed symptoms in the first year as in any other period (Scott and Kellaway 1958). These findings strongly suggest that the factors responsible for the genesis of the abnormality were operant in a very early stage of development.

The demonstration that spike foci may arise as a consequence of a pathological process acting peripherally (on the sense organ) is the first evidence we have that such foci, which have classically been considered a sign of a palpable brain lesion, may be engendered by an agent which does not act directly at the site of the focus. Clearly, spike foci elsewhere, for which no etiologic cause can now be specified, might also have their origin in defects of afferent input or other pathophysiological mechanisms presently unidentified. The recognized causes of focal electrical abnormalities (trauma, tumor, infection, etc.) may in fact account for a minority of the EEG spike foci seen in children.

The Critical Period in Human Infants

Our own serial findings do not yield a clear picture of the upper extent of the age limit of the critical period in which the human infant brain is vulnerable to aberrations of visual input. At the low end, the implications of the anophthalmos group are obvious. The upper age limit and whether there are circumscribed epochs within a more general critical period in which there is a supersensitivity to a given type of alteration of sensory input have not been established. The period of high susceptibility to monocular deprivation in the rhesus monkey is birth to 12 weeks (von Noorden 1973a). However, chromatic and binocular vision are not fully developed until the end of early childhood (4 to 5 years) and, on the basis of clinical experience, ophthalmologists usually set this as the age limit for any significant restoration of vision with forced use of an argamblyopic eye. von Noorden's (1973a) studies of children rendered amblyopic by disease at various ages during the first few years of life indicate that the sensitive period is much more prolonged than in the monkey, possibly extending beyond the age of four years (see also von Senden 1960).

Early Experience and the Neural Organization of the Brain

The model I have employed to illustrate the role of afferent input as a determinant of ontogenetic development may serve as a basis for extrapolation to more comple aspects of early experience and higher levels of behavioral integration. The neurobiologists have already achieved another level in the analysis of the problem by demonstrating, in a cogent manner, that in the immature brain experience is necessary for the appropriate organization of the sensory system in terms of the environment in which the organism lives. Appropriate organization may be achieved by the making of "S-S" connections, which Hebb (1949) has postulated must precede "S-R" learning. The structural and functional changes consequent to monocular deprivation and spatial disparity of binocular inputs are consonant with this postulate and with the concept that a developing axon will make contact preferentially with a cell when the activity of the axon and the target cell are correlated (Marr 1970).

It was previously thought that some neurons of the visual cortex of visually inexperienced kittens have all of the specific properties of the adult animal (Hubel and Wiesel 1963, 1970; Wiesel and Hubel 1965a). However, Barlow and Pettigrew (1971) have shown that many cells in the visually naive cortex can be activated through either eye by a stimulus moving along a particular axis. They further showed that the mechanisms for disparity and orientational selectivity require visual experience. Whereas in a normal adult cat, 68 percent of cells are disparity-selective, no cells with disparity-selectivity could be detected in the cortex of visually deprived kittens. The immature neuron shows marked binocular facilitation, with the binocular response being many times greater than the response to either eye alone, and with no clear left-right optimum.

These observations were the prelude to a series of experiments that demonstrate that the neuronal organization of a sensory system during the critical period of development is evolved, in terms of adaptation, to match the probability of occurrence of features in its sensory experience. Thus, when kittens were reared with one eye viewing vertical stripes and the other eye horizontal stripes, all cortical neurons with elongated receptive fields could, after a period, be monocularly driven, and the receptive-field orientations were coincident with the stripe pattern to which the eye had been exposed (Hirsch and Spinelli 1970, 1971; Hirsch 1972). When kittens were raised from birth to four and one-half months in a visual environment limited only to vertical or horizontal stripes, they exhibited normal behavioral and neurophysiological responses only to stimuli presented in the orientation of the visual environment in which they had been raised. When stimuli were presented in an orthogonal orientation, behavioral blindness was evident, and no responsive neurons could be detected in the visual cortex. "Not one neuron had its optimal orientation within 20-degrees of the inappropriate axis, and there were in-toto only twelve within 45-degrees of it" (Blakemore and Cooper 1970). Similar effects have recently been achieved during the critical period with quite brief exposure to a specifically oriented environment (Blakemore and Mitchell 1973).

An analogous situation has been shown to occur in human subjects with pronounced, uncorrected astigmatism dating from early life. Such individuals may show considerable differences in the visual resolution of vertical as compared to horizontal gratings. Evidence has been adduced to show that these meridional-resolution discrepancies are central in origin (Freeman, Mitchell, and Millodot 1972). It is not known if such experiential modifications of neuronal organization and function have an electrical signature. The behavioral and physiological changes are as profound as those seen, for example, in monocular deprivation, but the conditions essential for the generation of focal spike activity may not necessarily be present.

Summary

Prospective and retrospective studies are described which demonstrate that children rendered amblyopic during infancy develop occipital foci of abnormal electrical activity in the EEG. The character of this activity and its evolution over time are quite similar in blind infants regardless of the nature of the pathological process involving the end organ and optic nerve. The abnormal activity initially consists of single or polyspike discharges of rapid time course, which may initially only be demonstrable during slow-wave sleep. The voltage and incidence of the spikes tend to increase with age. The duration of the individual spikes also increases with age, and spike and slow-wave complexes tend to replace the rapid single and polyspike discharges seen initially. This type of progression is generally conceived as consequent to increased synchronization of the activity of involved neurons and increase in the size of the involved neuronal aggregate.

This evolving pattern is characteristic regardless of the nature of the pathologic process underlying the defect in the peripheral visual system. Thus, deafferentation or enucleation, or consequent to optic atrophy, has the same electroencephalographic consequences as pattern deprivation (cataracts). Of special interest is the finding that esotropia or exotropia dating from infancy may also give rise to occipital spike foci.

The evidence from a prospective study of 21 infants with retrolental fibroplasia indicates that the foci of abnormal occipital activity require a certain time to develop, or at least to reach a degree of synchronization at which they become manifest at the scalp. The data is not entirely adequate, but it would appear that the time of earliest development is about 7 to 10 months. Individual patients with other causes for deafferentation (enucleation, optic atrophy and anophthalmos), who have been followed prospectively, show a similar evolution.

On the basis of these EEG observations it is suggested that the fundamental pathophysiologic mechanism underlying the generation of the abnormal activity in the occipital cortex is the same for deafferentation, pattern deprivation and asymmetry of visual input (strabismus). The essential factor is that the deprivation, attentuation or derangement of afferent input occur before a certain, yet to be determined, critical age.

Experimental evidence derived from animal studies during the past 15 years provides the basis for a rational explanation of the clinical phenomenology. The principle of "criticality" has been repeatedly demonstrated in the morphologic and functional development of the visual system. It is now known that significant alterations in the behavior of individual visual cortical neurons occur as a consequence of deprivation or derangement of visual afferent input if this occurs within a certain critical period of development. Such changes can be brought about by very brief periods of altered visual input during this critical epoch and the changes may be virtually permanent. The functional alterations appear to be largely a consequence of morphologic changes. The plasticity of the visual system appears to be due not only to the proliferation and rapid growth of neurons and increase in the number of synapses during this period, but also to changes in ultrastructure—changes in efficacy of individual synapses. Imaginative experiments in which infant animals were reared in special, restricted visual environments have provided evidence which strongly indicates that the neuronal organization of a sensory system during the critical period of development is evolved, in terms of adaptation, to match the probability of occurrence of features of its sensory experience. The heuristic implications of the clinical electrographic observations in the light of the animal investigations which provide the basis for their explanation should serve as a stimulus to the search for more subtle associations between behavior and brain electrical activity.

References

Ajmone Marsan, C. 1961. Electrographic aspects of "epileptic" neuronal aggregates. *Epilepsia* 2:22.

Ashton, N., Ward, B., and Serpel, G. 1953. Role of oxygen in the genesis of retrolental fibroplasia: a preliminary report. *Br. J. Ophthalmol.* 37:513.

Baker, F.H., Grigg, P., and von Noorden, G.K. 1974. Effects of visual deprivation and strabismus on the response of neurons in the visual cortex of the monkey, including studies on the striate and prestriate cortex in the normal animal. *Brain Res.* 66:185.

Barlow, H.B., Blakemore, C., and Pettigrew, J.D. 1967. The neural mechanism of binocular depth discrimination. *J. Physiol. (Lond.)* 193:327.

Barlow, H.B., and Pettigrew, J.D. 1971. Lack of specificity of neurones in the visual cortex of young kittens. *J. Physiol. (Lond.)* 218:98P.

Baxter, B.L. 1966. Effect of visual deprivation during postnatal maturation on the electroencephalogram of the cat. *Exp. Neurol.* 14:224.

Berger, H. 1900. Experimentell-anatomische Studien über die durch den Mangel optischer Reize veranlaBten Entwicklungshemmungen im Occipitallappen des Hundes und der Katze. *Arch. Psychiatr. Nervenkr.* 33:521.

Bishop, P.O., Henry, G.H., and Smith, C.J. 1971. Binocular interaction fields of single units in the cat striate cortex. *J. Physiol. (Lond.)* 216:39.

Blakemore, C., and Cooper, G.F. 1970. Development of the brain depends on the visual environment. *Nature (Lond.)* 228:477.

Blakemore, C., and Mitchell, D.E. 1973. Modification by very brief exposure to the visual environment. *Nature (Lond.)* 241:467.

Campbell, K. 1951. Intensive oxygen therapy as a possible cause of retrolental fibroplasia: a clinical approach. *Med. J. Aust.* 2:48.

Cannon, W.B., and Rosenblueth, A. 1949. *The Supersensitivity of Denervated Structures.* New York: Macmillan.

Cohen, J., Boshes, L.D., and Snider, R.S. 1961. Electroencephalographic changes following retrolental fibroplasia. *Electroencephalogr. Clin. Neurophysiol.* 13:914.

Coleman, P.D., and Riesen, A.H. 1968. Environmental effects on cortical dendritic fields. I. Rearing in the dark. *J. Anat.* 102:363.

Conel, J.L. 1939. *The Postnatal Development of the Human Cerebral Cortex*, vol. I. Cambridge, Mass.: Harvard University Press.

Conel, J.L. 1941. *The Postnatal Development of the Human Cerebral Cortex*, vol. II. Cambridge, Mass.: Harvard University Press.

Conel, J.L. 1947. *The Postnatal Development of the Human Cerebral Cortex*, vol. III. Cambridge, Mass.: Harvard University Press.

Cook, W.H., Walker, J.H., and Barr, M.L. 1951. A cytological study of transneuronal atrophy in the cat and rabbit. *J. Comp. Neurol.* 94:267.

Cragg, B.G. 1971. The fate of axon terminals in visual cortex during transsynaptic atrophy of the lateral geniculate nucleus. *Brain Res.* 34:53.

Detwiler, S.R. 1936. *Neuroembryology: An Experimental Study*. New York: Macmillan.

Dews, P.B., and Wiesel, T.N. 1970. Consequences of monocular deprivation on visual behaviour in kittens. *J. Physiol. (Lond.)* 206:437.

Dichter, M., and Spencer, W.A. 1969. Penicillin-induced interictal discharges from the cat hippocampus. II. Mechanisms underlying origin and restriction. *J. Neurophysiol.* 32:663.

Doty, R.W. 1970. Modulation of visual input by brain-stem systems. In F.A. Young, and D.B. Lindsley (eds.), *Early Experience and Visual Information Processing in Perceptual and Reading Disorders*, p. 143. Washington, D.C.: National Academy of Sciences.

Echlin, F.A. 1959. The supersensitivity of chronically "isolated" cerebral cortex as a mechanism in focal epilepsy. *Electroencephalogr. Clin. Neurophysiol.* 11:697.

Freedman, D.A. 1971. Congenital and perinatal sensory deprivation: Some studies in early development. *Am. J. Psychiatry* 127:1539.

Freedman, R.D., Mitchell, D.E., and Millodot, M. 1972. A neural effect of partial visual deprivation in humans. *Science* 175:1384.

Ganz, L., Fitch, M., and Satterberg, J.A. 1968. The selective effect of visual deprivation on receptive field shape determined neurophysiologically. *Exp. Neurol.* 22:614.

Gary, L.J., and Powell, T.P.S. 1971. An experimental study of the termination of the lateral geniculo-cortical pathway in the cat and monkey. *Proc. R. Soc. Lond. [Biol]* 179:41.

Gibbs, E.L., Fois, A., and Gibbs, F.A. 1955. The electroencephalogram in retrolental fibro-plasia. *N. Engl. J. Med.* 253:1102.

Gibbs, F.A., and Gibbs, E.L. 1952. *Atlas of Electroencephalography, Vol. 2, Epilepsy*, p. 223. Cambridge, Mass.: Addison-Wesley Press.

Glees, P. 1961. Terminal degeneration and trans-synaptic atrophy in the lateral geniculate body of the monkey. In R. Jung and H. Kornhuber (eds.), *The Visual System: Neurophysiology and Psychophysics*, p. 104. Berlin: Springer-Verlag.

Globus, A., and Scheibel, A.B. 1967. The effect of visual deprivation on cortical neurons—a Golgi study. *Exp. Neurol.* 19:331.

Goldensohn, E.S., and Purpura, D.P. 1963. Intracellular potentials of cortical neurons during focal epileptogenic discharges. *Science* 139:840.

Goldensohn, E.S., Zablow, L., and Stein, B. 1970. Interrelationships of form and latency of spike discharge from small areas of human cortex. *Electroencephalogr. Clin. Neurophysiol.* 29:321.

Guillery, R.W. 1972. Binocular competition in the control of geniculate cell growth. *J. Comp. Neurol.* 144:117.

Guillery, R.W., and Stelzner, D.J. 1970. The differential effects of unilateral lid closure upon the monocular and binocular segments of the dorsal lateral geniculate nucleus in the cat. *J. Comp. Neurol.* 139:413.

Gyllensten, L.J., and Hellstrom, B.E. 1952. Retrolental fibroplasia: Animal experiments. Effect of intermittently administered oxygen and postnatal development of eyes of full-term mice. *Acta Paediatr.* 41:577.

Harlow, H.F., Harlow, M.K., and Suomi, S.J. 1971. From thought to therapy: Lessons from a primate laboratory. *Am. Sci.* 59:538.

Hebb, D.O. 1949. *The Organization of Behavior: A Neuropsychological Theory*. New York: John Wiley & Sons.

Hirsch, H.V.B. 1972. Visual perception in cats after environmental surgery. *Exp. Brain Res.* 15:405.

Hirsch, H.V.B., and Spinelli, D.N. 1970. Visual experience modifies distribution of horizontally and vertically oriented receptive fields in cats. *Science* 168:869.

Hirsch, H.V.B., and Spinelli, D.N. 1971. Modification of the distribution of receptive field orientation in cats by selective visual exposure during development. *Exp. Brain Res.* 13:509.

Horn, G., Rose, S.P.R., and Bateson, P.P.G. 1973. Experience and plasticity in the central nervous system. *Science* 181:506.

Hubel, D.H., and Wiesel, T.N. 1963. Receptive fields of cells in striate cortex of very young, visually inexperienced kittens. *J. Neurophysiol.* 26:994.

Hubel, D.H., and Wiesel, T.N. 1965. Binocular interaction in striate cortex of kittens reared with artificial squint. *J. Neurophysiol.* 28:1041.

Hubel, D.H., and Wiesel, T.N. 1970. The period of susceptibility to the physiological effects of unilateral eye closure in kittens. *J. Physiol. (Lond.)* 206:419.

Hyden, H. 1943. Protein metabolism in the nerve cell during growth and function. *Acta Physiol. Scand.* 6(Suppl. 17):3.

Jacobson, M. 1970. *Developmental Neurobiology*. New York: Holt, Rinehart and Winston.

Kasamatsu, T., and Adey, W.R. 1974a. Immediate effects of total visual deafferentation on single unit activity in the visual cortex of freely behaving cats. I. Tonic excitability changes. *Exp. Brain Res.* 20:157.

Kasamatsu, T., and Adey, W.R. 1974b. Immediate effects of total visual deafferentation on single unit activity in the visual cortex of freely behaving cats. II. Rhythmic EEG burst and PGO waves. *Exp. Brain Res.* 20:171.

Kellaway, P., Bloxsom, A., and MacGregor, M. 1955. Occipital spike foci associated with retrolental fibroplasia and other forms of retinal loss in children. *Electroencephalogr. Clin. Neurophysiol.* 7:469.

Kupfer, C., and Palmer, P. 1964. Lateral geniculate nucleus: Histological and cytochemical changes following afferent denervation and visual deprivation. *Exp. Neurol.* 9:400.

Marr, D. 1970. A theory of cerebral neocortex. *Proc. R. Soc. Lond. [Biol.]* 176:161.

Mason, W.A., Davenport, R.K., Jr., and Menzel, E.W., Jr. 1968. Early experience and the social development of rhesus monkeys and chimpanzees. In G. Newton, and S. Levine (eds.), *Early Experience and Behavior*, p. 1. Springfield, Ill.: Charles C Thomas.

Matsumoto, H., Ayala, G.F., and Gumnit, R.J. 1969. Neuronal behavior and triggering mechanisms in cortical epileptic focus. *J. Neurophysiol.* 32:688.

Matthews, M.R. 1964. Further observations on transneuronal degeneration in the lateral geniculate nucleus of the macaque monkey. *J. Anat.* 98:255.

Matthews, M.R., Cowan, W.M., and Powell, T.P.S. 1960. Transneuronal cell degeneration in the lateral geniculate nucleus of the macaque monkey. *J. Anat.* 94:145.

Nikara, T., Bishop, P.O., and Pettigrew, J.D. 1968. Analysis of retinal correspondence by studying receptive fields of binocular single units in cat striate cortex. *Exp. Brain Res.* 6:353.

Owens, W.C., and Owens, E.U. 1949. Retrolental fibroplasia in premature infants. *Am. J. Ophthalmol.* 32:1.

Patz, A., Hoeck, L.E., and DeLaCruz, E. 1952. Studies of the effect of high oxygen administration in retrolental fibroplasia. *Am. J. Ophthalmol.* 35:1248.

Pettigrew, J.D., Nikara, T., and Bishop, P.O. 1968. Binocular interaction on single units in the cat striate cortex: Simultaneous stimulation by single moving slit with receptive fields in correspondence. *Exp. Brain Res.* 6:391.

Prince, D.A. 1968. The depolarization shift in "epileptic" neurons. *Exp. Neurol.* 21:467.

Purpura, D.P. 1964. Relationship of seizure susceptibility to morphologic and physiologic properties of normal and abnormal immature cortex. In P. Kellaway, and I. Petersen (eds.), *Neurological and Electroencephalographic Correlative Studies in Infancy*, p. 117. New York: Grune & Stratton.

Purpura, D.P., and Housepian, E.M. 1961. Morphological and physiological properties of chronically isolated immature cortex. *Exp. Neurol.* 4:377.

Ramon y Cajal, S. 1959. *Degeneration and Regeneration of the Nervous System.* New York: Hafner.

Rayport, M. 1968. The Jacksonian hypothesis: An appraisal in the light of single unit recording in focal epileptogenic gray matter in man. *Proc. Rudolph Virchow Med. Soc. City N.Y.* Suppl. 26:301.

Rose, D., and Blakemore, C. 1974. An analysis of orientation selectivity in the cat's visual cortex. *Exp. Brain Res.* 20:1.

Sakakura, H., and Doty, R.W. 1969. Bizarre EEG of striate cortex in blind squirrel monkeys. *Electroencephalogr. Clin. Neurophysiol.* 27:734.

Schmidt, R.P., Thomas, L.B., and Ward, A.A., Jr. 1959. The hyperactive neuron. Microelectrode studies of chronic epileptic foci in monkey. *J. Neurophysiol.* 22:285.

Scott, J.P. 1962. Critical periods in behavioral development. *Science* 138:949.

Scott, J.S., and Kellaway, P. 1958. Epilepsy of focal origin in childhood. *Med. Clin. North Am.* 42:415.

Sharpless, S.K. 1969. Isolated and deafferented neurons: Disuse supersensitivity. In H.H. Jasper, A.A. Ward, Jr., and A. Pope (eds.), *Basic Mechanisms of the Epilepsies*, p. 329. Boston: Little, Brown.

Shlaer, R. 1971. Shift in binocular disparity causes compensatory change in the cortical structure of kittens. *Science* 173:638.

Sluckin, W. 1972. *Imprinting and Early Learning*, 2nd. ed. London: Methuen.

Smith, J.M.B., and Kellaway, P. 1964a. The natural history and clinical correlates of occipital foci in children. In P. Kellaway, and I. Petersen (eds.), *Neurological and Electroencephalographic Correlative Studies in Infancy*, p. 230. New York: Grune & Stratton.

Smith, J.M.B., and Kellaway, P. 1964b. Central (Rolandic) foci in children: an analysis of 200 cases. *Electroencephalogr. Clin. Neurophysiol.* 17:460.

Stillerman, M.L., Gibbs, E.L., and Perlstein, M.A. 1952. Electroencephalographic changes in strabismus. *Am. J. Ophthalmol.* 35:54.

Valverde, F. 1967. Apical dendritic spines of the visual cortex and light deprivation in the mouse. *Exp. Brain Res.* 3:337.

Valverde, F. 1968. Structural changes in the area striata of the mouse after enucleation. *Exp. Brain Res.* 5:274.

Valverde, F., and Esteban, M.E. 1968. Peristriate cortex of mouse: Location and the effects of enucleation on the number of dendritic spines. *Brain Res.* 9:145.

von Gudden, B. 1869. Experimentaluntersuchungen über das peripherische und zentrale Nervensystem. *Arch. Psychiatry.* 2:693.

von Noorden, G.K. 1973a. Experimental amblyopia in monkeys. Further behavioral observations and clinical correlations. *Invest. Ophthalmol.* 12:721.

von Noorden, G.K. 1973b. Histological studies of the visual system in monkeys with experimental amblyopia. *Invest. Ophthalmol.* 12:727.

von Noorden, G.K., and Dowling, J.E. 1970. Experimental amblyopia in monkeys. II. Behavioral studies in strabismic amblyopia. *Arch. Ophthalmol.* 84:215.

von Senden, M. 1960. *Space and Sight. The Perception of Space and Shape in the Congenitally Blind Before and After Operation.* Glencoe, Ill.: The Free Press.

Ward, A.A., Jr. 1969. The epileptic neuron: Chronic foci in animals and in man. In H.H. Jasper, A.A. Ward, Jr., and A. Pope (eds.), *Basic Mechanisms of the Epilepsies,* p. 263. Boston: Little, Brown.

Ward, A.A., Jr., and Schmidt, R.P. 1961. Some properties of single epileptic neurons. *Arch. Neurol.* 5:308.

Wiesel, T.N., and Hubel, D.H. 1963a. Effects of visual deprivation on morphology and physiology of cells in the cat's lateral geniculate body. *J. Neurophysiol.* 26:978.

Wiesel, T.N., and Hubel, D.H. 1963b. Single-cell responses in striate cortex of kittens deprived of vision in one eye. *J. Neurophysiol.* 26:1003.

Wiesel, T.N., and Hubel, D.H. 1965a. Comparison of the effects of unilateral and bilateral eye closure on cortical unit responses in kittens. *J. Neurophysiol.* 28:1029.

Wiesel, T.N., and Hubel, D.H. 1965b. Extent of recovery from the effects of visual deprivation in kittens. *J. Neurophysiol.* 28:1060.

cerebral physiology of the aged: relation to psychological function

Walter D. Obrist, Ph.D.

Duke University Medical Center
Durham, North Carolina

The purpose of this paper is to examine the relationship of altered cerebral physiology to impairment of intellectual function in old age. Although behavioral changes in senescence are well-documented, little attention has been paid to cerebral physiologic variables, primarily because of the limitations of directly observing such phenomena. An attempt will be made here to review some of the evidence available from electroencephalographic (EEG) and cerebral circulatory studies.

Brain rhythms as recorded from the human scalp undergo progressive changes with age from birth through senescence. Following a period of rapid development associated with physical growth, EEG patterns become stabilized in early maturity, but then undergo further alterations in the senium. Although it is hazardous to draw sweeping conclusions regarding senescent EEG changes, certain overall trends emerge that are worth noting. Outstanding among the age-related changes are shifts in the frequency spectrum. Relative to young adult standards, the average senescent EEG is shifted to the slow side, so that its frequency content resembles that of childhood. Specifically, there is a decrease in frequency of the dominant alpha rhythm (8 to 12 cycles per second), accompanied by an increase in the abundance of slower theta (4 to 7 cps) and delta (1 to 3 cps) waves. This regression of EEG frequency to an earlier level follows the general trend of many growth curves, including those for brain weight and intellectual function.

Because of variable rates of change, individual differences in EEG pattern become greater during senescence. As reviewed elsewhere (Obrist 1974), both longitudinal and cross-sectional studies suggest that health and institutionalization are critical variables related to the occurrence and rate of EEG change. Thus, elderly subjects who live in the community and maintain good health continue to reveal tracings that deviate only slightly from young adult standards, while institutionalized subjects and patients suffering from illnesses that directly or indirectly affect the nervous system undergo more pronounced EEG alterations. It is clear from this that characterization of specific EEG changes and their relation to intellectual function will depend on the particular population of elderly persons studied.

The most common age-related EEG change in senescence is a slowing down of the dominant alpha rhythm from a mean frequency of 10 cps to approximately 8 or 9 cps (Otomo 1966). The magnitude of this slowing is significantly related to both health status and longevity, being greatest among individuals with chronic illness, particularly cardiac and cerebrovascular disease (Obrist 1974). It is the presence or absence of such pathological factors that determines the relationship between alpha frequency and psychological function. As in the case of young adults, EEG findings bear little or no relationship to intelligence-test performance in healthy old subjects in whom both alpha frequency and cognitive function are well preserved (Birren et al. 1963). Significant correlations between EEG and mental function are obtained, however, in subjects with clinically evident disorders of the circulatory system, where alpha frequency and intelligence test performance undergo parallel declines (Obrist et al. 1962).

The EEG shows more pronounced alterations in aged patients with organic brain syndrome (OBS). Slow waves below the alpha range (theta and delta activity) usually predominate, appearing bilaterally and diffusely over the head. Figure 1 contrasts a normal with a diffusely slow EEG in two elderly patients of approximately the same age. The upper tracing, which has a normal alpha rhythm of 9 cps, was obtained from a physically well-preserved patient with paranoid tendencies but no obvious intellectual impairment. The lower tracing, which is dominated by diffuse delta and theta activity, was recorded from a patient with long-standing arteriosclerotic heart disease, who underwent progressive mental deterioration over a six-year period. Using a psychiatric rating scale, McAdam and Robinson (1962) obtained a correlation of +0.79 between the severity of intellectual impairment and degree of EEG slowing, quantitatively determined. The extent of the frequency shift occurring with mental deterioration is illustrated in Figure 2, in which 45 elderly patients with organic brain syndrome are compared with 47 healthy aged controls studied by the present author and co-workers. Not only is the dominant (peak) frequency

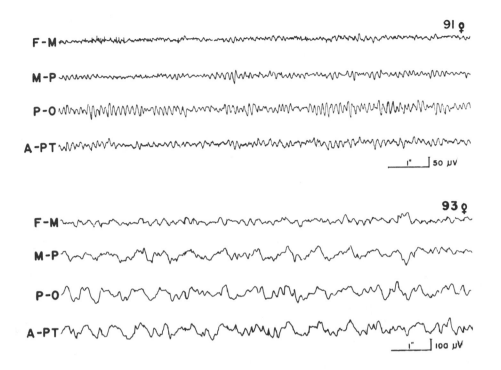

Figure 1. Top four lines: 91-year-old woman with paranoid reaction. Bottom four lines: 93-year-old woman with chronic brain syndrome. F = frontal, M = motor area, P = parietal, O = occipital, A-PT = anterior to posterior temporal. Only recordings from the left hemisphere are shown. From Obrist and Henry 1958a.

slower in the patient group, but there is a general increase in slow waves below 8 cps, with a corresponding decrease in faster activity.

Because diffuse slow activity is correlated with mental deterioration, its presence or absence has permitted a rough differentiation between organic and functional psychiatric disorders in old age (Frey and Sjögren 1959). Table 1 presents the EEG findings in two groups of hospitalized elderly psychiatric patients studied by Obrist and Henry (1958a, 1958b). A comparison is made between organic brain syndrome and "functional" disorders, the latter consisting primarily of depressions and paranoid reactions. Whereas diffuse slow activity is present in 30 of the 45 cases with OBS, it was found in only two patients with functional disorders. In contrast, normal tracings were recorded in 28 of the 45 functional cases and in only four patients with OBS. A slow occipital alpha rhythm of less than 8 cps distinguished the patients, although less clearly. Focal slow activity, on the other hand, failed to differentiate the groups. As shown in Table 1, EEG indices were also predictive of the outcome of illness one year later. Most

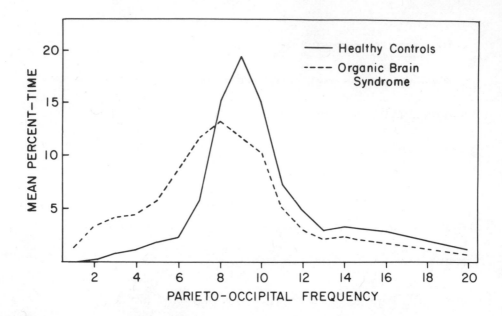

Figure 2. Mean EEG frequency spectra for two groups of elderly subjects: 47 healthy community volunteers (average age, 71), and 45 hospitalized patients with organic brain syndrome (average age, 76). The curves indicate the percentage of time that waves of a given frequency are present in the parieto-occipital tracing, as determined by manual frequency analysis. From Obrist 1974.

TABLE 1. Relation of EEG Findings to Diagnosis and Prognosis in
90 Aged Psychiatric Patients

Number of Cases with Different EEG Findings	Diagnosis		Outcome after One Year	
	Functional Disorder (N = 45)	Organic Brain Syndrome (N = 45)	Discharged or Convalescent (N = 47)	Hospitalized or Died (N = 43)
Normal tracing	28	4	23	9
Diffuse slow activity	2	30	9	23
Focal slow activity	8	7	8	7
Slow alpha rhythm*	8	16	10	14

*Not mutually exclusive with diffuse and focal slow activity

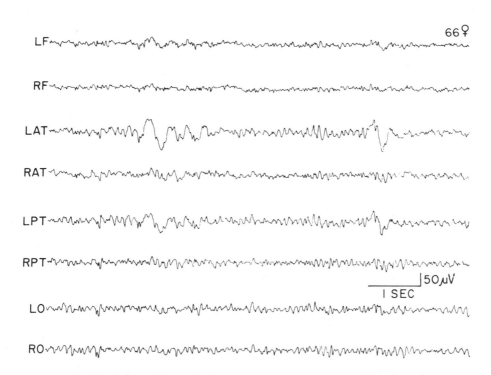

Figure 3. A left anterior temporal delta-wave focus in a 66-year-old woman who is in good health and living in the community. L = left, R = right, F = frontal, AT = anterior temporal, PT = posterior temporal, O = occipital. From Busse and Obrist 1965.

patients with diffuse slow activity either died or remained hospitalized, while those with normal tracings tended to be discharged. Similar reports on the prognostic significance of EEG findings in geriatric psychiatry have appeared elsewhere (Pampiglione and Post 1958, McAdam and Robinson 1962, Cahan and Yeager 1966).

In contrast to diffuse slowing, sharply localized EEG abnormalities are rarely associated with senescent intellectual decline. This is especially true of slow activity that is restricted to the anterior temporal region, a phenomenon observed in almost one third of normal elderly subjects, and manifested as early as middle age (Kooi et al. 1964, Busse and Obrist 1965). Figure 3 displays a left temporal focus recorded from a healthy old person. In an unpublished study by the author and S.H. Davis, 13 aged community volunteers with severe anterior temporal foci (delta waves) were compared with 13 age- and education-matched subjects having normal EEGs. Neurological findings were negative in all subjects except one in each group who had evidence of cerebrovascular disease. As shown in Table 2, no

TABLE 2. Psychological Function in Elderly Community-Living Subjects with
Two Types of EEG (Means and Standard Deviations)

	Normal Tracing (N = 13)	Severe Ant. Temp. Focus (N = 13)
Matching Variables		
Chronological age	71.0 ± 5.4	71.3 ± 5.0
Education (grade)	12.2 ± 4.9	13.4 ± 3.5
Paired Associate Learning		
Total no. errors	68.8 ± 37.6	65.4 ± 39.8
48-hr. retention	4.12 ± 2.26	6.12 ± 2.32
Wechsler Memory Scale		
Total raw score	50.2 ± 10.0	49.6 ± 8.0
Intelligence Test (WAIS)		
Total scaled score	79.3 ± 17.0	80.8 ± 14.9
12-Yr. Survival		
No. living/dead	8/5	6/7

differences were found between the normal and focal EEG groups in learning ability, 48-hour retention, memory scale performance, or intelligence test scores. A follow-up study 12 years later revealed that the two groups were similar with respect to health and longevity; eight and six subjects, respectively, survived.

Although temporal slow activity is prevalent among patients with cerebrovascular disease (Bruens, Gastaut, and Giove 1960; Frantzen and Lennox-Buchthal 1961), and is also commonly associated with diffuse slowing in mentally deteriorated patients (Obrist and Henry 1958a), a temporal focus per se cannot be considered pathognomonic of a psychological or neurological deficit in an elderly person. It is only when the slow waves become diffuse in their distribution, involving several regions of the brain bilaterally, that EEG frequency is correlated with intellectual deficit.

An exception to the general decline in EEG frequency during senescence is an increase in rhythmic beta activity (fast waves) over the precentral areas in middle-aged and elderly females (Busse and Obrist 1965). Such fast activity becomes prevalent in the fifth and sixth decades, possibly in association with menopause (McAdam, Tait, and Orme 1957), and then decreases at older age levels. It is consistent with the preservation of normal mental function (Obrist 1974).

The relation of EEG slowing to circulatory disorders suggests that vascular disease may play a role in the development of senescent EEG

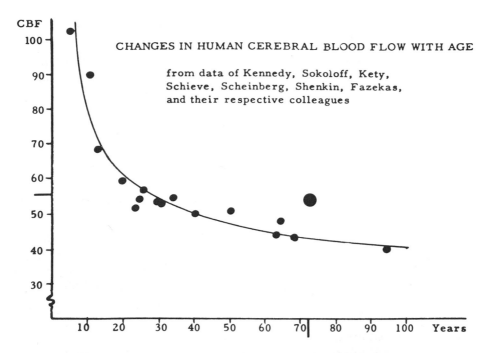

Figure 4. Cerebral blood flow (ml/100 g/min) plotted against age, as shown by Kety (1956). The large circle has been added to represent the mean blood flow for a select healthy aged sample (Dastur et al. 1963).

changes, just as it has been implicated in the etiology of senile mental deterioration (Corsellis 1962). In old age both cerebral blood flow and oxygen consumption undergo reductions, the magnitude of which is a function of health status. Figure 4 shows the relationship between age and cerebral blood flow, taken from an earlier review by Kety (1956). A large circle has been added to the graph to indicate the mean of a select healthy aged sample (Dastur et al. 1963), whose blood flow is comparable to that of young adults. Consistently lower cerebral blood flows have been found in elderly patients with various chronic illnesses (small circles on the graph), in aged community volunteers (Wang et al. 1972), and in patients with senile and presenile dementia (Obrist et al. 1970).

As in the case of intellectual function, the relationship of EEG to cerebral blood flow and metabolism depends on the existence of pathology. Little or no correlation between EEG frequency and these variables is found in well-preserved elderly subjects whose cerebral blood flow is in the normal young-adult range (Birren et al. 1963). Aged patients with organic brain syndrome, on the other hand, reveal a high correlation between diffuse EEG slowing and reductions in both cerebral blood flow and oxygen uptake (Obrist et al. 1963).

Because EEG frequency and oxygen uptake have been found to covary, the possibility arises that senescent EEG slowing and the accompanying intellectual changes are due to some rate-limiting factor in cerebral metabolism (Obrist 1972). Whether this limiting factor is tissue hypoxia resulting from circulatory insufficiency remains to be established. Although cerebral blood flow usually parallels oxygen uptake in the dementias of old age, it is not known whether the reduced blood flow causes the metabolic deficit or is a consequence of it. Given adequate autoregulatory mechanisms, it seems just as likely that blood flow is reduced because of the lesser metabolic demands of the tissue as that metabolism is impaired because of an insufficient delivery of oxygen. Based on studies of normal old people, Sokoloff (1966) has argued that blood flow reductions precede cerebral metabolic disturbances, thereby serving as a pacemaker for aging processes in the brain. Support for this argument is derived from recent studies on the relationship of cerebral blood flow to metabolism in early and late stages of cerebrovascular disease (Géraud et al. 1969). The role of brain atrophy and diffuse neuronal degeneration is, of course, crucial in any consideration of these pathophysiologic events.

In reviewing the relationship between spontaneous brain rhythms and psychological function in old age, emphasis has been given to the importance of pathological factors. The lack of correlation between resting EEG potentials and behavior in healthy old persons should not, however, discourage investigation of other electrophysiologic variables. There is now clear evidence that potentials evoked by sensory stimulation are subject to age variation (Dustman and Beck 1969, Thompson and Marsh 1973), and that electrical sleep patterns also undergo significant age changes (Feinberg, Koresko, and Heller 1967; Kales et al. 1967). It is possible that these more dynamic tests of electrocortical function will provide further insight into behavioral processes in senescence, particularly among healthy individuals.

References

Birren, J.E., Butler, R.N., Greenhouse, S.W., Sokoloff, L., and Yarrow, M.R. (eds.) 1963. *Human Aging: A Biological and Behavioral Study*. PHS Publication No. 986. Washington, D.C.: U.S. Govt. Printing Office.

Bruens, J.H., Gastaut, H., and Giove, G. 1960. Electroencephalographic study of the signs of chronic vascular insufficiency of the Sylvian region in aged people. *Electroencephalogr. Clin. Neurophysiol.* 12:283.

Busse, E.W., and Obrist, W.D. 1965. Pre-senescent electroencephalographic changes in normal subjects. *J. Gerontol.* 20:315.

Cahan, R.B., and Yeager, C.L. 1966. Admission EEG as a predictor of mortality and discharge for aged state hospital patients. *J. Gerontol.* 21:248.

Corsellis, J.A.N. 1962. *Mental Illness and the Ageing Brain.* London: Oxford University Press.

Dastur, D.K., Lane, M.H., Hansen, D.B., Kety, S.S., Butler, R.N., Perlin, S., and Sokoloff, L. 1963. Effects of aging on cerebral circulation and metabolism in man. In J.E. Birren, R.N. Butler, S.W. Greenhouse, L. Sokoloff, and M.R. Yarrow (eds.), *Human Aging: A Biological and Behavioral Study,* p. 57. PHS Publication No. 986. Washington, D.C.: U.S. Govt. Printing Office.

Dustman, R.E., and Beck, E.C. 1969. The effects of maturation and ageing on the wave form of visually evoked potentials. *Electroencephalogr. Clin. Neurophysiol.* 26:2.

Feinberg, I., Koresko, R.L., and Heller, N. 1967. EEG sleep patterns as a function of normal and pathological aging in man. *J. Psychiatr. Res.* 5:107.

Frantzen, E., and Lennox-Buchthal, M. 1961. Correlation of clinical electroencephalographic and arteriographic findings in patients with cerebral vascular accident. *Acta Psychiatr. Scand.* 36 (suppl. 150):133.

Frey, T.S., and Sjögren, H. 1959. The electroencephalogram in elderly persons suffering from neuropsychiatric disorders. *Acta Psychiatr. Scand.* 34:438.

Géraud, J., Bes, A., Delpha, M., and Marc-Vergnes, J.P. 1969. Cerebral arteriovenous oxygen differences. In J.S. Meyer, H. Lechner, and O. Eichhorn (eds.), *Research on the Cerebral Circulation,* p. 209. Springfield, Ill.: Charles C Thomas.

Kales, A., Wilson, T., Kales, J.D., Jacobson, A., Paulson, M.J., Kollar, E., and Walter, R.D. 1967. Measurements of all-night sleep in normal elderly persons: Effects of aging. *J. Am. Geriatr. Soc.* 15:405.

Kety, S.S. 1956. Human cerebral blood flow and oxygen consumption as related to aging. *Res. Publ. Assoc. Res. Nerv. Ment. Dis.* 35:31.

Kooi, K.A., Guvener, A.M., Tupper, C.J., and Bagchi, B.K. 1964. Electroencephalographic patterns of the temporal region in normal adults. *Neurology (Minneap.)* 14:1029.

McAdam, W., and Robinson, R.A. 1962. Diagnostic and prognostic value of the electroencephalogram in geriatric psychiatry. In H.T. Blumenthal (ed.), *Medical and Clinical Aspects of Aging,* p. 557. New York: Columbia University Press.

McAdam, W., Tait, A.C., and Orme, J.E. 1957. Initial psychiatric illness in involutional women—III. *Journal of Mental Science* 103:824.

Obrist, W.D. 1972. Cerebral physiology of the aged: Influence of circulatory disorders. In C.M. Gaitz (ed.), *Aging and the Brain,* p. 117. New York: Plenum Press.

Obrist, W.D. 1974. Problems of aging. In A. Remond (ed.), *Handbook of Electroencephalography and Clinical Neurophysiology,* vol. 6. Amsterdam: Elsevier Publishing Co. (in press).

Obrist, W.D., Busse, E.W., Eisdorfer, C., and Kleemeier, R.W. 1962. Relation of the electroencephalogram to intellectual function in senescence. *J. Gerontol.* 17:197.

Obrist, W.D., Chivian, E., Cronqvist, S., and Ingvar, D.H. 1970. Regional cerebral flood flow in senile and presenile dementia. *Neurology (Minneap.)* 20:315.

Obrist, W.D., and Henry, C.E. 1958a. Electroencephalographic findings in aged psychiatric patients. *J. Nerv. Ment. Dis.* 126:254.

Obrist, W.D., and Henry, C.E. 1958b. Electroencephalographic frequency analysis of aged psychiatric patients. *Electroencephalogr. Clin. Neurophysiol.* 10:621.

Obrist, W.D., Sokoloff, L., Lassen, N.A., Lane, M.H., Butler, R.N., and Feinberg, I. 1963. Relation of EEG to cerebral blood flow and metabolism in old age. *Electroencephalogr. Clin. Neurophysiol.* 15:610.

Otomo, E. 1966. Electroencephalography in old age: Dominant alpha pattern. *Electroencephalogr. Clin. Neurophysiol.* 21:489.

Pampiglione, G., and Post, F. 1958. The value of electroencephalographic examinations in psychiatric disorders of old age. *Geriatrics* 13:725.

Sokoloff, L. 1966. Cerebral circulatory and metabolic changes associated with aging. *Res. Publ. Assoc. Res. Nerv. Ment. Dis.* 41:237.

Thompson, L.W., and Marsh, G.R. 1973. Psychophysiological studies of aging. In M.P. Lawton, and C.E. Eisdorfer (eds.), *The Psychology of Adult Development and Aging*, p. 112. Washington, D.C.: American Psychological Association.

Wang, H.S., Obrist, W.D., Eisdorfer, C.E., and Busse, E.W. 1972. Regional cerebral blood flow (rCBF) of community aged persons determined by the 113-xenon inhalation method. *Gerontologist* 12 (no. 3, part II):44 (abstract).

changes in evoked responses during maturation and aging in man and macaque

Edward C. Beck, Ph.D.
Robert E. Dustman, Ph.D.

Veterans Administration Hospital and
University of Utah
Salt Lake City, Utah

The evoked response, or evoked potential, is the electrical response of the brain to a brief, peripherally applied stimulus. A pulse of light, a shock, or brief touch, or a click will elicit an evoked cerebral response by way of the respective sensory pathways. Single evoked response recordings have a long history and should not be confused with summed or averaged evoked responses. Single evoked responses were seen on cathode oscilloscopes or directly in the electroencephalogram (EEG). From these "older" methods it was concluded for years that the response of the brain to an instantaneous stimulus is a simple biphasic or triphasic wave lasting only a small fraction of a second. With the averaging or summing of evoked responses, the response that emerges is more complex, consisting of as many as fifteen phase shifts rather than two or three, and the response endures for several hundred milliseconds. Thus the technique of averaging or summing, whereby previously obscure cerebral electrical changes to stimuli can be extracted by computer from the brain's background "noise" or ongoing electrical activity by relating them to the time of the stimulus, provides a closer look at the brain's electrophysiology.

While the exact source and nature of the evoked response is still being debated, the technique is enjoying widespread acceptance as a research tool as well as a rapidly developing diagnostic and evaluative procedure. One reason for this widespread acceptance is that, in contrast to the EEG, evoked responses are under stimulus control, and they, thereby, provide additional information about the different sensory systems and the functionally different pathways and brain areas involved in the response. Another advantage is that evoked responses lend themselves to more quantifiable analyses than does the EEG trace; amplitudes, latencies, and wave component differences of evoked responses may be accurately measured and compared.

The technique is, in addition, extremely promising as a tool in research and subsequent diagnostic procedures since some components of the response seem to be determined or affected by different cerebral systems or brain structures. If the source and nature of the components of the evoked potential were definitive, one could identify with reasonable certainty from the waveform configuration of the evoked potential the area of the brain most affected by disease or injury.

Understanding of the evoked potential has been the main interest of this laboratory over the past decade. Our efforts have developed in a more or less organized fashion, although fortuitously and not as a result of careful planning. Still we have followed what seems to be an orderly itinerary directed toward certain critical questions about the evoked response. This paper will summarize a number of these experiments, including studies of the reliability and stability of the evoked response, some normative or developmental studies directed toward describing the "normal" evoked potential (visual, auditory, and somatosensory) at different age levels, and clinical application of the technique. We shall also report on use of the technique for studying the developmental electrophysiology of the stump-tailed macaque.

Procedure and Equipment

Evoked responses were recorded from most human subjects while they were seated in a comfortable padded chair, in a sound-deadened, darkened room which was electrically shielded. Nonambulatory patients were frequently seated in wheel chairs during recording procedures and infants on their mothers' laps. Although electrode placements varied slightly from one study to another, electrodes were usually placed at F_3, F_4, C_3, C_4, O_1, and O_2 according to the International Ten-Twenty System. All recordings were unipolar, both ear lobes combined serving as reference. Stimuli (flashes, clicks, or shocks) were triggered manually at two- to three-second intervals during artifact-free periods of EEG. Brain waves were amplified by an eight-channel Grass EEG machine and, together with pulses accompanying stimuli, were stored on magnetic tape by a seven-channel magnetic data recorder. The stored EEG was then played into an analog-digital converter of a Digital Equipment Corp. PDP-9 computer. Responses were averaged and plotted with a digital plotter. The sampling rate employed was usually 500/sec. In some of the earlier studies a computer of average transients (CAT) was used.

Visual stimuli of 10-μsec duration were generated by a photic stimulator. With few exceptions the setting of the stimulator was 2 on an intensity scale of 1 to 16. The stimulator lamp was enclosed in a fiberglas and foam-rubber container to muffle clicks accompanying the flashes. The lamp was positioned behind and directly above the subject's head and was aimed at a reflecting hemisphere 70 cm in diameter. The hemisphere was used to insure a relatively constant level of retinal illumination regardless of the position of the subject's head. At a stimulator setting of PS=2 the measured luminance at the center of the hemisphere, 40 cm from the subject's eyes, was 12 lux.

Auditory stimuli were clicks of 0.25-msec duration and 80-db intensity with reference to 0.0002 microbars delivered to subjects binaurally through earphones. These relatively low-intensity stimuli were used to decrease the possibility of myogenic contamination of the auditory responses.

Somatosensory potentials were evoked by 0.25-msec electrical pulses. Stimulus intensity for each subject was based on his subjective threshold, which was determined by the method of ascending and descending limits. Stimulus intensities employed in these studies varied from 1.5 to 3.5 times the threshold values obtained. Stimuli were delivered to the subject's left or right index finger through two silver clip electrodes; a copper cuff was placed on the forearm to ground the spread of shock artifact.

Figure 1 illustrates typical responses evoked by the presentation of stimuli in each of the three sensory modalities. As may be seen in Figure 1, the visual evoked response (VER) was the most complex, consisting of eight waves or components and an afterdischarge lasting several hundred milliseconds. The auditory response (AER) was composed of six components, the somatosensory (SER) of seven. In the studies to be reported all components were present in young children, and although some were missing or distorted in some subjects, all were seen throughout the life span of subjects in the study.

The results of the studies reported are concerned with three types of measurement: peak delay, wave component amplitude, and an overall amplitude measure encompassing a specified time segment of an evoked response. Peak delays were measured in milliseconds from the beginning of an evoked response (time zero) to the peaks shown in Figure 2. Wave component amplitudes, measured in microvolts, were determined by measuring the vertical distance between two peaks of opposite polarity. The overall amplitude measure was obtained by tracing the wave form of responses with a map-reading wheel which yielded measurements in centimeters, or by using the PDP-9 computer to calculate the actual total voltage change (regardless of the direction, positive or negative) occurring within a time segment of the response.

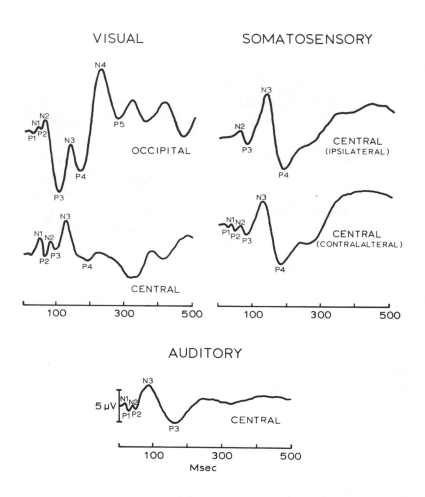

Figure 1. Typical visual, somatosensory, and auditory evoked responses. Differences in waveform of the visual response when recorded from central and occipital areas may be seen in the upper left of the figure. Additional components in the somatosensory response when recorded contralaterally may be seen by comparing somatosensory responses in the upper right of the figure. A downward deflection in this and subsequent figures indicates a positive change. From Dustman, Schenkenberg, and Beck 1974 (in press). In R. Karrer (ed.), Developmental Psychophysiology in Mental Retardation and Learning Disability. Springfield, Ill.: Charles C Thomas. Courtesy of the publisher.

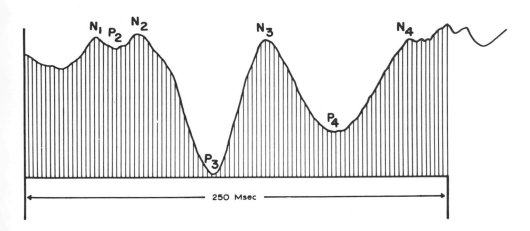

Figure 2. A summed VER showing seven wave components (N1 through P4) in the first 250 msec of the response. The figure also illustrates a method for measuring amplitudes of phase changes as explained in the text. From Dustman and Beck 1969. Courtesy of the editor, Electroencephalography and Clinical Neurophysiology.

Reliability

The reliability of the averaged evoked response was an early concern for us and others. To determine evoked response reliability we proceeded as follows: A baseline for each response was established by drawing a horizontal line below the base of the largest positive deflection that occurred within the first 250 msec. One hundred vertical lines, equally spaced within the first 250 msec of the response, were drawn from the baseline to the point of intersection with the response (Figure 2). The distance in millimeters between the baseline and each intersection was determined for each of the 100 lines. These amplitude values describing the contours of one evoked response could then be correlated (Pearson product-moment correlation) with similarly derived values from a second response (Dustman and Beck 1963).

The reliability data to be reported are from three groups of normal subjects and are concerned with visual and somatosensory responses. The first group participated in five recording sessions while the other two groups participated in two sessions. The interval between sessions was about a month.

For a particular recording site, the two or five responses obtained from each subject were intercorrelated, thus yielding 10 correlations for each member of Group 1, $\frac{N(N-1)}{2}$, and a single correlation for members of the remaining two groups. The correlations were converted to Fisher Z scores,

which have a normal sampling distribution, before computing the group
mean reliability coefficients shown in Table 1.

TABLE 1.
Mean Evoked Response Reliability Coefficients for
Three Groups of Normal Subjects

Group	N	Age	Stimulus	Left Central	Right Central	Left Occipital	Right Occipital
1	10	26-36	Flash	.88	.89	.86	.87
2	20	10-11	Flash	.84	.87	.92	.92
3	24	5-16	Flash	.81	.84	.91	.88
3	24	5-16	Shock	.87	.86	—	—

From Dustman, Schenkenberg, and Beck 1974 (in press). In R. Karrer (ed.), *Developmental Psychophysiology in Mental Retardation and Learning Disability*. Springfield, Ill.: Charles C Thomas. Courtesy of the publisher.

In Figure 3, three of the five VERs recorded from left occipital scalp of
each of four subjects in Group 1 are superimposed to illustrate the marked
reproducibility of the evoked responses of most subjects. The mean correlations for subjects W.M., M.R., I.A., and B.B. were 0.92, 0.92, 0.90, and 0.94,
respectively. Also of interest are the individual differences reflected among
the four sets of responses. Even though the major waves in the responses of
different individuals occur at approximately the same time, the overall configurations of the responses are noticeably different.

To determine the degree of evoked response similarity (homogeneity)
among subjects, the responses from each brain area of the ten subjects in
Group 1 were intercorrelated. The mean intersubject correlations for left and
right central scalp were 0.58 and 0.63, and for left and right occipital scalp
they were 0.51 and 0.52. These correlations, although much smaller than the
reliability coefficients, are fairly respectable positive correlations, again at-
testing to the fact that there is a reasonable degree of similarity among the
evoked response waveforms of different individuals.

To observe gross differences between the evoked responses of two
groups of subjects, or before and after a treatment has been imposed on a
single group, averaged group composites are often useful. These are obtained
by averaging all of the responses of all members of a group. Figure 4 illustrates overlays of three composites for responses from each of four scalp
areas of the ten subjects in Group 1. Thus each tracing represents the responses to 1000 flashes of light, that is, 100 flashes per subject. The mean

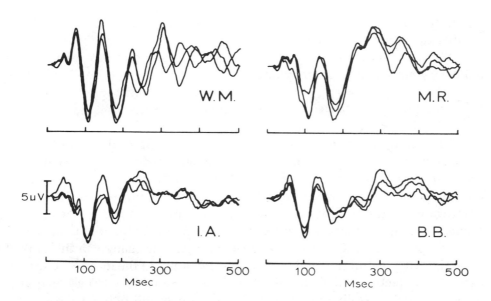

Figure 3. Reliability of visually evoked responses. The four illustrations show the super-imposition of averaged visually evoked responses recorded at monthly intervals for four subjects. From Dustman, Schenkenberg, and Beck 1974 (in press). In R. Karrer (ed.), Developmental Psychophysiology in Mental Retardation and Learning Disability. Spring-field, Ill.: Charles C Thomas. Courtesy of the publisher.

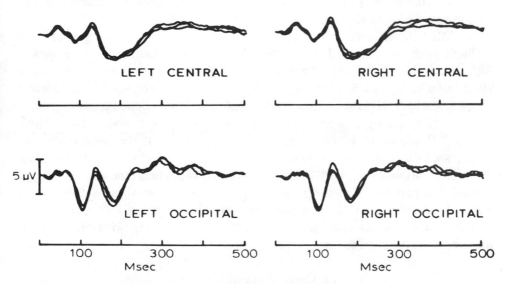

Figure 4. Reliability of group visual evoked responses. The figure illustrates overlays of three group composite responses for each of four scalp areas. The group was composed of ten subjects. Superimposed group composites are from responses separated by one month.

month-to-month reliability coefficient for these responses was 0.97, indicating that they are extremely stable over time.

With evidence that the averaged evoked response was reliable and unique we moved on to other studies.

Life Span Changes as Reflected in the Evoked Response

The use of the averaged evoked response as an approach to the study of the electrophysiology of the developing and aging brain represents the first major departure beyond simple EEG analysis. Despite its promise and its repeated application in other areas of brain research, few studies have been reported using the evoked response technique in a description of cerebral changes during the formative years and in later life. Unlike the situation in the early period of EEG research, knowledge regarding changes in the evoked potential with maturation and aging is meager, limiting the diagnostic usefulness of this technique. While the evoked response of infants has been adequately described (Ellingson 1958 and 1960, Engel and Butler 1963, Barnet and Goodwin 1965, Ferriss et al. 1967), any thorough description of evoked response changes and their relation to increasing age during the formative years is lacking. Similarly little is known about changes in the evoked response during later life. In an effort to satisfy the need for standard information we have directed our efforts toward the study of changes in the evoked response from infancy to senescence in 425 normal subjects whose age distribution spans 85 years.

With 160 subjects, visual, auditory, and somatosensory responses were studied; with the remainder only the visual evoked response was recorded. Age, hemisphere, and sex comparisons were made on the basis of response amplitudes and peak delays. Some of these results are reported in greater detail elsewhere (Dustman and Beck 1966 and 1969, Schenkenberg 1970).

Striking changes were seen during development and aging. These changes, fluctuations in both amplitude and latency of the various components, seemed to follow obvious developmental and aging transitions. Thus the child, adolescent, and aged subject showed characteristic responses. Figure 5 illustrates typical visual evoked responses at these different age levels. While the most obvious changes were seen in the visual and somatosensory responses, all systems demonstrated unique transitions with increasing age. A description for each sense modality follows.

The Visual Evoked Response

It is readily apparent from Figure 6 that the visual response changes drastically with increasing age and, in fact, continues to change over the entire life span. These changes show interesting phases or transitions, depicted in Figures 5, 7, and 8.

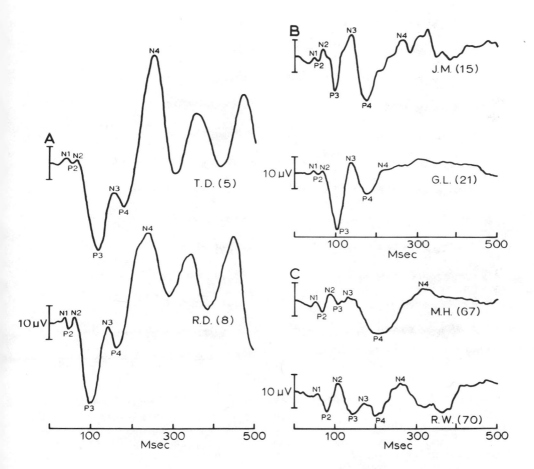

Figure 5. VERs of six subjects of different ages illustrating typical responses during (A) childhood, (B) adolescence and young adulthood, and (C) senescence. The large amplitude of late components, P3-P4, during formative years may be seen in (A) and the potentiation of early components (N1-N2) in senescence is illustrated in (C). From Dustman and Beck 1969. Courtesy of the editor, Electroencephalography and Clinical Neurophysiology.

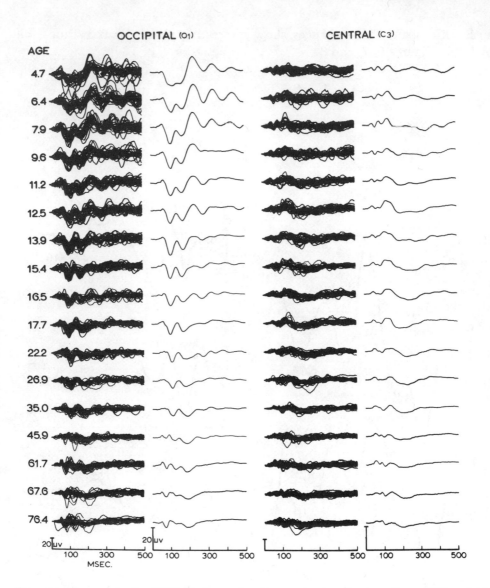

Figure 6. Changes in the VER during maturation and aging. Portrayed are VERs of 425 individuals ranging in age from 4 to 86. Each of the 17 age groups, designated by mean age at the left of the figure, is composed of 25 subjects (rather equally divided, male and female). It may be seen that the configuration of the VER changes with age and that the trend of these changes is obvious both in the individual and the group.

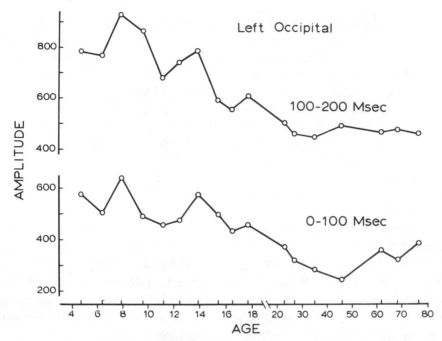

Figure 7. Changes in VER amplitude of early and later components during maturation and increasing age. Two epochs were measured, the first 100 msec and from 100 to 200 msec. Amplitudes for each epoch were obtained by summing the absolute values of all points within that interval. The VER segments had previously been reduced to a zero baseline by subtracting the means of the total epoch from each point.

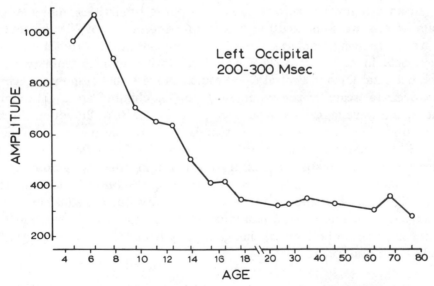

Figure 8. Age-related changes in amplitude of late components of the VER, those occurring from 200 to 300 msec after the stimulus. Groups and recordings are the same as in Figures 6 and 7. See Figure 7 legend for description of amplitude measurement.

Amplitude increases markedly from infancy to ages 6 to 8. The mean amplitude in children of this age is more than twice that of the adult. Following this period there is a decline in amplitude until ages 13 to 14, at which times there is a surge in amplitude in the first 200 msec of the response, apparently peculiar to pubescence (Figure 7). From age 15 on there is a continuous and decided decline in amplitude until age 45; from then on, early components, those in the first 100 msec, increase in amplitude (Figure 7). It should be noted that there is a rapid decline in amplitude of late components of the response, those from 200 to 300 msec, from childhood to young adulthood (Figure 8). Reciprocal amplitude changes seem to appear in old age, with late components attenuated and the early response potentiated.

Latency of various components of the VER also shows age-related changes. Generally speaking, peak delays of three early components, N1, P2, N2 (Figure 5), arrive significantly later in infancy, remain stable during childhood and young adulthood, then increase significantly from middle age throughout senescence. Late components, P3-N4, decrease in latency from infancy to late childhood, stabilize during adolescence, gradually increase in middle age, and continue to increase through senescence.

Comparisons of Homogeneity of Evoked Responses at Different Age Levels

In an attempt to examine evoked response similarities among subjects of similar age, we compared the visual evoked responses of 25 subjects in 17 age groups (ranging from age 4 to 70) by computing intercorrelations among all subjects in each group. This was done with responses from two scalp areas, occipital O_1 and central C_3. Results indicate that responses recorded from occipital scalp of the youngest group of children are highly similar. That is, the wave and phase relationship of the VERs of 25 young children, when correlated with one another (that is, 300 correlations), yield a mean r of 0.73. As may be seen in Figure 9, this relationship rapidly decreases with increasing age, up to about age 12. From that point there is a gradual change in homogeneity. With VERs from central scalp the *opposite* is true. There are negligible relationships in the youngest groups but a gradual increase in relationship reaching a peak at adolescence. It should be noted that these relationships (from both areas) change rapidly from infancy to puberty, then stabilize (see also Figure 10).

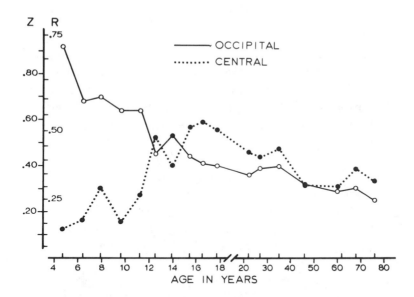

Figure 9. Age-group intercorrelations of VERs recorded from occipital and central scalp illustrating trends in group homogeneity with maturation and aging. Each point on the graph is the intercorrelation of 25 subjects of a certain age range, that is, the mean of 300 correlations.

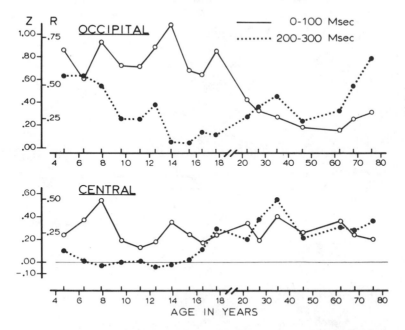

Figure 10. Age-group intercorrelations of two segments or epochs of VERs recorded from occipital and central scalp. Intercorrelations are computed for those components occurring early in the response, 0-100 msec, and those arriving late in the response, 200-300 msec. Each point on the graph is the intercorrelation of 25 subjects as in Figure 9.

The Auditory Evoked Response

Changes with maturation and aging in AERs are illustrated in Figure 11. Interestingly this sensory modality does not follow the same trend as that seen in responses of the visual and somatosensory systems. Amplitude and latency of early components of AERs change significantly from early childhood to adolescence but remain stable from then on. No changes were noted peculiar to senescence. Peak delays of various components decrease from childhood to adolescence but remain stable throughout the rest of life. Figure 11 shows an interesting change in AER configuration from childhood to adolescence. A late component, a negative wave following P3, is present in groups aged 7, 9, and 11; it disappears in late adolescence.

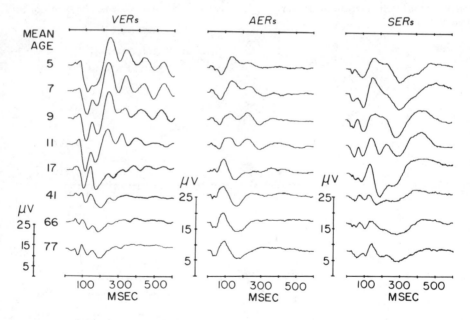

Figure 11. A comparison of group VERs, AERs, and SERs during maturation and aging. Each trace was obtained by averaging the evoked responses of the 20 subjects, 10 males and 10 females, in each group. VERs are from O_1; AERs and SERs are from C_3. The mean age of each group is shown at the left of the figure. From Dustman, Schenkenberg, and Beck 1974 (in press). In R. Karrer (ed.), Developmental Psychophysiology in Mental Retardation and Learning Disability. Springfield, Ill.: Charles C Thomas. Courtesy of the publisher.

The Somatosensory Response

There is minimal change in latency and amplitude of early components of SERs throughout all ages tested. However, postprimary portions of the response increase in amplitude from early childhood to adolescence, then decrease in middle age and senescence, following a trend very similar to that of the visual response. This may be seen in Figure 11. Peak delays of SERs, like VERs, gradually increase in middle age and continue to increase through senescence.

Hemispheric Asymmetry

VERs recorded from the right hemisphere are consistently larger than those from the left for all age groups when responses recorded from central scalp are compared. This is also true with responses recorded from occipital areas during formative years and through adolescence. These differences derive mainly from late components, N3 and P4; although consistent, they are rather small, 1 to 5 μV in most individuals. Interestingly no asymmetry of late components is seen with AERs or SERs.

Sex Differences

In comparing 80 males with 80 females ranging in age from 4 to 86, we found the responses of males during childhood to be larger than those of females. The reverse characterizes responses recorded during adolescence and adulthood, that is, the females' responses are larger. These sex differences emerge as a general difference. They are not specific to any particular sensory system, electrode placement, or component, although they are seen more clearly in the visual response.

The Evoked Response and Intelligence

For years investigators have looked for a relationship between brain wave patterns and level of intelligence. While some have reported significant correlations between various parameters of the EEG and intelligence test scores, others have been unable to demonstrate such a relationship. In recent years these contradictory findings have been interestingly summarized and debated by Vogel and Broverman (1964 and 1966) and Ellingson (1966). While Ellingson argues that the evidence concerning the relationship between EEG waves and intelligence is contradictory and inconclusive, Vogel and Broverman stress that there is reliable evidence to support the existence of such a relationship.

The evoked response seemed to offer a promising approach to the problem, since its wave configuration is more easily measured than that of spontaneous EEG waves.

We screened a population of about 800 school children, selecting from among them two groups of 10- and 11-year-old children. The first group was composed of 20 bright children who had Full Scale Wechsler Intelligence Scale for Children (WISC) IQ scores that ranged from 120 to 140, mean 130, while the second group consisted of 20 dull children, age- and sex-matched with the brighter group. The latter group had Full Scale WISC IQ scores that ranged from 70 to 90, mean 79. All of the low-IQ children were adapting satisfactorily to school and none had any known history of brain damage or emotional disturbance. See Rhodes, Dustman, and Beck (1969) for a complete description of the study.

Visually evoked responses to 100 flashes of light were recorded from each subject as previously described, in two recording sessions separated by about one month. Flash intensity was set at PS=2 for the first session, while two additional intensities were used in the second session, one dimmer (PS=1 + filter), the other brighter (PS=8).

Peak delays and amplitudes of all major waves occurring within the first 300 msec were scored. The mean peak delays of waves N2 through P5 are listed in Table 2.

Only one peak delay differentiated the two groups. Peak N4 in responses recorded from occipital scalp occurred significantly later in the VERs of low-IQ children ($p<0.01$). Interestingly, this wave, when recorded from central leads, arrived earlier in the response of the low-IQ group.

The excursion measures of the late waves (about 100 to 250 msec) from both central and occipital VERs were reliably larger in the responses from the high-IQ children ($p<0.05$ central; $p<0.01$ occipital). The amplitude differences can be seen in Figure 12 in which the composite VERs of the two groups are superimposed.

The high-IQ group also differed from the low-IQ group with respect to amplitude asymmetry in VERs recorded from central leads (Figure 13). The graph in Figure 13 is based on VER wave excursion measures which encompassed waves P3 through P5 in responses evoked by three different flash intensities. At each intensity setting late waves in the right central VERs of the high-IQ group were reliably larger than they were in responses from left central scalp. The responses of the low-IQ children did not show an amplitude asymmetry.

Consistent with the findings mentioned above, the responses of the bright children were significantly larger than those of the low-IQ children across all three intensities.

A correlational study was undertaken with two additional groups of

TABLE 2.
Mean Peak Delays (msec) of Late VER Waves Recorded
from High- and Low-IQ Children

Groups by Area	N2	P3	Peaks N3	P4	N4	P5
Left occipital						
high IQ	67	105	140	172	226	281
low IQ	66	106	146	180	244	291
Right occipital						
high IQ	65	106	143	176	227	284
low IQ	67	109	146	182	243	290
Left central						
high IQ	81	105	146	196	234	284
low IQ	84	109	142	182	220	269
Right central						
high IQ	81	106	148	198	232	280
low IQ	84	110	142	183	216	270

From Dustman, Schenkenberg, and Beck 1974 (in press). In R. Karrer (ed.), *Developmental Psychophysiology in Mental Retardation and Learning Disability*. Springfield, Ill.: Charles C Thomas. Courtesy of the publisher.

children to determine the relationship of IQ to VER wave amplitude and peak delay in subjects whose ages and IQs spanned a continuum. Group 1 was composed of 57 normal children whose IQ scores were between 70 and 131, mean IQ=110. Group 2 included 114 children whose parents were either on welfare rolls or were economically qualified to receive welfare assistance. The IQs of this group ranged from 62 to 133 with a mean IQ of 88. Subjects in both groups ranged in age from 4 to 15 years. Full Scale WISC intelligence tests were administered to all children except those in Group 1 who were 12 years of age or older (17 children). The older children in Group 1 were tested with the Culture Fair Intelligence Test (Cattell and Cattell 1960).

Visually evoked responses to 100 flashes of light (PS=2) were recorded from C_3, C_4, O_1, and O_2 of each subject. After the responses were plotted, the peak delays and amplitudes of waves N1 through N4 were measured. For each group the peak delays and amplitudes of each of the seven waves were correlated with IQ by means of the Pearson product-moment correlation technique. This procedure was followed for VERs from each scalp area, yielding 28 correlations of IQ with wave amplitude and an equal number with peak delay.

As can be seen in Figures 14 and 15, few correlations, only 6 of 112, were significantly different from zero and these were relatively small and showed no consistent trends.

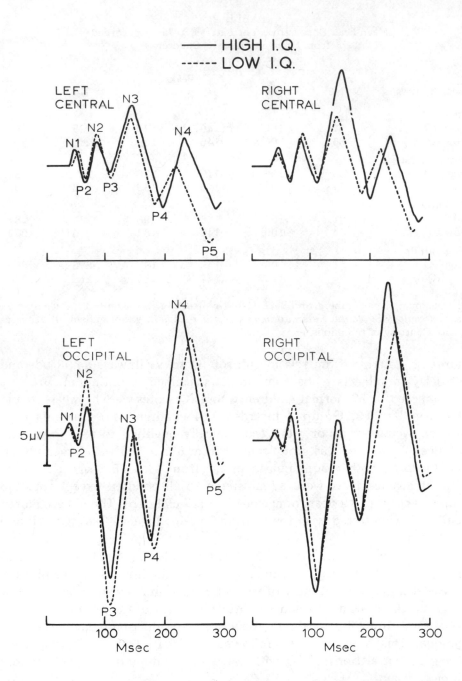

Figure 12. Visual evoked responses of bright and dull children. Composite VERs recorded from left and right central and occipital scalp of 20 high-IQ and 20 low-IQ children illustrating amplitude differences between groups. From Rhodes, Dustman, and Beck 1969. Courtesy of the editor, Electroencephalography and Clinical Neurophysiology.

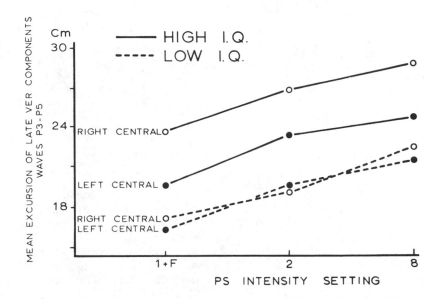

Figure 13. Hemispheric differences of high- and low-IQ children. Mean hemispheric amplitudes of VERs of high-IQ and low-IQ children at three levels of stimulus intensity showing interhemispheric asymmetry for the high-IQ children only. From Rhodes, Dustman,
and Beck 1969. Courtesy of the editor, Electroencephalography and Clinical Neurophysiology.

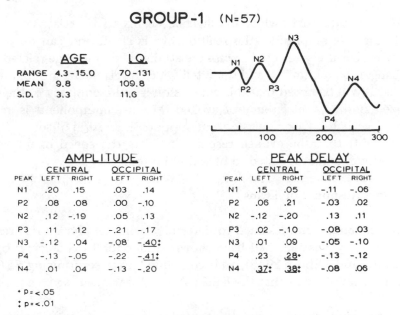

GROUP-1 (N=57)

	AGE	IQ
RANGE	4.3-15.0	70-131
MEAN	9.8	109.8
S.D.	3.3	11.6

AMPLITUDE

	CENTRAL		OCCIPITAL	
PEAK	LEFT	RIGHT	LEFT	RIGHT
N1	.20	.15	.03	.14
P2	.08	.08	.00	-.10
N2	.12	-.19	.05	.13
P3	.11	.12	-.21	-.17
N3	-.12	.04	-.08	-.40‡
P4	-.13	-.05	-.22	-.41‡
N4	.01	.04	-.13	-.20

PEAK DELAY

	CENTRAL		OCCIPITAL	
PEAK	LEFT	RIGHT	LEFT	RIGHT
N1	.15	.05	-.11	-.06
P2	.06	.21	-.03	.02
N2	-.12	-.20	.13	.11
P3	.02	-.10	-.08	.03
N3	.01	.09	-.05	-.10
P4	.23	.28•	-.13	-.12
N4	.37‡	.38‡	-.08	.06

• p=<.05
‡ p=<.01

Figure 14. Correlations of IQ with amplitude and peak delay of visual evoked response
components. Children in this group had a mean IQ of 110.

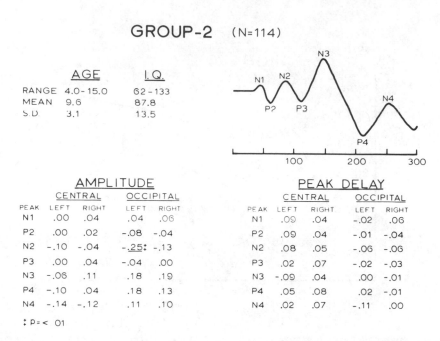

GROUP-2 (N=114)

AGE		I.Q.
RANGE	4.0-15.0	62-133
MEAN	9.6	87.8
S.D.	3.1	13.5

	AMPLITUDE					PEAK DELAY			
	CENTRAL		OCCIPITAL			CENTRAL		OCCIPITAL	
PEAK	LEFT	RIGHT	LEFT	RIGHT	PEAK	LEFT	RIGHT	LEFT	RIGHT
N1	.00	.04	.04	.06	N1	.09	.04	-.02	.06
P2	.00	.02	-.08	-.04	P2	.09	.04	-.01	-.04
N2	-.10	-.04	-.25‡	-.13	N2	.08	.05	-.06	-.06
P3	.00	.04	-.04	.00	P3	.02	.07	-.02	-.03
N3	-.06	.11	.18	.19	N3	-.09	.04	.00	-.01
P4	-.10	.04	.18	.13	P4	.05	.08	.02	-.01
N4	-.14	-.12	.11	.10	N4	.02	.07	-.11	.00

‡ p=< 01

Figure 15. Correlations of IQ with amplitude and peak delay of visual evoked response components. Children in this group came from an impoverished environment and had a mean IQ of 88.

We conclude that, while intelligence seems to be related to visually evoked response amplitude, the relationship is small and can only be observed when carefully selected groups are studied, in which age-related amplitude changes are minimized and the intelligence levels of the groups are quite different. It will be noted that this conclusion is quite contrary to the widely publicized finding that latency of evoked response components is inversely correlated with IQ. Our results *do not* support the notion of some (Ertl and Schafer 1969) that the evoked response reflects the speed of information processing and hence is related to behavioral intelligence.

The Evoked Response of Twins

Experiments were designed to determine whether the evoked response has a hereditary basis, as had been shown earlier for EEG tracings by Lennox, Gibbs, and Gibbs (1945), who concluded after scrutinizing EEG tracings of 71 pairs of twins that the EEG pattern does appear to be a hereditary trait.

We recorded visually evoked responses from 12 pairs of monozygotic twins, 11 pairs of dizygotic twins, and 12 pairs of unrelated children age-matched with the monozygotic pairs (Dustman and Beck 1965). Zygosity was determined by: identity of physical features, similarity of iris pigmentation, presence or absence of hair between the first and second joints of fingers, blood groups, M-N agglutination, Rh factor, and ridge count of finger patterns (Rife 1933a and 1933b).

The first 250 msec of the evoked responses of each pair of subjects were correlated using the methods described above. The correlations were made for responses from left central and left occipital scalp. After the correlations had been converted to Fisher Z scores, an analysis of variance was computed to test for differences between the mean correlations of the three groups (see Table 3 for a listing of mean correlations). The analysis of variance yielded an F ratio of 8.82, df 2/33, ($p<0.001$). A Duncan Multiple Range Test (to evaluate differences between means) showed that identical twin correlations were reliably larger than those of the other two groups ($p<0.01$). while the mean correlations of the nonidentical twins and age-matched controls were not different. An illustration of the striking similarity between the evoked responses of some pairs of identical twins is shown in Figure 16. The responses in this figure also demonstrate the unique qualities found in responses of different individuals.

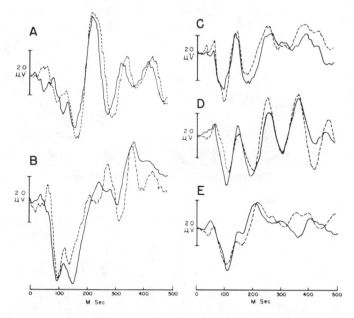

Figure 16. The visual evoked responses of twins. An illustration of the individuality and similarity of visually evoked responses of five sets of identical twins. (A) 11-year-old girls, r = 0.93; (B) 14-year-old boys, r = 0.90; (C) 15-year-old boys, r = 0.92; (D) 7-year-old girls, r = 0.93; (E) 9-year-old girls, r = 0.87. From Dustman and Beck 1965. Courtesy of the editor, Electroencephalography and Clinical Neurophysiology.

TABLE 3.

A Comparison of Coefficients of Correlation of Evoked Responses Among Identical Twins, Nonidentical Twins, and Children Matched for Age

Group	Number of Pairs	Mean Age (in years and months)	Age range (in years)	Region of Recording	Xr	Range
Identical twins	12	12,5	5-17	Occipital	0.82	0.41 — 0.93
				Central	0.74	0.29 — 0.94
Nonidentical twins	11	15,3	7.15	Occipital	0.58	-0.05 — 0.90
				Central	0.48	-0.24 — 0.75
Children matched for age	12	12,3	5-17	Occipital	0.61	-0.07 — 0.78
				Central	0.53	-0.20 — 0.82

From Dustman and Beck 1965. Courtesy of the editor, *Electroencephalography and Clinical Neurophysiology.*

Handedness and the Evoked Response

That bilateral symmetry in man and other mammals is often imperfect has long been recognized. The predominance of right-sidedness in man is a salient example. Related to this is the observation that handedness is associated with cerebral dominance for speech, with the left hemisphere almost always dominant among right-handed persons.

A few studies have investigated the relationship between handedness and laterality of EEG background activity. The comparisons have generally been based on the amplitude and frequency of alpha rhythm. Raney (1939), studying alpha rhythm in mirror-image twins, monozygotic twins discordant for handedness, found that right-handed twins had larger hemispheric differences in amount of alpha than did their left-handed counterparts. The tendency for increased alpha was generally toward the right or nondominant hemisphere.

Several investigators report asymmetrical amplitude with photic driving (Cornil and Gastaut 1951; Kooi, Eckman, and Thomas 1957; Hughes and Curtin 1960; Lansing and Thomas 1964). The results have been contradictory. While the majority of studies reported greater amplitude from the nondominant or minor hemisphere, Lansing and Thomas (1964) found the opposite, greater amplitude from the dominant hemisphere. Still others (Williams and Reynell 1945, Glandville and Antonities 1955) found no asymmetries.

To date no studies have reported on cerebral evoked responses recorded from the dominant and nondominant hemispheres of left- and right-handed subjects. Because the evoked response technique can provide for more precise hemispheric comparisons than the EEG, we decided to pursue the problem.

The subjects were 40 college students. Twenty were right-handed and 20 left-handed. Handedness was determined by a written test (Crovitz and Zener 1962) as well as by a number of physical tests for lateralization including relative coordination, grip strength, and reaction time.

Averaged cerebral evoked responses evoked by finger shock and light pulses were obtained from each subject. Somatosensory evoked responses were recorded from left and right central scalp. Stimulus intensity was 2.5 times subjective threshold. Two hundred shocks were delivered to the left or right index finger, selected randomly, followed by 200 to the other, so that from each of the two scalp locations two SERs were obtained, one contralateral and one ipsilateral to the shocked hand. Visual evoked responses to 100 flashes were also recorded from occipital and central scalp as previously described. To preclude any amplitude bias due to possible differences in amplification characteristics associated with the various EEG channels, the channels employed for recording brain potentials were randomly paired with the scalp electrodes of each subject.

A striking result was observed in the somatosensory responses. Amplitudes of the late waves P3-N3 and N3-P4 were much larger in the responses of the right-handed subjects, regardless of the scalp area from which records were made, or whether the responses were contralateral or ipsilateral to the stimulated finger. For example the mean N3-P4 amplitudes for contralateral responses from the left- and right-handed groups were 6.2 and 13.8 microvolts respectively, 7.6 and 15.4 microvolts for ipsilateral responses (Figure 17). The means in both pairs were statistically different ($p < 0.001$). Evoked response wave amplitudes from left central scalp were not significantly different from amplitudes of corresponding waves from right central scalp. Hence, while somatosensory responses showed differences between the right- and left-handed subjects, the differences were not related to asymmetry.

The visually evoked responses yielded still different results. While handedness was not related to VER wave amplitudes, significant differences between left and right VERs recorded from central scalp were found for *both* groups. Waves N2-P3, P3-N3, and N3-P4 were all reliably larger for responses recorded from the right side ($p < 0.01$, 0.001, and 0.01 respectively). Figure 18 shows that although these differences were seen in the responses of both right- and left-handed subjects, they were more pronounced for the right-handed group. It should be emphasized that these differences were confined to evoked responses recorded from central scalp leads; no differences were noted from occipital recordings.

From the above findings it was concluded that there are no evoked response hemispheric asymmetries peculiar to handedness. Handedness was, however, reflected in the somatosensory response as related to "whole" brain functioning, left-handed subjects showing, as a group, more variable and smaller somatosensory evoked responses bilaterally. Asymmetry in VERs recorded from central scalp is commonly seen in most normal subjects regardless of handedness, but the hemispheric difference is not as pronounced in left-handed subjects as it is in right-handed subjects.

Evoked Responses from Children with Down's Syndrome

It will be recalled that we emphasized earlier the unique quality of the evoked response, pointing out that the waveform configuration of a person's evoked response is individualized. Pertinent to this was the observation that the evoked responses of monozygotic twins were often nearly identical, suggesting that individuals with similar sensory systems and similar brains have similar evoked responses. In a number of instances an identical twin's visually evoked response was more like that of his twin than like his own

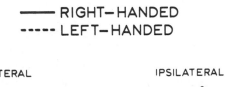

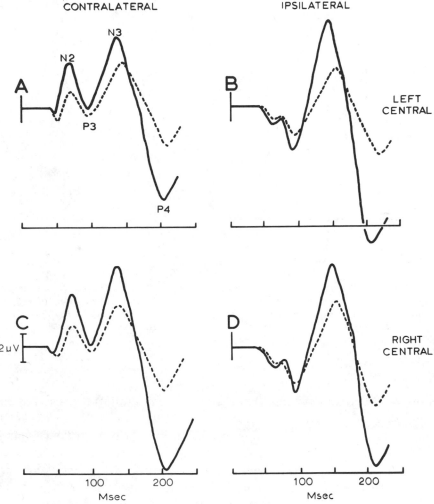

Figure 17. Composite somatosensory responses of 20 right- and 20 left-handed subjects. Responses are from left and right (C_3 and C_4) central scalp, contralateral and ipsilateral to shocked finger. The group responses were constructed by plotting the mean peak delays and amplitudes of waves N2 through P4 on graph paper and drawing interconnecting lines through the graphed points. Earlier components, P1-N1, by nature of the somatosensory system occur only in the contralateral response and hence were not included. From Dustman, Schenkenberg, and Beck 1974 (in press). In R. Karrer (ed.), Developmental Psychophysiology in Mental Retardation and Learning Disability. Springfield, Ill.: Charles C Thomas. Courtesy of the publisher.

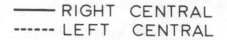

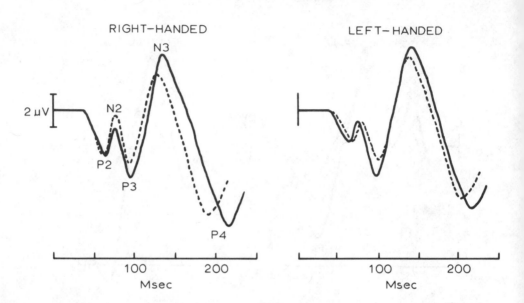

Figure 18. Composite visual evoked responses recorded from central scalp. The responses were constructed from the individual responses of 20 right- and 20 left-handed subjects in the same manner as those described in Figure 17. From Dustman, Schenkenberg, and Beck 1974 (in press). In R. Karrer (ed.), Developmental Psychophysiology in Mental Retardation and Learning Disability. Springfield, Ill.: Charles C Thomas. Courtesy of the publisher.

response recorded at a different time. In view of the unique characteristics of several forms of mental retardation, it would be reasonable to expect that the electrical activity of the brains of such persons would reflect some specific manifestation of the disorder.

Of all the groups considered, those afflicted with Down's syndrome seemed to be the most promising for such an experiment. These children form a relatively homogeneous group exhibiting unique physical and psychological features. Neuroanatomical studies have reported consistently that the affected brain is not only different from the normal brain but is different in unique ways (Meyer and Jones 1939, Crome 1954, Benda 1960, Crome et al. 1966).

These considerations led us to compare the visual and somatosensory evoked responses of 24 children with Down's syndrome with those of 24 normal children who were matched with the affected group for sex, handedness, and age. Each group consisted of 15 girls and 9 boys and ranged in age from 6 to 16 years. All of the Down's children were enrolled in a day school for trainable, mentally handicapped children (Bigum, Dustman, and Beck 1970).

Recording electrodes were attached to the scalp as previously described. All subjects participated in two recording sessions separated by about one month. In the first session responses were obtained from two sets of flashes and two sets of shocks. Shock intensity was 2.5 times each subject's threshold. During the second session, in addition to one set of flashes, three sets of shocks, each set at a different intensity (1.5, 2.5, and 3.5 times threshold), were presented in a randomly determined order. One hundred stimuli were used for each set of VERs and SERs.

Visual Evoked Responses

While the VER waveforms of both sets of children were basically similar, several differences were observed. In centrally derived responses, wave P2 occurred earlier ($p<0.01$) and P4 appeared later ($p<0.001$) in responses from the normal group. Two significant amplitude differences were found. Wave P3-N3 was larger in the responses of the normal group while P4-N4 was larger in the retarded VERs. Once again an amplitude asymmetry was found in responses from the central areas, but only for the normal group. Waves P3-N3 and N3-P4 were reliably larger ($p<0.01$) in responses from right central scalp.

Visually evoked responses from occipital scalp differentiated the two groups primarily on the basis of peak delay. The three latest waves, N3, P4, and N4, occurred significantly later in the VERs of children with Down's syndrome.

Somatosensory Responses

The somatosensory responses of the two groups were quite different in appearance. The SERs of the affected children were characterized by two late waves (P4-N4 and N4-P5 in Figure 19), which were approximately three times the amplitude of those of the normal children. An illustration of the magnitude of these differences is shown in Figure 19, and Table 4 lists the mean peak delays, amplitudes, and significant differences. Although the shock thresholds of the affected group were higher than those of the normal children (12.4 and 9.5 volts respectively), this cannot be the explanation for the differences in amplitude. Waves P4-N4 and N4-P5 were considerably larger in the retarded children's SERs to low-intensity shock than they were in the normal children's SERs to high-intensity shock, despite the fact that

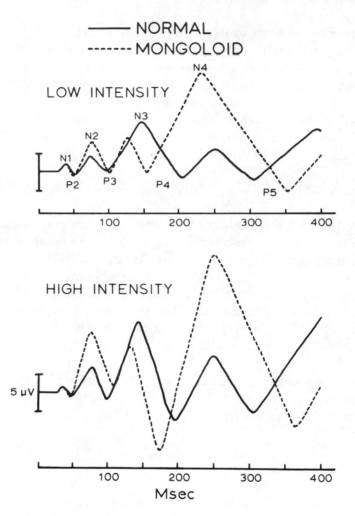

Figure 19. Composite somatosensory responses recorded from left central (contralateral) scalp of 24 normal and 24 mongoloid children. Low and high intensity refers to shock stimuli which were 1.5 and 3.5 times subjective threshold. From Bigum, Dustman, and Beck 1970. Courtesy of the editor, Electroencephalography and Clinical Neurophysiology.

TABLE 4.

Means and p Values Computed from the Peak Delays (msec) and Amplitudes (μV) of SER Components Recorded from Left and Right Central Scalp of 24 Mongoloid and 24 Normal Children

(A low-intensity (1.5 x threshold) shock stimulus was used.)

| Peak | Peak Delay | | | | p* |
| | Mongoloid | | Normal | | |
	C_3	C_4	C_3	C_4	
P2	50	60	53	62	
N2	76	78	74	81	
P3	101	101	98	111	
N3	127	138	148	157	<0.001
P4	155	189	206	214	<0.001
N4	232	260	250	261	
P5	352	366	305	308	<0.001

| Component | Amplitude | | | | p* |
| | Mongoloid | | Normal | | |
	C_3	C_4	C_3	C_4	
P2-N2	5.0	1.6	2.7	1.4	<0.05
N2-P3	4.6	1.7	2.5	2.5	
P3-N3	5.2	5.6	7.3	6.5	
N3-P4	5.1	7.1	8.1	8.9	
P4-N4	14.1	8.9	4.2	5.0	<0.001
N4-P5	16.8	12.6	4.5	3.4	<0.001

*p values were computed from the average of both hemispheres and thus indicate a significant difference between groups.

From Dustman, Schenkenberg, and Beck 1974 (in press). In R. Karrer (ed.), *Developmental Psychophysiology in Mental Retardation and Learning Disability.* Springfield, Ill.: Charles C Thomas. Courtesy of the publisher.

the normals received nearly twice as much voltage. As can be seen in Figure 19 and Table 4, the P4-N4-P5 wave complex was not only larger but was of longer duration in the responses of the retarded children.

Since recording sessions were separated by a month, it was possible to determine the reliability, or stability, of the two groups' evoked responses over time. With the procedure described in the Procedure and Equipment section, reliability coefficients were computed for VERs and SERs from each scalp area of the subjects in each group. The mean correlations of the retarded and the normals were relatively high, ranging from about 0.80 to 0.90 (Table 5), but they did not show group differences.

To determine the similarity of evoked responses within a group, a response from one scalp area of each subject within each group was intercorrelated with the responses from the same scalp area of the remaining 23 subjects. A mean of the intercorrelations obtained for each scalp area was then computed. These means, reflecting homogeneity of responses, are listed in Table 5. Both SERs and VERs of the Down's children were more homogeneous than those of the normals ($p < 0.001$).

In general then, the evoked responses of Down's children (both VERs and SERs), like their physical features, seem to be unique and characteristic of the group.

TABLE 5.
SERs of 24 Mongoloid and 24 Normal Children
Showing (1) Reliability Over One Month's Time and
(2) Intersubject Similarity (Homogeneity) of
Evoked Response Waveform

	VERs				SERs	
	C_3	C_4	O_1	O_2	C_3	C_4
Reliability						
Mongoloid	.86	.84	.91	.90	.89	.83
Normal	.81	.84	.91	.88	.87	.86
Homogeneity						
Mongoloid	.45	.43	.61	.61	.74	.63
Normal	.41	.43	.52	.47	.48	.49

From Bigum, Dustman, and Beck 1970. Courtesy of the editor, *Electroencephalography and Clinical Neurophysiology*.

The Effects of Socioeconomic Deprivation on Evoked Responses

As early environment and critical periods modify or fix later behavioral patterns, they are topics that have elicited the investigative interests of a wide spectrum of scientific specialties. The pervasiveness of early environmental stimulation or deprivation has been shown by the studies of the Berkeley group (Bennett et al. 1964) in their analyses of weight and chemical composition of rat brain after the animals were subjected to various environmental conditions. The stimulatory needs of human infants have been fairly well established by Spitz (1958), and the Harlows' well-known studies (1962) brought experimental quantification to maternal and other social deprivation effects on monkeys.

For a variety of reasons, not the least of which are social and political implications, there has been increasing concern regarding the effects, both immediate and long-term, of an impoverished environment on children. That such concern may be well founded is seen in the results of such studies as one recently published by Naeye et al. (1969), in which the authors measured the weight of several organs, including the brains of stillborn babies and infants who died shortly after birth. These were separated into two groups on the basis of the economic level of their families. It was found that the average weight of all organs sampled was less in the "poor" group than in the other.

The relationship between early social environment and brain development is poorly understood at present. A clearer understanding of the effect of early nutrition does seem to be emerging. One might well infer a nutritional factor in the results of Naeye et al. (1969). In addition both postnatal physical development and intellectual functioning have been shown to be impaired as a consequence of malnutrition (Stock and Smythe 1963, Cabek and Najdanvic 1965). Changes in EEG activity have also been seen in cases of malnutrition, for example, kwashiorkor syndrome (Engle 1956). Preliminary investigation with cerebral evoked response analysis suggests that this measure may also be sensitive to specific early nutritional deficits in both human beings (Mizuno et al. 1969) and animals (Mourek et al. 1967).

The study to be reported was undertaken to determine whether socioeconomic deprivation is reflected in altered brain function as measured by the evoked response.

Subjects for the investigation were 114 children selected from various economically depressed sections of Salt Lake City. They were principally identified through their participation in various government-sponsored, poverty-related programs such as Head Start, Office of Economic Opportunity Title I programs, or as recipients of state welfare assistance. Through these agencies and personal interviews information regarding each child's

TABLE 6.
Number, Age Range, Mean Age, IQ Range, and Mean IQ of Three
Groups of Children from Economically Deprived Families*

Group	N	Age (years) Range	Age (years) Mean	IQ Range	IQ Mean
Never	27	4.4–15.0	9.9	62–119	85
Intermittent	51	4.2–14.9	10.2	62–117	89
Always	36	4.0–13.6	8.8	62–113	89

*Groupings were based on the welfare history of each child's parents since the child's birth as follows: The parents (1) had *never* received welfare assistance, (2) had received welfare assistance on an *intermittent* basis, and (3) had *always* been receiving welfare assistance.

From Dustman, Schenkenberg, and Beck 1974 (in press). In R. Karrer (ed.), *Developmental Psychophysiology in Mental Retardation and Learning Disability*. Springfield, Ill.: Charles C Thomas. Courtesy of the publisher.

TABLE 7.
Mean Amplitudes (μV), Hemispheric Differences, and Probability Values
Computed for Two Late VER Waves Recorded from Scalp Areas C_3 and C_4
of Three Groups of Children Whose Parents Were Economically Deprived*

Group	Wave P3-N3 C_3	Wave P3-N3 C_4	Wave P3-N3 Diff	Wave P3-N3 p^{**}	Wave N3-P4 C_3	Wave N3-P4 C_4	Wave N3-P4 Diff	Wave N3-P4 p^{**}
Never	8.2	8.4	0.2		10.8	10.0	0.8	
Intermittent	7.9	10.3	2.4	<0.001	11.0	12.7	1.7	<0.05
Always	10.8	14.5	3.7	<0.001	15.5	18.7	3.2	<0.01
p†	<0.05	<0.001			<0.05	<0.001		

*Groupings were based on the welfare history of each child's parents since the child's birth as follows: (1) had *never* received welfare assistance, (2) had received welfare assistance on an *intermittent* basis and (3) had *always* been receiving welfare assistance.

**p values refer to differences between *hemispheres*.

†p values refer to differences between *groups*.

From Dustman, Schenkenberg, and Beck 1974 (in press). In R. Karrer (ed.), *Developmental Psychophysiology in Mental Retardation and Learning Disability*. Springfield, Ill.: Charles C Thomas. Courtesy of the publisher.

economic and health status was obtained.

Each child was assigned to one of three groups based on the welfare history of his parents as follows: (1) The parents had *never* received welfare assistance since the child's birth; they were "poor but proud" families, definitely deprived. (2) The parents had received welfare assistance on an *intermittent* basis since the child's birth. (3) The parents had *always* been receiving welfare assistance since the child's birth. The number of subjects in each group, as well as age and IQ information, is shown in Table 6. Analysis of variance indicated that neither the mean ages nor the IQs of the groups were reliably different.

For the sake of brevity we report only the amplitude data from the central scalp areas. The amplitudes of two late waves, P3-N3 and N3-P4, from both scalp areas (C3 and C4) were significantly larger in the VERs of the group whose parents had always been on welfare during the child's development. The mean amplitudes of these waves in the VERs of the remaining two groups were not different. Table 7 lists the mean amplitudes for the three groups and shows significant probability values. The mean differences between the *always* and the other two groups were largest for responses recorded from right central scalp. For example, while the largest difference for N3-P4 in C3 responses was 4.7 μV, the difference was 7.8 μV for C4 VERs.

Interestingly, we found that the VERs of two of the three groups showed an amplitude asymmetry favoring the right hemisphere (Table 7). Waves P3-N3 and N3-P4 in the responses of children whose parents had received welfare assistance were reliably larger from the right hemisphere than from the left. As can be seen in Table 7 and Figure 20, the asymmetry was most pronounced in the *always* group. Thus, in terms of amplitude asymmetry, the VERs of the two groups who had benefited from a welfare program were more like the responses of normal subjects reported in our earlier studies than were those of the children whose parents had not participated in a welfare program.

The Ontogeny of the Visual Evoked Response in the Infant Stump-Tailed Macaque

While the EEG patterns of the normal developing monkey have been systematically studied (Kennard and Nims 1942; de Ramirez de Arellano 1961; Caveness 1964; de Gallardo, Fleishman, and de Ramirez de Arellano 1964), and in the last ten years a number of studies have investigated evoked responses of the developing brain of other mammals, little is known of the evoked response of the infant monkey.

The EEG of the infant monkey at birth shows low voltage (10 to 40

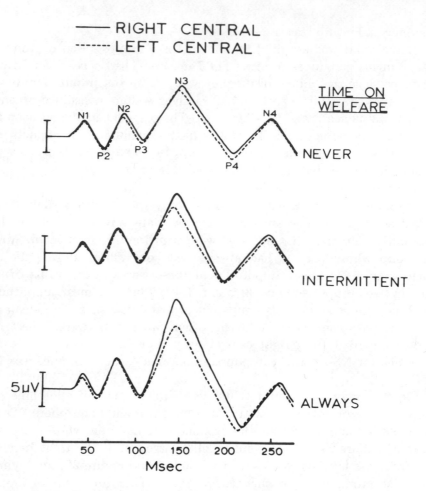

Figure 20. Composite visual evoked responses recorded from three groups of economically deprived children. Note that the amplitude asymmetry is most marked in the responses of children who have continuously received welfare benefits and is absent in the responses of those whose parents were never on welfare. From Dustman, Schenkenberg, and Beck 1974 (in press). In R. Karrer (ed.), Developmental Psychophysiology in Mental Retardation and Learning Disability. Springfield, Ill.: Charles C Thomas. Courtesy of the publisher.

μV), irregular waves at 2 to 3 sec with a few short bursts at 5 to 10-sec waves. This activity rapidly increases in amplitude by 1 to 2 months of age when the predominant pattern is one of generalized high voltage, up to 200 to 300 μV, sinusoidal waves, 4 to 6 sec in frequency. A gradual decline in amplitude begins at about 4 to 6 months and by 24 months has reached a level of 30 to 60 μV. The average frequency increases gradually to 8/sec at 20 weeks, 9/sec at 40 weeks and reaches the adult level of 10/sec at about 21 months.

While there is a general consistency in the results of a number of studies investigating the responsivity to sensory stimulation of the developing mammalian brain, certain differences emerge as one ascends the phylogenetic ladder. Changes in the evoked response to visual and/or auditory stimuli have been reported in the developing rat (Rose and Ellingson 1968), rabbit (Hunt and Goldering 1951, Farber 1968), cat (Ellingson and Wilcott 1960, Marty 1967, Rose and Lindsley 1965), and dog (Fox 1968). In the kitten, Rose and Lindsley first observed a long-latency, 165-msec, single negative wave in the contralateral (to the monocularly stimulated eye) visual cortex at about 4 to 5 days of age. The maximum amplitude of this wave was reached by 10 days while its latency became progressively shorter. At about this time a shorter latency negative wave appeared, often preceded by a positive wave. This diphasic wave shortened in latency (to 40 and 60 msec for the positive and negative components, respectively) and increased in amplitude until an age of about 30 days. The first observed negative wave during this time gradually merged with the earlier response, that is, the long-latency negative. Interestingly, lesions of the superior colliculus and the tectal area abolished the long-lasting negative wave, indicating that its origin may be the nonspecific sensory pathways. On the other hand lesions of the lateral geniculate affected the short-latency biphasic wave, suggesting its reflection of the specific visual pathways.

With such interesting developmental findings with the subprimates, one wonders what new information could be gained by studying visual evoked responses in the infant monkey. We agree with Doty, Kimura, and Mogenson (1964) who pointed out that the monkey's anatomical visual system nearly approximates that of man and thus makes these animals superior to other mammals as subjects in visual neurophysiological study.

An immediate advantage of using monkeys in developmental research is that they may provide longitudinal data and detail so lacking in research with human subjects. The close correspondence between the developmental phases of the brain and the anatomical similarities between man and monkey enable the experimenter to use the more accessible monkey as a model; the monkey's more rapid maturation makes possible longitudinal studies using single subjects, thereby reducing the variability found in cross-sectional studies. With this in mind we have undertaken the study of the development of the VER in the stump-tailed macaque *(Macaca arctoides)* from birth to adolescence.

These animals are much more docile than most other species, and it was found that fondling and handling them from birth resulted in a tractable animal. Young infants, up to six months or more, could be easily restrained by swaddling them in a towel and holding them on the experimenter's lap (a method found to be far superior to other seemingly more sophisticated procedures and apparatus that were tried).

Three infants, including one male, were removed from their mothers at birth and housed and nursed separately. They were tested the day of birth and subsequently three times weekly until the age of 28 days; thereafter once weekly until they were about 9 months old. Five other macaques, three of these males, were tested from 6 to 18 months of age. These older animals were taught to sit in a primate restraining chair and to fixate on a 30 x 40-inch stimulus card placed in a holder so that the card formed a curved surface with the center of the card 40 cm from the monkey's eyes. Although both ganzfeld (full field) and patterned light were presented, only the response to the white or ganzfeld will be discussed.

A Grass PS2D photic stimulator lamp, which was located behind and above the animal's head, illuminated the stimulus card reflecting into the animal's eyes. The monkeys' heads were shaved and kept clean to facilitate application of electrodes. Solder pellet electrodes were placed bilaterally over the occipital (O_1 and O_2) areas in accordance with the Ten-Twenty International System. The ear lobe leads, which were linked together, served as a common reference.

A Grass PS2D photic stimulator was used to generate a 10-microsecond pulse of light. The lamp of the photo stimulator was enclosed in a fiberglas box to muffle clicking sounds accompanying flashes. Electrocortical responses were amplified by a Grass Model 6 electroencephalograph and were recorded on an FM tape recorder. The frequency response limits of the recording system were ± 3dB 0.8 to 80 Hz. The ink-records from the EEG allowed the experimenter to monitor ongoing electrical activity and to trigger the stimuli during artifact-free periods and when the monkey was quiet and attending; consequently, interstimulus intervals varied from 2 to 20 or more seconds. The room was darkened throughout the experiment with the experimenter present, a situation to which the infant was habituated.

The visual evoked response of the monkeys showed dramatic age changes in amplitude as portrayed in Figure 21. The figure is a composite of three monkeys from birth to 35 weeks (Group 1) and a composite of five monkeys (Group 2) recorded regularly from age 6 to 18 months.

At this point in the study the data have not been fully analyzed; more infants should be studied before any definitive conclusions are reached. However, some reliable observations are possible.

We have arbitrarily labeled the waves or peaks most commonly observed as P2, N2, P3, N3, P4 on the assumption that these may be homologous to components seen in the human VER. Early components, P1 and N1,

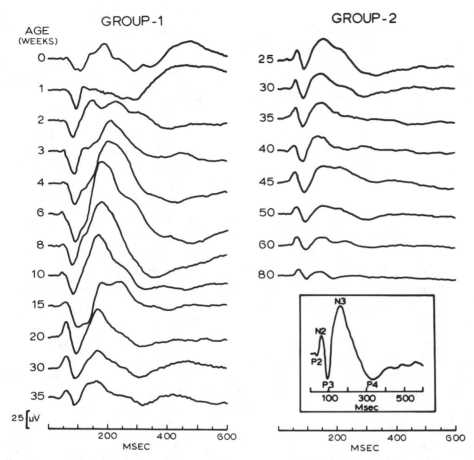

Figure 21. Composite visual evoked responses recorded from occipital scalp for two groups of developing stump-tailed macaques (Macaca arctoides).

which are difficult to see in man, were seen only occasionally in the macaque and so these have been ignored in our analysis. Similary, P2 was too small and variable for any reliable measurement, but it was seen occasionally, even in the first two weeks and persisting throughout. It becomes more obvious at about 8 to 10 weeks of age.

Two negative waves, N2 peaking at approximately 60 and N3 at 160 msec, and two positive waves, P3 at about 90 and P4 at 300 msec, were consistently seen. These waves were observed in about 95 percent of the recordings. A change in amplitude of these waves with increasing age was obvious and measurable. A horizontal baseline, established to coincide with the amplitude of the first points of the response, provided an arbitrary zero amplitude. Amplitude changes were measured in microvolts above and below this baseline. Wave N2, the negative wave peaking at about 60 msec, was particularly interesting. It slowly grew in size during the first 10 to 15 weeks and then suddenly increased in amplitude to reach its maximum 20 μV at 20 weeks of age. Amplitude of this wave then gradually decreased as the animal grew older. It is speculated that this wave stabilizes into an "adult" amplitude at about 24 months (Figure 21).

N3 at about 160 msec reached its maximum amplitude at 6 weeks, then declined rapidly and was still slowly declining in amplitude at 80 weeks. Of all the waves observed, N3 changes most rapidly and dramatically with maturation. Figure 22 shows an interesting correlation with N3 and changes in EEG amplitude. The amplitude of the N3 wave is plotted against the EEG amplitude of the rhesus monkey (Caveness 1964), suggesting a direct relationship between N3 and background EEG amplitude.

P4 follows a trend similar to N3; in fact, the two waves N3 and P4 increase rapidly in amplitude and peak together at 6 weeks, then decline together very rapidly from 6 to 18 weeks. P3 follows a different trend, declining in amplitude only after 20 weeks. These trends may be seen in Figure 21.

Latency changes have not as yet been analyzed but there seems to be a general decrease in latency of most waves from birth to adolescence.

While the visual evoked response of the infant macaque, like the human infant, shows marked changes throughout infancy and maturation, these changes seem to follow quite different time courses. For example, in both the human being and the monkey there are periods during maturation when the amplitude of the visual evoked response reaches its maximum. In the human being this appears to be at ages 6 to 8 years, in the monkey at about 6 weeks, a fiftyfold time difference. Yet the evoked response of the macaque seems to stabilize into an adult pattern at about 20 to 24 months as contrasted with the human at 16 to 18 years, only an eightfold time ratio. A striking difference was the lack of repetitive alphalike "after-discharge" or "ringing" which was rarely seen in the visual evoked responses of the developing monkey but is a salient characteristic of the human VER throughout maturation.

This study was initiated with the assumption that the similarities between the brains of man and macaque would allow for interesting extrapolations from the longitudinal study of the monkey to man. So far we have observed mainly differences. But even these remain to be confirmed and explained.

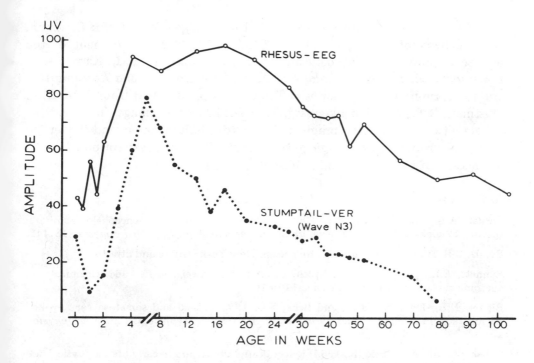

Figure 22. A comparison between the amplitude changes of a negative wave, N3, in the developing stump-tailed macaque and age changes in amplitude of the EEG of the developing rhesus.

Acknowledgments

1. Approved research projects 0864-02 and 1973-03 of the Veterans Administration, and supported in part by NIMH Research Grant 1 R01 DA00388-01 and NICHD Contract PH-43-67-1451.

2. Thanks to Dr. David Ditsworth for his valuable contribution to the study, The Effects of Socioeconomic Deprivation on Evoked Responses, while he was a medical student at the University of Utah College of Medicine. Thanks also to Albert S. Johnson who provided needed expertise in computer operation and analysis of the data, to Dr. Thomas Schenkenberg whose careful and tireless efforts contributed significantly to studies in development and aging, to Dr. David H. Groberg who conducted the experiments on handedness and the evoked response, to Dr. William Gibson and Mrs. Barbara Linde for their valuable help with the study of evoked responses in the infant monkey.

3. Parts of this paper are reprinted in abridged form from: Dustman, R.E., Schenkenberg, T., and Beck, E.C., 1974. The development of the evoked response as a diagnostic and evaluative procedure. In R. Karrer (ed.), *Developmental Psychophysiology in Mental Retardation and Learning Disability*. Springfield, Ill.: Charles C Thomas (in press). Also from Beck, E.C., Dustman, R.E., and Schenkenberg, T. 1974. Life span changes in the electrical activity of the human brain. In J.M. Ordy, K.R. Brizzee, and P. Gerone (eds.), *Neurobiology and Aging*. New York: Plenum Press (in press). With permission of the authors and publisher.

References

Barnet, A.B., and Goodwin,R.S. 1965. Averaged evoked electroencephalographic responses to clicks in the human newborn. *Electroencephalogr. Clin. Neurophysiol.* 18:441.

Benda, C.E. 1960. *The Child With Mongolism*. New York: Grune and Stratton.

Bennett, E.L., Diamond, M.C., Krech, D., and Rosenzweig, M.R. 1964. Chemical and anatomical plasticity of brain. *Science* 146:610.

Bigum, H.B., Dustman, R.E., and Beck, E.C. 1970. Visual and somatosensory evoked responses from mongoloid and normal children. *Electroencephalogr. Clin. Neurophysiol.* 28:202.

Cabek, V., and Najdanvic, R. 1965. Effect of undernutrition in early life on physical and mental development. *Arch. Dis. Child.* 40:532.

Cattell, R.B., and Cattell, A.K. 1960. *Handbook for Culture Fair Intelligence*. Champaign, Ill.: Institute for Personality and Ability Testing.

Caveness, W.F. 1964. Studies of the maturational changes in the EEG during sleep and wakefulness in the monkey. In P. Kellaway and I. Petersen (eds.), *Neurological and Electroencephalographic Correlative Studies in Infancy*, p. 168. New York: Grune and Stratton.

Cornil, L., and Gastaut, H. 1951. Note complémentaire sur l'étude électroencéphalographique de la dominance cérébrale (à propos de la gaucherie). *Ext. C. R. Congrès des Médécins Alienistes et Neurologistes*.

Crome, L. 1954. Some morbid-anatomical aspects of mental deficiency. *J. Ment. Sci.* 100:984.

Crome, L., Cowie, V., and Slater, E. 1966. A statistical note on cerebellar and brain stem weight in mongolism. *J. Ment. Defic. Res.* 10:69.

Crovitz, H.F., and Zener, K. 1962. A group test for assigning hand and eye dominance. *Am. J. Psychol.* 75:271.

Doty, R.W., Kimura, D.S., and Mogenson, G.J. 1964. Photically and electrically elicited responses in the central visual system of the squirrel monkey. *Exp. Neurol.* 10:19.

Dustman, R.E., and Beck, E.C. 1963. Long-term stability of visually evoked potentials in man. *Science* 142:1480.

Dustman, R.E., and Beck, E.C. 1965. The visually evoked potential in twins. *Electroencephalogr. Clin. Neurophysiol.* 19:570.

Dustman, R.E., and Beck, E.C. 1966. Visually evoked potentials: Amplitude changes with age. *Science* 151:1013.

Dustman, R.E., and Beck, E.C. 1969. The effects of maturation and aging on the wave form of visually evoked potentials. *Electroencephalogr. Clin. Neurophysiol.* 26:2.

Ellingson, R.J. 1958. Electroencephalograms of normal, full-term newborns immediately after birth with observations on arousal and visual evoked responses. *Electroencephalogr. Clin. Neurophysiol.* 10:31.

Ellingson, R.J. 1960. Cortical electrical responses to visual stimulation in the human infant. *Electroencephalogr. Clin. Neurophysiol.* 12:663.

Ellingson, R.J. 1966. Relationship between EEG and test intelligence: a commentary. *Psychol. Bull.* 65:91.

Ellingson, R.J., and Wilcott, R.C. 1960. Evoked responses in the visual and auditory cortices of kittens. *J. Neurophysiol.* 23:363.

Engel, R. 1956. Abnormal brain patterns in Kwashiorkor. *Electroencephalogr. Clin. Neurophysiol.* 8:489.

Engel, R., and Butler, B.V. 1963. Appraisal of conceptual age of newborn infants by EEG methods. *J. Pediatr.* 63:386.

Ertl, J.P., and Schafer, E.W.P. 1969. Brain response correlates of psychometric intelligence. *Nature* 223:421.

Farber, D.A. 1968. Evolution of specific visual reactions of the cerebral cortex in ontogenesis. *Fiziologicheski Zhurnal USSR* 54:778. Abstract in *Psychological Abstracts* 1969.

Ferriss, G.S., Davis, G.D., Dorsen, M. McF., and Hackett, E.R. 1967. Changes in latency and form of the photically induced averaged evoked response in human infants. *Electroencephalogr. Clin. Neurophysiol.* 22:305.

Fox, M.W. 1968. Neuronal development and ontogeny of evoked potentials in auditory and visual cortex of the dog. *Electroencephalogr. Clin. Neurophysiol.* 24:213.

deGallardo, F.O.E., Fleishman, R.W., and de Ramirez de Arellano, M.R. 1964. Electroencephalogram of the monkey fetus in utero, and changes in it at birth. *Exp. Neurol.* 9:73.

Glandville, A.D., and Antonities, J.J. 1955. Relationship between occipital alpha activity and laterality. *J. Exp. Psychol.* 49:249.

Harlow, H.F., and Harlow, M.K. 1962. Social deprivation in monkeys. *Scient. Am.* 207:137.

Hughes, J.R., and Curtin, M.J. 1960. Usefulness of photic stimulation in routine clinical electroencephalograph. *Neurology* 10:777.

Hunt, W.E., and Goldring, S. 1951. Maturation of evoked response of the visual cortex in the post-natal rabbit. *Electroencephalogr. Clin. Neurophysiol.* 3:465.

Kennard, M.A., and Nims, L.F. 1942. Changes in normal electroencephalogram of Macaca mulatta with growth. *J. Neurophysiol.* 5:325.

Kooi, K.A., Eckman, H.G., and Thomas, M.H. 1957. Observations on the response to photic stimulation in organic cerebral dysfunction. *Electroencephalogr. Clin. Neurophysiol.* 9:239.

Lansing, R.W., and Thomas, H. 1964. Laterality of photic driving in normal adults. *Electroencephalogr. Clin. Neurophysiol.* 16:290.

Lennox, L.G., Gibbs, E.L., and Gibbs, F.A. 1945. Brain wave patterns: an hereditary trait. *J. Hered.* 36:233.

Marty, R. 1967. Maturation post-natale du système auditif. In A. Minkowski (ed.), *Regional Development of the Brain in Early Life*, p. 327. Oxford: Blackwell.

Meyer, A., and Jones, J.B. 1939. Histological changes in the brain in mongolism. *J. Ment. Sci.* 85:206.

Mizuno, T., Chiba, F., Sakai, M., Watanabe, S., Tamura, T., Arakawa, T., Tatsumi, S., and Coursin, D.B. 1969. Frequency analysis of electroencephalograms and latency of photically induced averaged evoked responses in children with Riboflavinosis: Preliminary report. Presented by D.B. Coursin to Palo Alto NIH Conference, June 1969.

Mourek, J., Himwich, W.A., Myslivecek, J., and Callison, D.A. 1967. The role of nutrition in the development of evoked cortical potentials in the rat. *Brain Res.* 6:241.

Naeye, R.L., Diener, M., Dellinger, W.S., and Blanc, W.A. 1969. Urban poverty: Effects on prenatal nutrition. *Science* 166:1026.

deRamirez de Arellano, M.R. 1961. Maturational changes in the electroencephalogram of normal monkeys. *Exp. Neurol.* 3:209.

Raney, E.T. 1939. Brain potentials and lateral dominance in identical twins. *J. Exp. Psychol.* 24:21.

Rhodes, L.E., Dustman, R.E., and Beck, E.C. 1969. The visually evoked response: A comparison of bright and dull children. *Electroencephalogr. Clin. Neurophysiol.* 27:364.

Rife, D.C. 1933a. Genetic studies of monozygotic twins: Diagnostic formula. *J. Hered.* 24:339.

Rife, D.C. 1933b. Genetic studies of monozygotic twins: Finger patterns and eye-color as criteria for monozygosity. *J. Hered.* 24:407.

Rose, G.H., and Ellingson, R.J. 1968. The comparative ontogenesis of visually evoked responses in rat, cat, and human infant. Proc. Amer. Enceph. Soc., *Electroencephalogr. Clin. Neurophysiol.* 24:284 (abstract).

Rose, G.H., and Lindsley, D.B. 1965. Visually evoked electrocortical responses in kittens: Development of specific and nonspecific systems. *Science* 148:1244.

Schenkenberg, T. 1970. Visual, auditory, and somatosensory evoked responses of normal subjects from childhood to senescence. Unpublished doctoral dissertation, University of Utah.

Spitz, R.A. 1958. An inquiry into the genesis of psychiatric conditions in early childhood. In *The Psychoanalytic Study of the Child*, vol. I. New York: International Universities Press.

Stock, M.V., and Smythe, P.M. 1963. Does undernutrition during infancy inhibit brain growth and subsequent intellectual development? *Arch. Dis. Child.* 38:546.

Vogel, W., and Broverman, D.M. 1964. Relationship between EEG and test intelligence: A critical review. *Psychol. Bull.* 62:132.

Vogel, W., and Broverman, D.M. 1966. A reply to "Relationship between EEG and test intelligence: a commentary." *Psychol. Bull.* 65:99.

Williams, D., and Reynell, J. 1945. Abnormal suppression of cortical frequencies. *Brain* 68:123.

brain potentials
and prediction of performance

Enoch Callaway, M.D.

Langley Porter Neuropsychiatric Institute, and
Department of Psychiatry
University of California Medical Center
San Francisco, California

To test an idea, use it to predict something. Only when we try to predict can we discover that we are wrong and the possibility of disproof is the principal distinction between scientific and theological concepts. One has almost to begin a paper on the use of brain potentials to measure IQ with such an apology. An applied goal often suggests commercial exploitation and extravagant claims. I hope to illustrate that an applied goal such as this has theoretical as well as practical merit, that prediction of performance from brain potentials is a real possibility, and that some novel approaches are waiting for exploitation.

Brain waves have always had a curious attraction for off-beat students of the mind-brain. The brain produces patterns of electrical potentials and patterns of thought. We should be able to relate one to the other. Berger, the father of electroencephalography, was a psychiatrist with an interest in extrasensory perception and that interest was closely connected to his interest in brain waves. I suspect that Berger, like some of the rest of us, must have felt frustrated and lonely at being excluded from the minds of others. Each of our minds is locked in its own bony prison and is able to communicate only by the crude prison telegraph system that the sensory and motor pathways provide. The appeal of extrasensory perception lies in its promise of a direct mind-to-mind communication. To more pragmatic souls, the electroencephalogram seems to offer a sort of "window" onto the mind.

473

Unfortunately, right from the beginning it seemed as though brain waves were more related to what the mind was not doing than they were to what the mind was doing. Berger observed that the alpha waves appeared from over the visual cortex when one ceased to use the visual apparatus. Instead of being windows on the mind, brain waves seemed to be sort of "not-operating" signals. Of course, the neurologists discovered that various sorts of diseases produced rather characteristic "not-operating" signals and so the EEG found its niche in the study of things like epilepsy, coma, brain tumors, sleep, and death. Ever hopeful, the psychological types continued to try to find relationships between brain waves and more subtle mental functions, and in particular attempted to use brain waves to measure intelligence.

The results were disappointing, to say the least. For example, when Ellingson (1966) reviewed the literature on correlations between EEG and intelligence, he decided that most of the correlations were due to the fact that very sick brain waves (for example, those reflecting epilepsy and brain damage) were likely to go with low IQs. I could argue with some of the details of Ellingson's conclusions, but they serve our purpose here. We need to underline the fact that brain waves by and large tell us what the mind is not doing. Alpha waves at the occiput appear when we cease to use the visual cortex. Alpha waves over the left hemisphere disappear when we read. Even the slow waves of deep sleep disappear when we dream. I oversimplify, but not excessively, when I say that averaged evoked potentials were the first demonstration that brain potentials could be positively related to mental function.

Intriguing parallels between thought processes and brain electrical processes revealed by the evoked potential suggest that Berger's dream may indeed come true some day and that the electrical potentials of the head may provide a window on the mind. Further, these parallels suggest that brain potentials may even be serving a purpose in the brain and not just reflecting gross metabolic states.

Let us assume that the brain is usually doing many things at the same time—with brisk potential changes playing a role in data processing, while obvious rhythmic activity arises from idling areas. This humming, blooming confusion is tamed by averaging, and we see signs of those effective signals that were previously swamped by the idling noise. But there is a cost. To make averaging work, we must have the mind do more or less the same thing repeatedly so we can average the electrical potentials associated with the repeated act. Anything the mind does repeatedly tends to be banal, particularly if the repetition rate is fast enough for practical work in an evoked response laboratory.

So now we have a window on the mind, but to use it we must set the mind to banal repetitive activities.

For the moment, let that sour note hang, for banal or not, we can use evoked responses to measure intelligence. Indeed, the processing of banal data may be a major factor in school performance, and that, of course, is what many IQ tests are about. There are a number of evoked potential measures that correlate with IQ, but four will serve the purposes of illustration. References for what follows may be found in a recent review (Callaway 1973). First, let us consider two latency measures.

By now, we are familiar with "neural efficiency." Flash a light repeatedly, record the averaged evoked potential (AEP) from P4-F4, and in general, one will find shorter latencies in brighter subjects. Even better, trigger the flash when the brain wave goes negative through zero, and count the time to the third negative going line-cross, average 100 of these 3 cross periods, and one will also have a measure that correlates with IQ. Studies using different electrode placements have found no such correlations, but replications have now come from at least three different laboratories.

Ertl's original idea was that fast neuronal responses would go with fast AEP responses (that is, short latencies) and fast mental responses (high IQ) (Ertl and Schafer 1969). There are several reasons for rejecting that pleasantly straightforward idea. Early on, Shucard and Horn (1972) found that visual latency-IQ correlations were better when the subject was bored than when the subject was attending to flashes. More recently, accumulating data on auditory AEP latencies show, at least on occasion, the opposite sort of relationship. Long auditory latencies go with higher IQ. In other words, if fast neurons produce fast AEPs and fast minds, then this is true only for neurons in the visual pathways and not for those in auditory pathways. Even in the visual system the apparent requirement seems to be that the stimuli be uninteresting. There are a number of alternatives to the neural-efficiency hypothesis. For example, perhaps dull subjects stay involved with unimportant stimuli longer than do bright subjects. There is some evidence that with increasing boredom, visual AEP latencies shorten. Thus, bored bright subjects might have shorter latencies.

In summary, visual latencies and auditory AEP latencies both are correlated with IQ, but with opposite signs. Short visual and long auditory latencies go with high IQ. There are a number of technical points that I have omitted here but that will be of great importance in replicating these results. The more crucial point of my arguments is that by manipulating such things as electrode placement and stimulus significance, we can make these correlations come and go. In this way, we can check our theory about why such correlations should exist at all, and perhaps in the long run learn more about the structure of intelligence than the factor analysts with their rotating matrices have been able to discover. I doubt the answers will be quite so neat as the neural-efficiency hypothesis—but then again, who knows?

Although, as noted above, a variety of other AEP measures also correlate with intelligence, I will deal only with two—AEP variability and AEP asymmetry—because they lead us toward some speculation about the future.

Variability came to occupy our attention by the back door. Through a long, circuitous series of experiments, we arrived at the somewhat unremarkable finding that the perceptual responses of schizophrenics are less stable than those of normals, and that this perceptual/cognitive instability leaves its imprint both on task performance and on evoked cortical potentials. Children also show more AEP variability—again a somewhat unsurprising finding. But then we found that, with due technical precautions, measures of stability or variability are, in themselves, relatively stable over time in a given individual. If age is held constant, AEP variability is inversely correlated with performance on tasks that give good scores for stable accurate performance (as opposed to imaginative and creative performance). More recently, Laurian (1973) showed that demanding tasks cause AEP variability to increase in the period after the task has been completed. Does the correlation between AEP variability and IQ simply reflect the association between generally stable cognitive performance and good IQ test scores? Does it reflect a correlation between maturity and intelligence? If AEP variability reflects fatigue, does the increased AEP variability of schizophrenics and individuals with low IQ reflect stresses to which such persons are subject? Could, for example, a person whose problems in life were in part the result of unstable cognitive functioning be trained to cognate in a more stable way? These questions have both practical and theoretical interest; what is more, there is even reason to assume they can be examined empirically.

The last AEP correlate of IQ to be considered is asymmetry. The correlation between AEP asymmetry and IQ was first noted by Dustman and Beck (1972), although Rémond's group (Lairy et al. 1969) had noted that alpha averages were more asymmetrical in bright than in dull subjects. Since that first report, Beck's group has also noted that alcoholics and persons retarded by Down's syndrome have more symmetrical visual AEPs than do normals (Lewis, Dustman, and Beck 1970; Bigum, Dustman, and Beck 1970). We have found this asymmetry/IQ correlation in two studies, but not in the third. We are not absolutely certain, but it seems that too much interest in the stimulus makes the IQ/asymmetry correlation disappear. Using a short sitting, or directing the subject's attention to the stimulus seems to make the AEPs less asymmetrical and to abolish the asymmetry/IQ correlation. The sort of attention one can most easily direct to a light flash is usually what Bogen (1969) calls appositional—that is to say, the nonverbal spatial sort of operation characteristic of the right hemisphere. In general, we know that right-brain tasks suppress EEG and AEP from the right hemisphere unless, in the case of AEPs, the evoking stimulus is itself a part of the right-brain task. The same is true for the left brain. To take some left-brain examples, letter trigrams and phonems cause large left visual and auditory AEPs, but reading a book suppresses both AEP and EEG on the left. Perhaps the AEP/IQ asymmetry correlation reflects the fact that when a person sits and watches repetitive light flashes, he tends to amuse himself with his own thoughts, and people who use their left (verbal) hemisphere more than their right do better on IQ tests.

I am suggesting that waves in the EEG are an indication that something is not happening in the mind, and although AEPs indicate something happening, that something must be repetitive and hence rather banal. Can we find some measure of the ongoing EEG that does not depend on the extended wavelike properties of the EEG, and that can be applied when more natural nonrepetitive thought processes are going on? I have a candidate to be considered, one that could be applied straightaway to the measurement of both variability and asymmetry (Callaway and Harris 1974).

The method I suggest involves examining the contingency between electrical activities arising from different areas of the brain moment by moment.

If the EEG reflects messages going back and forth between parts of the brain, then any messages that have to do with complex mental functions must say their piece and be done quickly. An alpha wave which takes 100 msec to announce itself is too slow by orders of magnitude. We can, however, describe brain potentials in some detail by specifying their polarity and derivatives. One might also suspect that the cells of the brain use potentials and rates of change in potentials for high-speed data processing, and gross frequency data for specifying more enduring states.

To explore this idea we simply decoded brain waves by specifying polarity and derivative and measured the contingency of the decoded signals from pairs of areas (Figure 1). We reasoned that if two brain areas increased their functional relationships, we should see this reflected in an increase in their electrical relationship—that is, by an increase in the contingency of signals recorded in the two areas in question and decoded or classified according to the potential and derivation scheme described.

We felt reasonably sure that visual data involved the occipital area. Propositional processing (such as reading) should couple occiput and left hemisphere, while appositional processing (such as attempting to engage oneself in the sensual aspects of a picture) should couple occiput and right hemisphere. That is exactly what happened.

As our measure of contingency we used information transmission, which has some nice mathematical and computational properties and a suggestive (even if potentially misleading) name. For simplicity, information transmission (or uncertainty reduction) can be considered as analogous to chi-square computed using logarithms of averaged probability. In our examples there are four cells on each margin. Uncertainty for the X margin (H_X) is computed as follows:

$$H_X = -\sum_{i=1}^{4} P_{x_i} \log_2 P_{x_i}$$

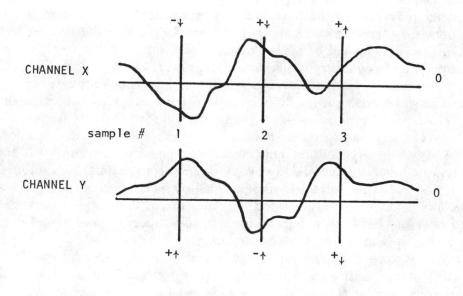

Figure 1. Example of polarity and first derivative decoding with contingency table showing entries based on three samples.

Where P_{x_i} is the probability of an event in the ith cell on the X margin. We also compute X_y and H_{xy}, the latter being computed using the 16 cells inside the matrix. Uncertainty reduction ($H_{\widehat{xy}}$) is then

$$H_{\widehat{xy}} = H_x + H_y - H_{xy}$$

The computational advantage comes from the fact that, if epoch size is small and constant, an exhaustive $P \log_2 P$ table can be stored in the computer, and all computation is done by retrieval from a stored log table and addition.

We are now doing more parametric studies of this measure, but we have some speculations about what one could hope for unless some unexpected flaw in the logic or in the supporting experiments comes to light.

One might imagine that people of differing temperaments, abilities, and cognitive styles might show differences in both magnitude and stability of brain-area coupling at rest, and differences in the way such couplings could be altered by varying task demands. Do people of differing abilities couple their brain areas differently when approaching the same problem? Could training alter these brain-potential differences? Do dyslexic children show some characteristic inter-area relationships? Do children who become "ready" to learn reading show increased inter-area coupling on the left?

Suppose left hemisphere dominance is reflected in higher left inter-hemispheric coupling than right inter-hemispheric coupling. Do such drugs of abuse as alcohol and marijuana release the right hemisphere from left hemisphere domination? Could biofeedback of information-transmission measures enable the drug user to achieve the state he desires without drugs? The method is simple, and computationally well within the reach of the smaller minicomputers. We shall see.

In summary, then, we have complained that the temporally extended and wavelike qualities of the EEG are principally useful for diagnosing disease. When we want positive information about mental processes, we can average evoked potentials. Studying correlations between averaged evoked potentials and intelligence will surely improve our understanding of both these poorly understood things, and it may even have immediate practical value. Averaged evoked potentials offer considerable hope that brain potentials may be related to complex mental processes, but averaging has inherent limitations. Various routes to freedom from the bondage of the repetitive banal mental processes required by averaging are being explored, and one of these is a measure of inter-hemispheric coupling described above.

Acknowledgments

This work was supported chiefly by Office of Naval Research Contract

N00014-69-A-0200-2007, and aided by National Institute of Mental Health General Research Support Grant FR 05550 and U.S. Army Medical Research and Development Command Contract DADA17-73-C-3146.

References

Bigum, H.B., Dustman, R.E., and Beck, E.C. 1970. Visual and somatosensory evoked responses from mongoloid and normal children. *Electroencephalogr. Clin. Neurophysiol.* 28:576.

Bogen, J.E. 1969. The other side of the brain I, II, III, *Bulletin of the Los Angeles Neurological Society* 34:73, 135, 191.

Callaway, E. 1973. Correlations between evoked potentials and measures of intelligence: An overview. *Arch. Gen. Psychiatry* 29:553.

Callaway, E., and Harris, P.R. 1974. Coupling between cortical potentials from different areas. *Science* 183:873.

Dustman, R.E., and Beck, E.C. 1972. Relations of intelligence to visually evoked responses. *Electroencephalogr. Clin. Neurophysiol.* 33:254.

Ellingson, R.J. 1966. Relationship between EEG and intelligence: A commentary. *Psychol. Bull.* 65:91.

Ertl, J., and Schafer, E.W.P. 1969. Brain response correlates of psychometric intelligence. *Nature* 223:421.

Lairy, G.C., Rémond, A., Rieger, H., and Lesèvre, N. 1969. The alpha average. III. Clinical application in children. *Electroencephalogr. Clin. Neurophysiol.* 26:453.

Laurian, S. 1973. AER variability and mental load. In *Activités Evoquées et Leur Conditionnement chez l'Homme Normal et en Pathologie Mentale.* Proceedings of Colloque de Neurophysiologie Humaine Appliquée à la Psychologie et à la Psychiatrie, Tours, September 1972. Paris: Éditions INSERM.

Lewis, E.G., Dustman, R.E., and Beck, E.C. 1970. The effects of alcohol on visual and somatosensory evoked responses. *Electroencephalogr. Clin. Neurophysiol.* 28:202.

Shucard, D.W. and Horn, J.L. 1972. Evoked cortical potentials and measurement of human abilities. *J. Comp. Physiol. Psychol.* 78:59.

evoked potentials in psychopathology and psychiatric treatment

Charles Shagass, M.D.

Temple University Medical Center and
Eastern Pennsylvania Psychiatric Institute
Philadelphia, Pennsylvania

Electrical signals that reflect several kinds of cerebral responses can be recorded from the intact human scalp by the use of time-coherent signal averaging. Sensory evoked potentials are the best known of these phenomena, but several other kinds of activity are encompassed under the more generic term of "event-related potentials" (ERP) (Vaughan 1969). ERPs also include the time-coherent cerebral electrical events related to motor acts (Vaughan, Costa, and Ritter 1968), the slow potential shifts associated with such phenomena as expectancy (Walter et al. 1964) and with the intention to move (Kornhuber and Deecke 1965), and potentials accompanying such complex psychological processes as those involved in stimulus recognition (Sutton, Braren, and Zubin 1965). In addition to ERPs of cerebral origin, there are several that originate outside of the brain; the sources of some of these are ocular movements, muscle twitches, aspects of the electrocardiogram, movements of the tongue, and galvanic skin responses (GSR). Special precautions, sometimes of rather complex nature, must be taken to distinguish between the desired signals of brain origin and those arising in extracerebral structures.

Some aspects of all the major kinds of cerebral ERPs have been investigated in psychiatric populations. There have also been a number of studies of the effects on these potentials of drugs commonly used for psychiatric treatment. In this paper an attempt will be made to review the main findings obtained in psychiatric investigations of ERPs. A substantial portion of the material to be presented has been gathered in the author's laboratory, in which the main effort since 1958 has been research on evoked potentials in psychiatry.

In order to restrict its scope, the review will deal primarily with results obtained in studies of psychiatric patient populations. Evoked potential investigations more directly concerned with normal psychological processes, such as perception, attention and consciousness, all of which may be highly relevant to psychopathology, will receive only peripheral consideration. Some of these topics have been reviewed recently in a monograph (Shagass 1972).

Methodology

Comprehensive discussions of evoked potential methodology may be found in the monographs by Perry and Childers (1969), Regan (1972), and Shagass (1972). The purpose of this section is to highlight certain methodological issues of particular relevance to the application of the techniques in psychiatric research.

Instrumentation

The essential equipment includes a stimulating device, EEG amplifiers, timers and trigger pulse generators, and an instrument for summing or averaging the EEG samples. There are many kinds of averaging instruments, the most favored being those of digital type. Special-purpose digital averaging computers have been in common use for over a decade, but small general-purpose laboratory computers are becoming increasingly popular. Although averages may be obtained "on-line," there are advantages to storing the EEG in analog form on magnetic tape for later playback into the averaging computer. A device for accurate amplitude calibration is probably the most important of the various accessory instruments used in ERP recording. In our laboratory we have used Emde's (1964) low level calibrator for many years.

Among the many issues to be considered in selecting equipment for average response recording, the degree of temporal resolution in the various components of the system merits priority. The temporal resolution required will depend upon the nature of the events to be studied; slow potentials, such as the contingent negative variation (CNV), can be recorded with reasonable accuracy by using a computer that provides only one data point for

10 or 20 msec, whereas the rapid early events of the auditory evoked response may require one data point per 20 μsec for accurate measurement (Jewett, Romano, and Williston 1970). The frequency response of the amplifiers and tape recorders should be compatible with the desired resolution. The selection of a stimulator is obviously governed by the evoked response phenomenon of interest. Because of the nature of the averaging process, the main requirement is that stimulus onset be sharply defined in time, so that the averaging computer can be set into action with minimal temporal "jitter" in relation to the response of interest.

General Factors in Recording

Averaging requires repeated presentation of stimuli. The individual responses in an averaging sequence may vary considerably because of order effects, habituation, and such other changes in subject state as alertness and boredom. If a meaningful complex stimulus is used, repetition may cause it to have a different meaning at the end of the averaging sequence. The interval between stimuli (repetition interval) may have to be quite long to reduce overlap with the effects of the preceding stimulus; ideally, stimuli after the first in a sequence should be administered after full recovery of responsiveness. In practice, to avoid making the recording session too long and fatiguing for the subject, the investigator usually must compromise; he may administer fewer stimuli than the number that would assure a stable, noise-free average and he may employ a shorter repetition interval than needed for unattenuated responses. These considerations are of particular importance in studies of psychiatric patients, who are frequently tense and restless.

In working with patients it is necessary to keep the duration of single averaging sequences to a minimum and perhaps to fractionate the sequence into several parts in order to permit the subject to rest, and to provide reassurance. Furthermore, with some subjects it may be necessary to engage in special maneuvers to reduce muscle tension. Voluntary and involuntary movements of the tongue and frequent eye blinking and eye movement are troublesome sources of artifact. Nevertheless, with patience and persistence, well-trained technicians have been able to obtain satisfactory recordings from many disturbed patients in our laboratory. In recent years their work has been facilitated by the installation of a device for halting the stimulating sequence when artifactual potentials, usually originating in a muscle, exceed an arbitrarily set amplitude. Clearly, the shorter the duration of the experimental session, the easier it is for the subject to maintain cooperation; however, in most of our experiments we successfully employed designs that require the subject to be in the laboratory for two to three hours.

Display and Quantification

ERPs are most frequently displayed by writing the average on paper with devices like an XY plotter. They may also be displayed on a cathode ray oscilloscope and photographed. The characteristics of these waveforms must be quantified for most research purposes, since qualitatively distinctive responses for specific psychiatric conditions have not been demonstrated. Measurements may be made visually by locating the points of interest and measuring the time from stimulus (latency) and the amplitude. Amplitude measurements may be made between two identified peaks or between one peak and some estimate of the isoelectric or base line. Quantification can be greatly facilitated by a general-purpose computer. In recent years we have most often measured amplitude in terms of the average deviation around the mean of set time epochs that are identified as likely to contain events of interest; for example, the epoch from 15 to 30 msec after median nerve shock contains the initial negative-positive complex of the somatosensory response (Figure 1). Peak-to-peak or deviation from baseline amplitude measurements can be made automatically by computer if the peaks are clearly the maximal or minimal values in a given time epoch; when peaks can be clearly identified in this way, latency measurements can also be made.

Recovery Functions

Recovery functions are determined by applying pairs of stimuli separated by an interval that is changed for each averaging sequence. When interstimulus intervals are brief, the two responses will overlap; to visualize the response to the second stimulus of the pair (R2), we have intermixed unpaired and paired stimuli in the same averaging sequence. The response to a single, unpaired stimulus (R1) is entered into two channels of the averaging computer in opposite polarity. One R1 is retained for measurement, but the R1 entered in inverse polarity is added to the responses to the paired stimuli in the other channel, thus being subtracted from them; R2 is then visualized because R1 + R2 − R1 = R2. Ordinarily, in recovery function determinations, the two stimuli of the pair are of equal intensity. In our recent work, however, we employed a modified somatosensory recovery function procedure, in which we varied the strength of the first, or conditioning, stimulus, while keeping the intensity of the second, or test, stimulus constant (Shagass, Overton, and Straumanis 1971). We also employed a train of nine stimuli, in addition to a single conditioning stimulus, in the same procedure. Figure 1 shows sample responses obtained with two intensities of conditioning stimuli. The test stimulus was a 0.1-msec-duration median nerve shock at 10 mA above sensory threshold. Average responses to single test stimuli and

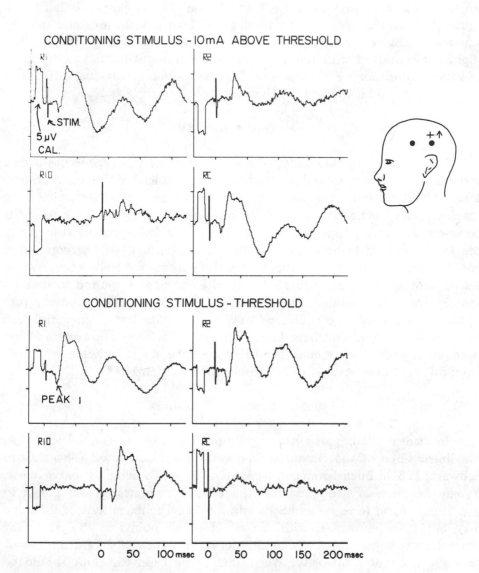

Figure 1. Somatosensory evoked responses obtained with the modified recovery function procedure for one subject in two averaging sequences with conditioning stimulus intensity at 10 mA above sensory threshold and at threshold. Test stimulus 10 mA above threshold. Relative positivity at presumably active electrode gives upward deflection. R1 (R1T) is average response to 50 stimuli of test intensity. RC (R1C) is average response to 50 stimuli of conditioning intensity. R2 is response to 50 paired conditioning and test stimuli (interstimulus interval, 10 msec) minus 50 RC. R10 is response to 50 trains composed of 9 conditioning stimuli and 1 test stimulus (interval between stimuli 10 msec) minus 50 trains of 9 conditioning stimuli. Initial negative deflection is designated as peak 1. Note suppression of R2 and R10 with 10 mA conditioning stimuli, and slight augmentation of R2 and R10 with threshold conditioning stimuli.

single conditioning stimuli, as well as R2 and R10 responses obtained by subtraction, are displayed. The tracings of Figure 1 demonstrate marked suppression of test responses with the intense conditioning stimulus, and slight augmentation with the threshold conditioning stimulus. The purpose of varying conditioning stimulus intensity was to assess individual differences in inhibitory and facilitatory reactivity.

Wave Shape Stability

The stability, or variability, of evoked response wave shape has been a variable of interest in several psychiatric studies (Callaway, Jones, and Layne 1965; Lifshitz 1969). The most common procedure for determining wave shape stability has been to compute product-moment correlation coefficients between the corresponding successive data points following the stimulus in the two responses being compared. For statistical analysis, the correlation coefficients, which are not normally distributed, are generally converted to the Zr transform. Figure 2 illustrates application of the method to somato-sensory responses obtained in the context of the modified recovery procedure. The Zr value can also be used to compute the mean correlation coefficient when several have been obtained. The correlation method has been employed to determine similarity of wave shape between responses from different head areas (Rodin, Grisell, and Gottlieb 1968).

Intensity-Response Functions

In studies relating response amplitude or latency to stimulus intensity, the linear slope of the curve has frequently been computed (Shagass and Schwartz 1963a, Buchsbaum and Silverman 1968). To make the curve linear, it may be necessary to transform the evoked response measurements to logarithmic form (Shagass and Schwartz 1963a). The magnitude of the slope may be highly correlated with the mean of all points in the curve; for example, the higher the mean amplitude, the greater the slope from lowest to highest stimulus intensity. When this is the case, the slope should be corrected for its covariance with the mean, in order to obtain a slope value independent of mean level (Soskis and Shagass 1974). We have used the same covariance adjustment with recovery function data to obtain test response measures that are independent of the general response level obtained when no conditioning stimuli are applied (Shagass 1968).

Subject Variables

The two most critical subject variables to be controlled in comparing

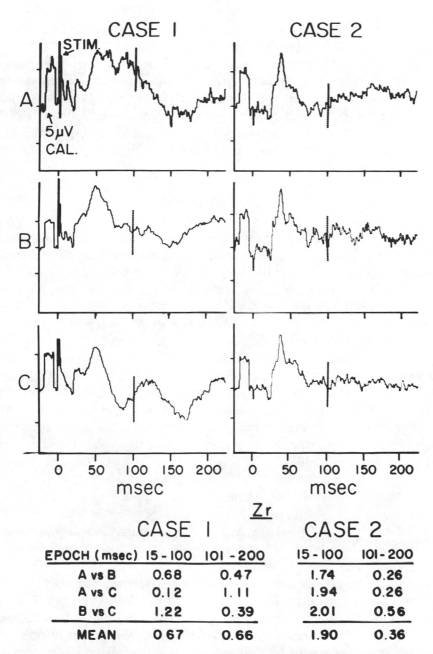

Figure 2. R1T tracings from the modified recovery function tests of two subjects, selected to illustrate how variations in wave shape are reflected in the index of similarity (Zr), derived from product-moment correlations between corresponding, successive data points. Each R1T is average of 50 sweeps with stimulus 10 mA above threshold. Vertical lines in middle of tracings at 100 msec from stimulus. Zr values shown at bottom for data points from 15 to 100 msec and 101 to 200 msec after stimulus. Note lack of correspondence between the Zr values for the two analysis epochs.

clinical groups are probably age and sex, since evoked response characteristics may vary considerably with both of these factors (Shagass 1972). In recent work we have demonstrated sex and age differences in somatosensory responses within psychiatric populations that were absent in matched control groups (Shagass, Overton, and Straumanis 1972 and 1974). Handedness may be a factor in some kinds of visual evoked responses (Eason et al. 1967). For some purposes it may be necessary to equate clinical groups on intelligence in order to control for this variable (Ertl and Schafer 1969; Rhodes, Dustman, and Beck 1969).

Transitory Subject Factors

In addition to such more or less consistent subject variables as age and sex, which can affect evoked response characteristics and lead to fallacious conclusions concerning psychopathology, a number of transitory factors can also produce effects. Some of these factors, such as time of day, are relatively easy to control (Heninger et al. 1969). Other factors, like smoking habits and time since the last cigarette, may be more difficult to control (Hall et al. 1973). Still others, like minor fluctuations in level of alertness, may be virtually impossible to control with certainty. Although gross evoked potential changes occur with sleep, this can be detected in the EEG, which should be monitored constantly during evoked response recordings. However, minor variations in attention are capable of producing marked effects on the components of the evoked response that occurs after about 100 msec and may be extremely difficult to control even with sophisticated experimental designs (Sutton 1969).

Drugs

All drugs commonly used for psychiatric treatment have the capacity for altering level of alertness; changes related to altered alertness may combine or interact with more specific pharmacological effects on evoked responses. Such drug effects are of interest in themselves, but they pose a formidable methodological problem in comparative clinical studies. Since it is rare for an investigator to be able to study psychiatric patients who have not received drugs for several months, it is always possible that differences between clinical groups may be due to the drug treatment of one group. There can be greater confidence in the results when both the groups compared have an equivalent drug history. Even under such circumstances, however, it would still be possible for the differences to be determined more by differential responsiveness to the same drugs, or to their withdrawal, in one or another group than by essential neurophysiological differences.

One useful strategy in psychiatric investigations is to study patients serially before and during somatic therapy. The evoked response changes in patients responding to treatment can then be compared with those in patients who did not respond to the same treatment; this can be of help in sorting out drug effects on the ERPs from those related to the psychopathology (Shagass 1973; Saletu, Saletu, and Itil 1973). Also, if successful treatment causes the evoked response measurements to return toward normal, initial deviations from normal in the patients can be attributed to their illness (Shagass and Schwartz 1962).

Results of Clinical Group Comparisons

Evoked Responses to Unpaired Stimuli

Using several intensities of stimulation, we found the amplitude of somatosensory evoked responses to be generally greater in psychiatric patients than in controls (Shagass and Schwartz 1963a, 1963b). The slope of the intensity-response function was significantly greater in most patient groups, the exception being "dysthymic" neuroses characterized by anxiety, depression, and somatic complaints. In these studies, however, the computed slopes were not adjusted for variations in mean amplitude level, so that the slope results could indicate no more than differences in mean amplitude. In a subsequent study of somatosensory recovery functions, using a single stimulus intensity, amplitude differences between clinical groups were not found (Shagass 1968), but we have recently confirmed some of the earlier findings within the context of the modified recovery function procedure, which employs several stimulus intensities. These recent data show higher amplitudes of the early portion (up to 50 msec) of the somatosensory response in schizophrenic patients with the chronic undifferentiated, chronic paranoid, and schizo-affective subtypes of the disorder than in normals or in patients with acute or latent subtypes of schizophrenia (Shagass, Overton, and Straumanis 1974). Figure 3 shows intensity-response curves comparing age- and sex-matched groups of chronic and acute schizophrenics with nonpatients. Although amplitudes were lower in the acute schizophrenics than in the controls, the significant differences were between the chronic schizophrenics and the other groups.

We have recently studied the relationships between somatosensory evoked response amplitude measurements, obtained within the modified recovery procedure context, and clinical assessments of symptom patterns in a heterogeneous schizophrenic population. The main findings were obtained with ratings based on the Brief Psychiatric Rating Scale (Overall and Gorham 1962). Schizophrenic patients who were rated high on depressive mood, but

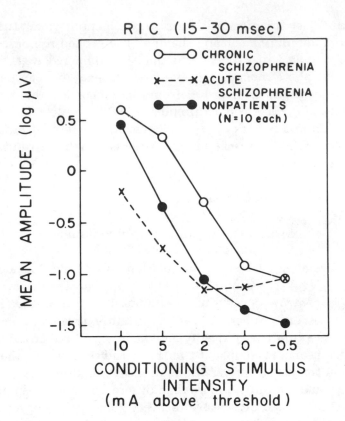

Figure 3. Curves relating somatosensory response amplitude to stimulus intensity in chronic schizophrenic, acute schizophrenic, and nonpatient subject groups. Amplitude measurements are the average deviation from the mean value for the epoch 15 to 30 msec after the stimulus, expressed as natural logarithms. Data obtained in the context of the modified recovery function experiment.

low on such overt psychotic symptoms as hallucinations, suspiciousness, and unusual thought content, tended to have a lower amplitude of evoked responses; in contrast, patients with high ratings on psychotic symptoms and low ratings for depression tended to have high-amplitude evoked responses (Shagass, Overton, and Straumanis 1974). Although these results were in general agreement with the findings shown in Figure 3, which indicate that chronic schizophrenics tend to have higher-amplitude responses, our data suggested that the symptom pattern ratings were more closely related to the evoked response measurement than was the diagnostic subtype of schizophrenia. Furthermore, the patients in the different symptom pattern groups had similar drug histories, so that the evoked response differences were less likely to be a function of previous drug use than patient-control differences.

Parenthetically, in this study, no patients were tested while receiving drugs, and the period of freedom from drug administration averaged ten days.

Several workers have found the amplitudes of auditory responses to be lower in schizophrenic patients than in nonpatients (Cohen 1973; Jones and Callaway 1970; Saletu, Itil, and Saletu 1971). Satterfield (1972) compared auditory response amplitudes in depressed patients and controls; although the amplitudes of the patients tended to be somewhat greater, the differences were not significant.

Comparing a heterogeneous group of psychiatric patients with controls, flash-evoked response amplitudes were found to be greater and latencies shorter in the patients (Shagass and Schwartz 1965; Shagass, Schwartz, and Krishnamoorti 1965). Within the patient population, amplitudes were greater in nonpsychotics, while schizophrenics tended to have faster latencies for the initial positive peak of the response. The amount of rhythmic after-activity in the responses to flash was also measured by the method indicated in Figure 4. Significantly less after-activity was found in schizophrenic patients. However, this finding is not specifically related to schizophrenia, since similar results were obtained in elderly patients with chronic brain syndromes (Straumanis, Shagass, and Schwartz 1965). The group differences found by us in the earlier components of the response were not replicated by the data of Speck, Dim, and Mercer (1966) and Floris et al. (1967), who compared nonpatients with psychiatric patient groups composed mainly of schizophrenics. Unfortunately, nearly all studies of visual evoked responses in schizophrenic patients have been done without fixation of the pupil. The importance of this factor is indicated by the results of Rodin et al. (1964) and Rodin, Grisell, and Gottlieb (1968). In the earlier study these workers found significant differences between normals and schizophrenic patient subgroups differing in lactate-pyruvate ratio, but the group differences were no longer present when responses were recorded later with the diameter of the pupil controlled. Rodin's results suggest caution in interpreting visual evoked response data obtained with mobile pupils.

Evoked Potential Tests of Augmenting-Reducing

Petrie (1967) formulated a dimension of perceptual responding along which people could be classified as stimulus augmenters or reducers. Phenomena such as pain tolerance provided an important source for Petrie's concepts; reducers tolerated pain to a greater extent than did augmenters. She placed considerable emphasis upon a test measuring degree of kinesthetic figural after-effect (KFA) in classifying people on the augmenter-reducer dimension. Buchsbaum and Silverman (1968) were able to show that the slope of the intensity-response curve for flash-evoked responses was sig-

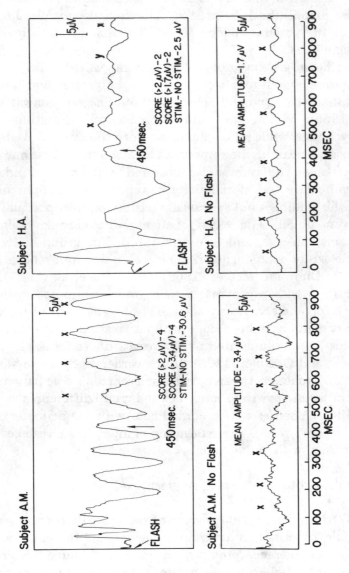

Figure 4. Method used to measure rhythmic after-activity in flash-evoked responses (Straumanis, Shagass, and Schwartz 1965). Upper traces, responses to flash; lower traces, summation of EEG with flash in same subjects. X and Y indicate waves meeting criteria of duration between 60 and 140 msec in activity 450 msec or more after stimulus. Waves designated Y did not meet criteria of amplitude; that is, they were not either greater than 2 μv or greater than the mean amplitude of similar duration waves in the record without flash.

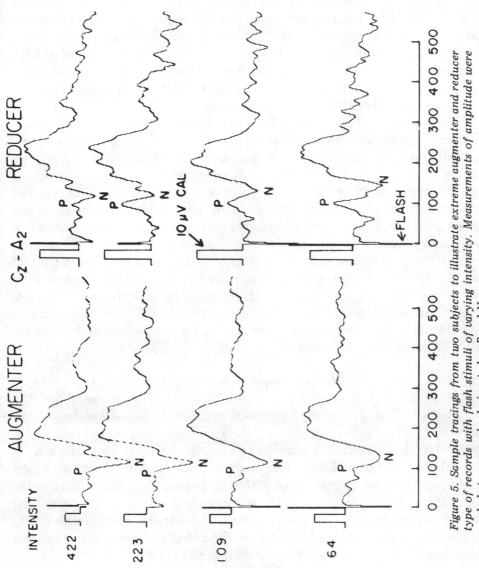

Figure 5. Sample tracings from two subjects to illustrate extreme augmenter and reducer type of records with flash stimuli of varying intensity. Measurements of amplitude were made between peaks designated as P and N.

nificantly correlated with KFA performance, thus suggesting that sensory evoked responses could be used to measure a subject's position on the augmenting-reducing dimension. KFA augmenters showed increased evoked response amplitude with increasing light intensity, particularly in a component occurring from 90 to 150 msec after light flash in the recording from vertex to ear; the reverse was found for KFA reducers. Figure 5 shows tracings from clear augmenter and reducer subjects obtained in our laboratory. Sine wave-modulated light has been used as a stimulus instead of flash to measure augmenting-reducing, and has also been found to be correlated with KFA measurements (Spilker and Callaway 1969); variations in depth of modulation provided different stimulus strengths.

Buchsbaum and Silverman (1968) found marked reducing, that is, negative slope tendencies with increasing light intensity, in a group of male nonparanoid schizophrenic subjects who were not being treated with drugs. Blacker et al. (1968) found a similar tendency toward reducing in a group of chronic LSD users. Borge et al. (1971) and Buchsbaum et al. (1971) reported that bipolar manic-depressive patients (with both manic and depressive episodes) were augmenters, whereas unipolar depressive patients (depressive episodes only) were reducers. In a recent methodological study of both the flash and sine wave-modulated light tests of augmenting-reducing, we found that the two procedures gave unrelated results, but that the findings were relatively unaffected by fixation of the pupil in miosis (Soskis and Shagass 1974). This suggests that the clinical correlations found with the augmenting-reducing tests were probably unaffected by the failure of the investigators to immobilize the pupil.

Evoked Response Variability

Probably the first worker to use a measure of evoked response variability in a psychiatric study was Callaway (Callaway, Jones, and Layne 1965). He reasoned that schizophrenics would be more characterized by segmental set and should, therefore, pay more attention than normals to the differences between two tones of different frequencies. The similarity between the average responses to the two tones was compared by computing the product-moment correlation between corresponding successive data points. The findings supported the prediction that the responses to the two tones would differ more in schizophrenics than in normals. In a later study, however, it was found that similar differences in variability were obtained when only one tone frequency was used (Jones and Callaway 1970), indicating that variability in time was the key factor. Callaway's finding of increased auditory response variability in schizophrenics has been confirmed by Saletu, Itil, and Saletu (1971) and Cohen (1973); other data also indicate that variability may be greatest in schizophrenics when they are grossly disturbed (Jones, Blacker, and Callaway 1966). It is noteworthy that Cohen's (1973) verification of Callaway's findings was made in a schizophrenic population free of drugs, since Callaway's patients were receiving drugs when tested. Although increased auditory response variability appears to be a consistent finding in schizophrenics, it is not specific to these disorders; Malerstein and Callaway (1969) obtained similar results in patients with Korsakoff syndrome and senile psychosis.

Greater than normal variability of visual evoked responses in schizophrenics has been reported by Lifshitz (1969). Furthermore, in addition to greater temporal variability of responses recorded from the same electrodes, there is evidence of greater spatial variability in the visual evoked responses of schizophrenics, that is, greater differences between responses recorded from different parts of the head. Correlations between visual responses recorded from left and right occiput, left and right parietal, and right parietal and occipital areas were lower in schizophrenics than in normals (Rodin, Grisell, and Gottlieb 1968).

We have recently studied somatosensory evoked response variability. The basic data came from five average responses to single, unconditioned test stimuli obtained in the modified recovery function procedure. We computed the product-moment correlations for epochs from 15 to 100 and 101 to 200 msec after the stimulus (Figure 2). Most of the significant findings derived from the 15- to 100-msec epoch. Comparing nonpatients, nonpsychotic patients, and chronic schizophrenic patients matched for age and sex, the least variability of wave shape was found in the schizophrenics, while variability was about equal in nonpatients and nonpsychotics. A high degree of wave shape similarity for the first 100 msec was also found in major depressions, whether of manic-depressive or of psychotic depressive type, and in the schizo-affective subtype of schizophrenia (Shagass 1973). These data, suggesting a lower than normal degree of variability in the first 100 msec of the somatosensory response in chronic schizophrenias and other major psychoses, appear at first glance to be discrepant with the findings cited above for auditory and visual responses. It should be noted, however, that the measures of variability employed by these other workers were mainly determined by events that occurred after 100 msec. Consequently, our data indicating greater stability during the first 100 msec of the response are not really in conflict.

Our recent analysis of the modified recovery function data with respect to symptom patterns in the schizophrenic groups has provided evidence that indicates different clinical correlates of variability in the early and later portions of the somatosensory response. In accord with the diagnostic differences, patients with low depression ratings and high psychotic symptom ratings showed lower variability of the first 100 msec of the response than did patients high in depression and low in other psychotic symptoms. In the epoch from 101 to 200 msec, however, the patients high in psychotic symptoms and low in depression displayed greater variability than did patients low in psychotic symptoms and high in depression. This latter finding is in accord with the results of the workers who have studied auditory and visual responses, and it suggests that variability after 100 msec in responses of all modalities may be greater in seriously ill schizophrenic patients.

A significant factor which, if uncontrolled, could render the variability findings in schizophrenic patients rather meaningless, results from the fact that, in general, variability is less when evoked response amplitude is greater. Since the amplitude of auditory responses tends to be lower than normal and that of somatosensory responses tends to be higher than normal in schizophrenics, this could account for the variability findings. However, in both our data and those of Cohen (1973), the discrimination between clinical groups persisted after the effect of amplitude on the variability index was statistically removed.

Evoked Response Recovery Functions

In our first studies of somatosensory recovery functions we measured the responses evoked by stimulating the ulnar nerve at the wrist. Measurements of the initial negative-positive component amplitude yielded a biphasic recovery curve in normal subjects (Shagass and Schwartz 1961). In the initial phase the ratio of R2 to R1 amplitudes reached or exceeded 1.0, indicating complete amplitude recovery at one or more of the eight intervals measured between 2.5 and 20 msec. This initial phase of recovery was followed by a phase of reduced R2 amplitude, usually with intervals between 30 and 60 msec; the suppressed phase was succeeded by a second phase of recovery in which the R2/R1 ratio reached or exceeded 1.0 at about 100 msec. The main finding of clinical relevance was that degree of recovery in the initial phase (to 20 msec) was significantly less in patients with schizophrenias, psychotic depressions, and personality disorders; degree of recovery did not differ from normal in patients with dysthymic neuroses. These group differences were subsequently verified in a second cross-sectional investigation (Shagass and Schwartz 1963c). Serial recovery measurements in patients with psychotic depressions undergoing treatment revealed normalization of recovery as clinical improvement took place (Shagass and Schwartz 1962). Reduced recovery is thus not a fixed biological characteristic.

In a third cross-sectional study (Shagass 1968), a number of methodological refinements were applied to the recovery function determination and handling of the data. In addition to the initial negative-positive component, several later peaks of the somatosensory response were measured for both amplitude and latency. In this study the previously found differences between nonpatients and patients with the functional psychoses and personality disorders were once again verified, but significant differences were found also between nonpatients and patients with dysthymic neuroses. The amplitude values of nonpsychotic patients tended to fall intermediately between those of nonpatients and psychotics. The measurement of additional peaks added relatively little extra clinical discriminative power to that yielded by the amplitude recovery of the initial negative-positive component. The results for latency recovery were somewhat unexpected, being opposite in direction to amplitude recovery. The significant differences between patients and nonpatients indicated greater, or more rapid, latency recovery in the patient groups. The differences between the clinical correlates of latency and amplitude recovery suggest that they may be mediated or influenced by different mechanisms. Figure 6 shows mean amplitude recovery curves for selected subgroups from a population of 162 psychiatric patients and 54 nonpatients matched for age and sex; Figure 7 shows mean latency recovery curves for the entire group. These curves reflect the general trend of the results, although there were some additional differences of interest between nonpatients and patients in specific diagnostic groups (Shagass 1968).

Visual flash stimuli have been used in recovery function determinations by several workers. Our own study of visual evoked response recovery functions yielded rather poor discriminations between psychiatric groups (Shagass and Schwartz 1965). We did find delayed recovery of the latency of the initial visual peak (negative at about 30 msec) in the patients, particularly in nonpsychotic categories. Other workers have obtained more positive results with amplitude recovery of the visual response. Speck, Dim, and Mercer (1966) showed that recovery was reduced from normal in psychiatric patients, most of whom were schizophrenic. Heninger and Speck (1966) retested some of the schizophrenic patients and found that changes in the recovery ratio were related to clinical improvement. It is of interest that the highest correlation with an increase in the recovery ratio was found with respect to degree of improvement in hallucinatory activity. Floris et al. (1967, 1968, 1969) also found that visual evoked response recovery differed significantly between schizophrenics and nonpatients, the patients showing reduced recovery. In the data of Floris et al., patients with psychotic depressions did not differ from normals, but epileptics had greater than normal recovery. Ishikawa (1968) compared normals and schizophrenics with respect to visual evoked response recovery functions; he found differences mainly in relation to the presence of hallucinations. Schizophrenics with hallucinations had significantly later recovery than normals, whereas nonhal-

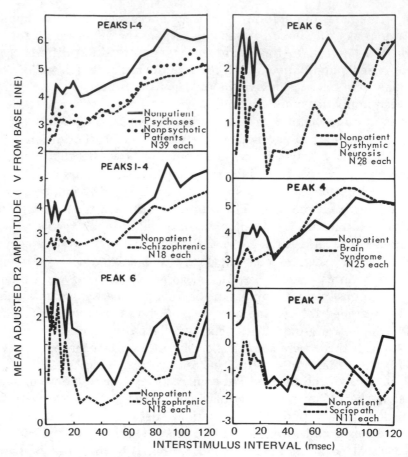

Figure 6. Mean somatosensory amplitude recovery curves for various groups. R2 values adjusted statistically for their covariance with R1. All group differences statistically significant. Note generally lower recovery in patient groups.

lucinating patients did not differ from nonpatients.

Satterfield (1972) compared depressive patients with nonpatients with respect to auditory recovery functions. The patient group had a wider distribution of recovery function measurements than the normals, i.e., there were patients outside the normal distribution at both the low and high ends. Comparing the extreme patient groups, the finding of greatest interest was that patients with low recovery gave a history of depressive illness in first-degree relatives, whereas none of the high-recovery patients had such a positive family history. This finding, which suggests that auditory evoked response recovery may be related to subtypes of depression, requires confirmation.

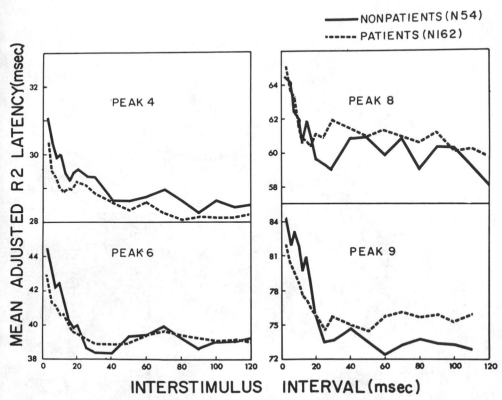

Figure 7. Mean somatosensory latency recovery curves for 54 nonpatients and 162 psychiatric patients matched for age and sex. All group differences statistically significant. Note more rapid latency recovery in patients.

Modified Somatosensory Recovery Function

The results so far yielded by the modified recovery function procedure have differed in nature from those obtained in the three earlier studies that employed the more conventional somatosensory recovery function determination. In general, greater discrimination between groups has been obtained with measures based on unconditioned responses, i.e., average responses to single test (R1T, Figure 1) or conditioning stimuli (R1C) than with the test responses following conditioning stimuli, i.e., R2 and R10. In an early comparison of unmatched groups, the results suggested that the conditioning train produced greater reduction of R10 amplitude in both schizophrenic and nonpsychotic groups than in nonpatients (Shagass, Overton, and Bartolucci 1969). In a study of drug abuse patients, evidence was obtained that schizophrenics and drug abusers with a history of psychotic reactions dif-

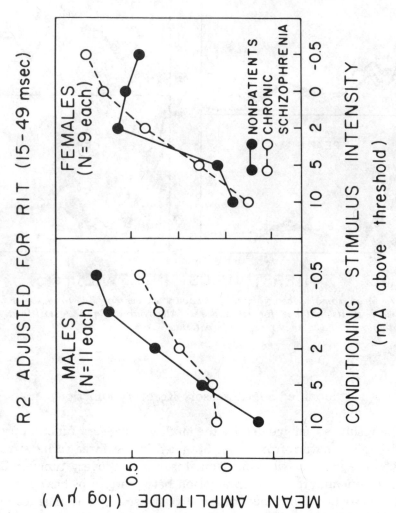

Figure 8. Mean curves based on data from modified somatosensory recovery function procedure, comparing nonpatients with chronic schizophrenic patients matched for age and sex. Note that patient-nonpatient differences depend on the sex of the subjects.

fered from drug abusers without psychotic reactions, and from nonpatients. The two psychotic groups showed less variation in R2 and R10 with different intensities of conditioning stimuli than did the nonpatients or nonpsychotic drug abuse patients (Shagass, Overton, and Straumanis 1971). The subjects in the drug abuse study were males matched for age, and subsequent results indicated that the findings for psychotic patients in this study were sex-specific (Shagass, Overton, and Straumanis 1972). Data for a larger sample of chronic schizophrenics of both sexes showed that male psychotic patients had significantly less recovery and less variation of R2 and R10 amplitude as a function of conditioning stimulus intensity than did male nonpatients, but reverse trends were found when female schizophrenic patients were compared with female nonpatients. Figure 8 provides an example of this kind of finding; it will be seen that the adjusted R2 values for the 15- to 49-msec epoch in the male schizophrenic patients tend to be lower and the slope less steep than in the male controls, whereas reverse trends occur in the female groups.

The interaction between sex and psychopathology, with respect to neurophysiological measurements as shown in Figure 8, extends to chronic schizophrenia a finding that we have previously obtained in two other, quite different, clinical populations. The sex differences in schizophrenics resemble those found in investigations of elderly patients with chronic brain syndromes (Straumanis 1964) and of young adults with Down's syndrome (Straumanis, Shagass, and Overton 1973). In all of these studies the sex differences within the matched nonpatient groups were minimal, whereas the females of the patient group displayed greater and the males showed less than normal responsiveness. No ready explanation for these interactions between sex and psychopathology is forthcoming. They do not seem to be due to factors related to menstruation.

Figure 9 shows an additional finding of interest obtained with the modified recovery function procedure. Latency recovery measurements for the initial negative peak (average latency about 20 msec) differed from normal in two psychotic patient groups. With the highest conditioning stimulus, the mean delay in R2, compared with R1T, for nonpatient subjects was nearly 2 msec, but there was no significant delay in chronic schizophrenic and manic-depressive, depressed patients of the same age and sex. These results are in agreement with the evidence for more rapid latency recovery in patients that was obtained with the conventional somatosensory recovery function procedure (Figure 7).

Contingent Negative Variation (CNV)

The CNV is the slow negative potential shift discovered by Grey Walter and his associates in a reaction time situation, involving an alerting tone followed by a series of light flashes at least 0.5 seconds later (Walter et al. 1964). The subject was instructed to terminate the light flashes by pressing a button. The slow negative shift started about 200 msec after the alerting tone. The termination of the CNV generally took place in association with the button press; there was a return to baseline, or an overswing toward positivity. The CNV must be recorded with DC or long time-constant amplifiers, in order to pick up the slow negative shift. Although there is little doubt that the CNV phenomenon is real, it is easily contaminated by a

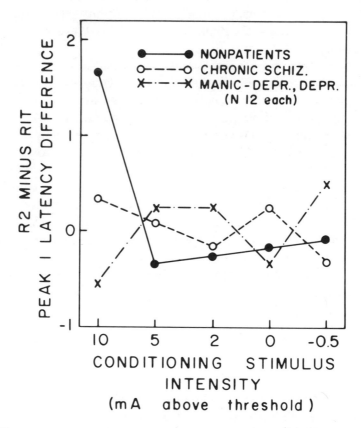

Figure 9. Mean somatosensory peak 1 latency recovery curves from modified recovery function procedure, comparing nonpatients, chronic schizophrenic patients, and manic-depressive, depressed patients matched for age and sex. Measure of recovery is the latency difference between R2 and R1. With conditioning stimulus intensity of 10 mA above threshold, the delay in peak 1 found in nonpatients was absent in the psychotic patient groups.

number of events, which have the same general appearance and are record-able at the same electrodes. Perhaps the most important of these contami-nants are the electrooculogram (EOG), which reflects eye movements and eye blinks, and the electrodermal response or galvanic skin response (GSR). GSR may be substantial at the mastoid area, which has been a favorite location for the reference lead used by CNV workers (Picton and Hillyard 1972). Although various means of correcting the CNV for EOG have been proposed (Walter 1967, Hillyard 1969), none are wholly satisfactory because they are based on the assumption that there is a uniform potential field gradient from the eye backward for both eye movement and eye blink. This assumption is incorrect; the fields for movement and blink are not identical (Overton and Shagass 1969, Corby and Kopell 1972). The problems of arti-fact control render psychiatric studies of CNV extremely difficult. There is also evidence suggesting that individual differences in CNV may vary con-siderably from one experimental paradigm to another (Straumanis, Shagass, and Overton 1969).

Despite the difficulties, a fairly large number of CNV studies have been carried out with psychiatric patients, and some of these have yielded inter-esting results. Walter (1966) noted that in autistic children the CNV was absent or appeared only occasionally. McCallum and Walter (1968) found that neurotics had smaller CNVs than did normals, and that the differences became much greater when distraction was introduced. With distraction, CNV amplitude in the neurotics decreased more than in the normals. Walter (1966) found that patients with psychopathic disturbances of antisocial type were virtually incapable of producing more than a trace of CNV. In patients with schizoid features, Walter observed greater than normal variability of CNV. McCallum (1969) found that results in schizophrenics were rather similar to those obtained in patients suffering from anxiety neuroses, in that the amplitudes tended to be somewhat lower than normal and decreased dramatically with distraction. Small and Small (1971) compared normals with manics, depressives, and schizophrenics. The manic and depressed pa-tients showed very little discrimination between recordings in which they were required to make a response and those in which this requirement was not imposed; in essence, patients with affective psychosis, on the average, gave no indication of a potential associated with response contingency. The results obtained by Small and Small in schizophrenic patients were more variable than those in the other groups; schizophrenics tended to have smaller CNVs, with a persistence of negativity after the motor response was made. McCallum (1973) has recently reported an investigation in which 23 drug-free schizophrenic patients were studied. The patients were divided according to Schneider's first-rank symptoms; these subgroups were com-pared with one another and with a small group of normal controls. The

Schneider-positive patients showed smaller CNVs and greater effects of distraction than did either the controls or the Schneider-negative patients, who did not differ significantly from one another.

Dongier and Bostem (1967) failed to find CNV amplitude differences between normals and neurotics; a condition of distraction was not employed in their experiment as in the study of McCallum and Walter (1968). In the same laboratory, Timsit et al. (1970) obtained psychiatrically significant findings with the CNV method by focusing on the duration of negativity following the response to the imperative stimulus. They found that the negativity lasted less than 1.5 sec after the imperative stimulus in 91 percent of 45 normals, 66 percent of 70 neurotics, but only 7 percent of 45 psychotics. The most prolonged durations of negativity were found in acute schizophrenic patients. In a group of psychotics retested after more than a 15-day interval, prolonged negativity was again found. Timsit-Berthier (1973) presented the data in a larger series of cases with essentially the same results. In addition, Timsit-Berthier's data showed that low-amplitude CNVs occur more frequently among psychotics than other groups, and slightly more frequently in hysteric than in obsessional neurotics. The results indicated that prolonged negativity occurred more frequently in schizophrenias considered to be of "process" than in those considered to be of "residual" type. McCallum (1973) reported that investigations in his laboratory had failed to reveal the prolonged negativity reported by Timsit-Berthier, but Dongier, Dubrovsky, and Garcia-Rill (1973) recently reported a high incidence of prolonged negativity in psychotics, and a greater frequency in neurotics than in normals. Dongier and his co-workers were unable to distinguish between manic, depressive, schizophrenic, and paranoid states; abnormalities appeared to be greatest in acute cases and to decrease with duration of illness. It is important to note that Dongier, Dubrovsky, and Garcia-Rill took great care to eliminate the effects of EOG and GSR on the slow potential recordings. The observations of Timsit et al. (1970) are also in accord with those of prolonged negative activity in schizophrenics made by Small and Small (1971).

Slow Potentials Associated with Movement

Timsit-Berthier (1973) has elaborated the CNV method to look more closely at long latency potentials following imperative stimuli, and motor potentials obtained by asking the subject to press a button repetitively. Long latency potentials were obtained both with and without instructions to press. In the data of 57 control subjects, 57 neurotics, and 76 psychotics, several variations in the form of the long latency potential following a sensory stimulus were described. The response to a series of 18 light flashes in 1 sec could involve either no after-potential, a positive deflection, a brief negative deflection, or a very prolonged negative deflection lasting more than 300 msec after the stimulus was stopped. The highest incidence of long-lasting after-negativity occurred in the psychotic patients. The difference between psychotic and nonpsychotic groups was of about the same magnitude with and without imperative responses, although the prolonged negativity was more frequent when an imperative response was required.

Motor potentials associated with button-pressing were also classified into a variety of types by Timsit-Berthier (1973). The classification was based on the presence or absence of the "readiness" potential corresponding to the phenomenon noted by Kornhuber and Deecke (1965) and a negativity persisting after the button-press. The negative intention wave occurred in only 23 percent of 80 psychotics, compared to 85 percent of controls and 71 percent of neurotics. On the other hand, persistent negativity following the button-press was found in 77 percent of psychotics, compared with only 15 percent of controls, and 20 percent of neurotics. A number of measures were taken to rule out the possibility of contamination of slow potential recordings by EOG and GSR artifacts, including subcutaneous injection of atropine to eliminate GSR in a subsample.

The concordance of findings obtained by Timsit-Berthier in Belgium and Dongier, Dubrovsky, and Garcia-Rill in Montreal strongly suggests that the slow negative potentials normally associated with movement may, indeed, be deviant in a large portion of patients with major functional psychoses.

P300 (P3) Wave

A long latency component, which appears usually from 300 to 500 msec after stimulus, seems to be related more to complex psychological variables than to the physical attributes of the stimulus. Sutton, Braren, and Zubin (1965) originally described the P300 wave as a correlate of stimulus uncertainty. It may also be elicited by the absence of the expected stimulus (Sutton et al. 1967). Ritter and Vaughan (1969) concluded that the P300 wave reflected a shift of attention associated with the orienting response.

Sutton's studies with the P300 wave involved careful attention to the details of instructions to the subject and control of stimulus frequency in order to restrict subject "options" (Sutton 1969). The emphasis on the instruction aspect would limit the applicability of the P300 measurements in a psychiatric context. However, Roth and Cannon (1972) have recently reported a psychiatric study under the rubric of passive attention, in which no response was required of the subject, and in which measurements of the P300 wave yielded significant clinical differences. Subjects were exposed to a

10-min sequence of frequent and infrequent auditory stimuli. In one part of the sequence, clicks occurred 15 times as often as tone bursts, and in the other the reverse was true. The average responses to the infrequent stimuli revealed P300 waves in the control subjects but not in the schizophrenics. Over the 10-min period of recording, the amplitude of the P300 wave decreased systematically in the controls, although the relative frequency of the clicks and tones was switched in the middle of the recording. The fact that the P300 phenomenon can be studied with subjects in a passive state makes it more feasible to investigate this event in psychiatric patients.

Effects of Drugs and Treatments

From a psychiatric point of view, concomitant study of the effects of drugs on evoked responses and clinical symptoms offers the exciting possibility of shedding some light on neurophysiologic changes associated with changes in psychopathology. The problem is by no means an easy one because drugs can exert a variety of electrophysiological effects unrelated to the amelioration of psychopathology. One important group of effects has already been mentioned, namely, the changes in alertness produced by most drugs used in psychiatric treatment. A second broad area of drug effects which must be separated out concerns nonspecific changes, probably unrelated to behavior, which may be called "tissue effects." Examples of these are the fast waves produced by barbiturates in the EEG, and the augmented negativity in somatosensory responses at about 35-msec latency, which we have observed with agents as diverse as barbiturates, amphetamines, phenothiazines, LSD, and even electroconvulsive therapy (ECT) (Shagass, Schwartz, and Amadeo 1962). Figure 10 gives an example of this nonspecific effect on somatosensory responses.

Electroconvulsive Therapy

Most of the patients in psychotic depressive states, whose somatosensory recovery functions were measured serially during the course of treatment in one of our early studies, received ECT (Shagass and Schwartz 1962). The early peak of recovery occurring with interstimulus intervals up to 20 msec, which was low prior to treatment, increased progressively toward normal as the patient's clinical condition improved.

Barbiturates and Minor Tranquilizers

Corssen and Domino (1964) found that secobarbital increased the amplitude of visually evoked responses in association with sleep. However, the amplitude of the initial somatosensory evoked response component was not significantly altered by intravenous amobarbital administered in doses insufficient to produce sleep (Shagass, Schwartz, and Amadeo 1962). Diaze-

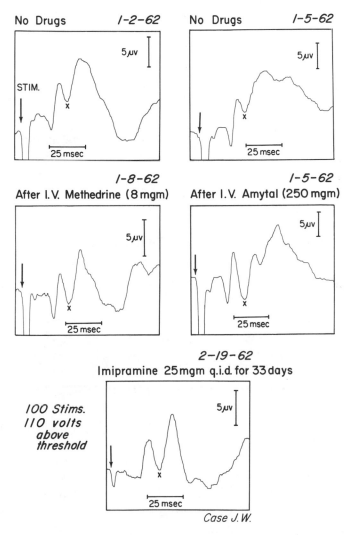

Figure 10. Somatosensory evoked responses of one patient, selected to illustrate that different kinds of drugs may augment the negative deflection occurring about 35 msec after stimulus (designated by X). Note similarity of the two "no drug" records taken on different days and the increased negativity with methedrine, amytal, and imipramine.

pam produces consistent reduction of amplitude in both somatosensory and visual responses and tends to increase the latency of somatosensory responses (Bergamasco 1966 and 1967; Ebe, Meier-Ewart, and Broughton 1967; Poire et al. 1967; Saletu, Saletu, and Itil 1972). Saletu, Saletu, and Itil (1972) demonstrated that chlordiazepoxide increased the latency of early somatosensory components and decreased the latency of the later components; this contrasts with the early negative findings concerning this drug reported by Corssen and Domino (1964). Oxazepam has been reported to produce a reduction of amplitude and slight increases in latency in the response to flash (Dolce and Kaemmerer 1967). Meprobamate, in a dose of 800 to 1200 mg, was found to have no effects on visual evoked responses (Prieto, Villar, and Bachini 1965).

Alcohol

In general, alcohol tends to reduce the amplitude of evoked responses. Gross et al. (1966) showed this effect in auditory evoked responses. Lewis, Dustman, and Beck (1970) reported that three ounces of alcohol reduced both visual and somatosensory response amplitudes; however, early components were relatively unchanged. It may be noted that the responses found by Lewis et al. to show amplitude reduction were recorded from central areas; these are generally considered to be unspecific with respect to sensory modality and are influenced markedly by state of alertness.

Excitants

The convulsive agent pentamethylenetetrazole (Metrazol) has been reported to increase the amplitude of visual evoked responses and to shorten the visual cortical recovery cycle (Bergamasco 1966). Studies with the amphetamines have yielded inconsistent results. Domino, Corssen, and Sweet (1963) found no significant effects of d-amphetamine on visual evoked responses, and we failed to find significant effects of intravenous methamphetamine on the initial components of the somatosensory response (Shagass, Schwartz, and Amadeo 1962). On the other hand, Crighel and Ciurea (1966) noted that visual evoked response amplitude and variability were increased by d-amphetamine, and a combination of dextroamphetamine and amobarbital was found by Bishop, Guthrie, and Hornsby (1969) to shorten the latency of visual responses. Single doses of amphetamine produced consistent decreases of latency of the somatosensory response in nonpatients (Saletu et al. 1972). The same workers found that the effects of dextroamphetamine and methylphenidate were not completely alike.

Major Tranquilizers

In considering the results on evoked responses obtained with the major antipsychotic agents, such as the phenothiazines, it is necessary to bear in mind the possibility that evoked response changes with these drugs may not be of the same nature in patients as in nonpatients. Recently Saletu et al. (1971a and 1971b) found that both fluphenazine and thiothixene reduced the amplitude of the initial somatosensory component in schizophrenic patients, whereas 50 mg of chlorpromazine, given in a single dose to nonpatient volunteers, tended to produce the opposite effect, i.e., increasing amplitude (Saletu, Saletu, and Itil 1972). On the other hand, amplitudes of later components tended to decrease in all subjects, and latencies, particularly of the later somatosensory peaks, tended to become prolonged. In early work with imipramine, we found that the amplitude of the initial somatosensory peak tended to be reduced in depressed patients treated with this agent; in contrast, nonpatient controls given the drug in therapeutic doses for several weeks showed an increase in amplitude (Shagass, Schwartz, and Amadeo 1962).

In our long-term studies of somatosensory and visual evoked response characteristics in psychiatric patients, we made repeated attempts to demonstrate consistent effects of phenothiazines. We were not able to demonstrate significant differences between patients who received some phenothiazines from one to seven days before testing, and patients who either had not received drugs at all or in whom drug administration had been stopped for periods longer than one week. The results of Saletu and his colleagues, as well as preliminary results from our laboratory, suggest that there may be great variability in the effects of drugs on somatosensory evoked responses, and that this variability may be of clinical significance. Employing the modified recovery function, we found that schizophrenic patients who responded well to phenothiazines differed in their pretreatment measurements from those who subsequently did not respond well to the drugs. Furthermore, the drugs had little effect on the measurements of those who did not respond, but exerted significant effects on the good responders. The findings of Saletu et al. (1971a, 1971b, and 1971c) are in general agreement with these results; they found that "good" clinical responders displayed somatosensory evoked potential changes with phenothiazines and haloperidol, while "poor" responders did not. In addition, they found pretreatment differences in the somatosensory evoked response measurements of the two clinical groups, with the "good" responders showing higher amplitudes.

Heninger and Speck (1966) showed visual response effects with phenothiazine medication in schizophrenic patients, but it appears that some of the changes could have been caused by drowsiness induced by the drugs. The possible effect of drowsiness is suggested by the fact that amplitudes were markedly increased early in drug treatment, but after 30 days of therapy there was little change from the pretreatment records. Helmchen and Kunkel (1964) demonstrated slowing of visual response after-rhythms with chronic administration of perazine. Chronic administration of fluphenazine, thiothixene, and haloperidol appears to reduce amplitude and prolong latency of somatosensory responses (Saletu et al. 1971a, 1971b, and 1971c). The results of Saletu et al., which were obtained in a population of schizophrenic patients, also indicate that there may be a rather prolonged effect of the drugs after they are stopped; the study demonstrated a "rebound" effect several weeks after placebo was substituted for chronic drug administration.

There is some evidence to suggest that phenothiazines tend to increase augmentation in evoked potential tests of augmenting-reducing; Silverman (1972) has recently reviewed the literature and suggested that schizophrenics tend to be reducers, so that phenothiazines may counteract this tendency. A reduction of the increased auditory evoked response variability obtained with the Callaway two-tone procedure has been demonstrated after effective phenothiazine therapy (Jones et al. 1965). Heninger and Speck (1966) found that visual recovery functions, which were significantly reduced in schizophrenics, tended to shift toward normal with phenothiazine therapy.

Lithium

Heninger (1969) reported that lithium carbonate increased the amplitude of the initial negative-positive component of the somatosensory response. Employing the modified recovery function procedure, we have confirmed and extended Heninger's findings (Shagass, Straumanis, and Overton 1973). Examples of responses to single, unpaired stimuli obtained before and during lithium therapy are shown in Figure 11; the increase in amplitude of the initial component is evident. Figure 12 shows the mean curves for modified recovery function measurements for 14 patients before and during lithium therapy. Lithium dosage ranged from 1200 to 1800 mg per day, and the curves were based on the amplitude of the initial negative-positive component automatically measured by computer. The increased amplitude of responses to single stimuli is clearly demonstrated. The results for both R2 and R10 show that amplitudes of test responses following single conditioning stimuli or trains of highest intensity were at about the same level as before treatment. However, the test responses following threshold-intensity conditioning stimuli were of considerably higher amplitude than before drug administration. The increased amplitudes following threshold-intensity conditioning stimuli indicate relative "facilitation." Since the amplitude of R1 was increased, the absence of change in R2 and R10 with the most intense conditioning stimuli suggests a relative "inhibition." Consequently, lithium appears to increase both inhibitory and facilitatory response tendencies; this may be described as an augmentation of the dynamic range of cerebral responsiveness. The results with the most intense conditioning stimuli seem to be similar to those obtained by Gartside, Lippold, and Meldrum (1966);

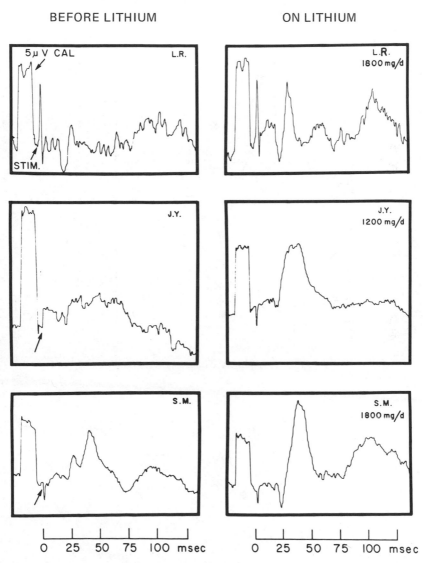

Figure 11. Somatosensory evoked responses from three patients before and during treatment with lithium carbonate. Note increased amplitude of initial portion of somatosensory responses when patients were receiving lithium.

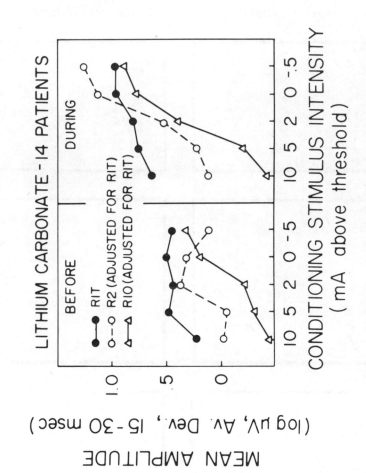

Figure 12. Mean curves obtained from modified recovery function experiment in 14 patients before and during lithium carbonate treatment. Lithium generally increased amplitudes, but in R2 and R10 these increases occurred only with conditioning stimulus intensities of 2 mA above threshold or less.

these workers measured somatosensory recovery function in nonpsychotic volunteers, and found that lithium carbonate caused suppression of the early portion of the recovery function curves.

A further analysis of the R1T data displayed in Figure 12 has been performed recently by subjecting the responses to digital filtering. The procedure employed performs a Fourier transform of the signals with a reconstitution by means of an inverse Fourier of the signals restricted to two frequency bands: 4 to 28 Hz, and 32 to 500 Hz. The data showed clearly that the lithium effect was confined to the 32- to 500-Hz portion of the signal, and that there was no effect on the 4- to 28-Hz portion. It appears therefore that the effect of lithium is restricted to early, rapid events in the somatosensory response. Since lithium tends to slow the EEG (Mayfield and Brown 1966), it might have been expected that the evoked events, if related to the EEG, should show greater changes in the slower frequency range. This was not the case.

Borge et al. (1971) have measured augmenting-reducing with a flash stimulus in unipolar and bipolar manic-depressive patients. They found that lithium therapy tended to decrease the amount of augmentation in both groups, that is, to reduce the slope of the intensity-response function. The effect of lithium on visual responses superficially appears opposite to that found with somatosensory responses. However, a much later and less specific aspect of the evoked response was being measured in the visual records.

Antidepressants

In our serial study of somatosensory recovery functions in psychotic depressive patients, some of the patients were treated with drugs; the data indicated that, like ECT, imipramine and tranylcypromine returned the recovery function toward normal (Shagass and Schwartz 1962). Recently, with the modified recovery function procedure, we found that amitriptyline reduced somatosensory evoked response amplitude (Shagass, Straumanis, and Overton 1973). The amplitude reduction effect was general, and it occurred in responses to single stimuli or to test stimuli preceded by conditioning stimuli or trains. The amplitude reduction tended to occur over the whole response. Analysis with digital filtering showed that the amplitude reduction with amitriptyline was almost entirely in the 4- to 28-Hz portion of the response; this contrasts with the lithium effect which was found in the 32- to 500-Hz range. The increases in dynamic range of responsiveness produced by lithium were not found with amitriptyline.

Psychotogenic Drugs

Ditran is an anticholinergic agent that produces delirium (Wilson and Shagass 1964). Brown, Shagass, and Schwartz (1965) studied the effect of Ditran on somatosensory and visual responses in 13 volunteer psychiatric patients. The main changes produced by the drug were in the later components and consisted of prolongation of latency. The after-rhythm of the flash response was abolished in all subjects. The early positive component of the somatosensory response (latency about 30 msec) decreased in latency and increased in amplitude. In the visual response, the latencies of the first four components also decreased. It seems that Ditran alters the later components of evoked responses in a manner similar to that observed in normal sleep, but the effects on the earlier components are of a different nature. An agent similar to Ditran, phencyclidine, appears to have variable effects on the visual evoked response (Rodin and Luby 1965). Psilocybin, in a dose of 10 mg p.o., was found by Rynearson, Wilson, and Bickford (1968) to have relatively little effect on the visual evoked response. Reduction of the after-rhythm was found in a few subjects.

Lysergic acid diethylamide (LSD) has been studied by several investigators. In a dose of 1 µg/kg i.v., we failed to find effects on the amplitude of the initial somatosensory response component (Shagass, Schwartz, and Amadeo 1962). Rodin and Luby (1965), giving the same dose by mouth, found some decrease in amplitude in the components of the visual response occurring in the first 250 msec, and also reduction in amplitude of after-rhythms. Chapman and Walter (1965), using a larger dose of LSD, also observed a striking reduction of after-rhythms. In our study of the visual and somatosensory response effects of 2.5 µg/kg i.v. of LSD, we recorded from multiple channels (Shagass 1967). LSD increased the amplitude of the early components of the visual responses and tended to increase the frequency of the after-rhythm. The results suggested that the after-rhythm was originating from a wider area of brain during the influence of LSD than before. Somatosensory evoked response changes included reduction of amplitude and latency of the early components. All effects were gone in 20 hours.

Marijuana

The effects of Δ^9-tetrahydrocannabinol (THC) have been studied by Lewis et al. (1973). They found no difference in the data from frequent and occasional users of this agent. The highest dose of THC significantly lengthened the latency of several evoked response waves, but it produced a consistent change in the amplitude of only one component. Lower doses of THC produced no significant evoked response changes. Rodin, Domino, and

Porzak (1970) found no significant evoked response changes after marijuana smokers had attained a social "high." The dose of THC appears to be a significant factor in determining electrophysiological effects; doses sufficient to produce clinical changes do not necessarily produce electrophysiological changes.

Discussion

Since some commentary has been included with the survey of research findings, this discussion will be confined to some general statements about the current status and future perspectives of ERP research in psychiatry.

The overall impression yielded by the review of results is that many ERP characteristics may differ from normal in the presence of psychopathology and be modified by psychoactive drugs. Although a number of individual findings require confirmation or repetition with better controls, it seems hardly disputable that ERP methods are capable of providing data of psychiatric relevance. It also seems clear that much more information must be accumulated before the degree of relevance can be established. There are two major sources of uncertainty. First, the correlations so far demonstrated lack precision; particular symptoms or syndromes have not been identified as close correlates of specific ERP deviations. Second, there is inadequate understanding of the neural mechanisms underlying ERP phenomena; without such understanding, the significance of even highly specific psychopathology-ERP correlations would be unclear. Resolution of the second source of uncertainty depends upon advances in neurophysiology. However, neurophysiological research cannot be expected to focus upon mechanisms of particular ERP phenomena unless they have been shown to have high clinical relevance. Demonstration of such relevance is the primary task of ERP research in psychiatry.

It is possible to discern two different viewpoints held by investigators of ERP in a psychiatric context. One viewpoint can be designated as psychophysiological; it assumes that an ERP event is closely correlated with a "normal" psychological function. For example, it may be considered that CNV amplitude reflects degree of attentive activity. Consequently, in a condition characterized by impaired attentiveness, e.g., severe anxiety or schizophrenia, CNV amplitude would be low; although reduced CNV amplitude could then be taken as an objective sign of poor attentiveness, it would also reflect a "normal" psychophysiological relationship. The second viewpoint can be designated as pathophysiological; it assumes that an abnormal physiological process underlies the deviant behavior. From the pathophysiological point of view, slowed recovery, which could result from such processes as metabolic defects of neurotransmitter substances, might lead to altered timing of neural activity underlying transmission and interpretation of sensory inputs. This could produce behavioral disturbances as a consequence of a physiological abnormality. These two general approaches are not necessarily incompatible with one another, and neither can presently be regarded as superior. Experimental designs and interpretation of data, however, will be affected by whether the investigator's orientation is psychophysiological or pathophysiological (Shagass 1972).

The rather embryonic state of ERP research in psychiatry is nowhere so clearly reflected as in the nature of the theoretical formulations made about research findings. Concepts commonly used to explain an ERP measurement in patients that differs from normal include: abnormal "arousal," with assumed variations in activity of the ascending reticular system; alterations of balance between inhibitory and excitatory systems in the Sherringtonian or Pavlovian sense; models or analogies based on electronics, for example, defective filters or relays; computer analogies, for example, inefficient comparators. Although such concepts have some heuristic merit, they await replacement by more adequate formulations that can emerge only from better understanding of underlying neural mechanisms.

In the particular sphere of ERP studies of psychopathology, three main areas can be identified in which methodological improvement could lead to significant advances. The first area concerns the clinical criterion variables. Although this is a universal problem in clinical psychiatric research, it seems worthwhile to reiterate that the relevant variables on the clinical side of clinical-physiological correlations require precise identification and measurement as much as do the physiological variables. The second area of deficit may possibly be related to the first. It concerns the stimuli or events to which potentials are related in ERP recording. Research to date has mainly used elemental stimuli, selected more for reasons of ease and convenience than because they were appropriate for testing specific hypotheses. Light flashes, auditory clicks, and nerve shocks are easier to manipulate and control than pictures of faces, speech sounds, and tactile forms, but the latter may be more meaningful events with which to study abnormalities in perceiving and interpreting the environment. In future ERP research we may expect more frequent use of complex stimuli, which may have a better chance of being relevant to the psychological abnormalities under investigation.

The third area of deficit concerns the ERP variables themselves. Methods for more sophisticated quantification of these are constantly being developed. In psychiatric studies, however, there has been relative neglect of the important parameter of spatial distribution of ERPs and of the interrelationships between ERP characteristics and those of the EEG in which they are embedded. The obvious reasons for the neglect of these factors is that much effort and complex equipment are required to investigate them. However, sophisticated use of general-purpose computers can be expected to overcome many of the practical difficulties. It seems likely that we shall see more data concerning spatial distribution of ERPs and ERP-EEG relationships and that these may contribute more significant information in relation to psychopathological variables than have single-channel ERP recordings.

The implication of the foregoing remarks is that a long, hard road awaits investigators in this field before they can achieve truly gratifying results. Nevertheless, in my opinion, the goals are sufficiently important and the evidence in hand encouraging enough to justify such an effort.

Acknowledgments

Drs. M. Amadeo, D.A. Overton, and J.J. Straumanis, Jr. have been collaborators in recent research. Thanks are due to H. Kosoff, A. McLean, T. McLean, W. Nixon, J. Pressman, S. Slepner, and G. Stam for computer and technical assistance.

Research supported (in part) by grant MH12507 from the U.S. Public Health Service.

References

Bergamasco, B. 1966. Study of the modification of cortical response in man induced by drugs acting on the CNS. *Sist. Nerv.* 18:155.

Bergamasco, B. 1967. Modifications of cortical responsiveness in humans induced by drugs acting on the central nervous system. *Electroencephalogr. Clin. Neurophysiol.* 23:191.

Bishop, M.P., Guthrie, M.B., and Hornsby, L.D. 1969. Objective and subjective tests in measuring response to CNS drugs in normal subjects. *J. Clin. Pharmacol.* 9:308.

Blacker, K.H., Jones, R.T., Stone, G.C., and Pfefferbaum, D. 1968. Chronic users of LSD: The "acidheads." *Am. J. Psychiatry* 125:341.

Borge, G.F., Buchsbaum, M., Goodwin, F., Murphy, D., and Silverman, J. 1971. Neurophysiological correlates of affective disorders. *Am. J. Psychiatry* 24:501.

Brown, J.C.N., Shagass, C., and Schwartz, M. 1965. Cerebral evoked potential changes associated with the Ditran delirium and its reversal in man. In J. Wortis (ed.), *Recent Advances in Biological Psychiatry*, vol. 7, p. 223. New York: Plenum Press.

Buchsbaum, M., Goodwin, F., Murphy, D., and Borge, G. 1971. AER in affective disorders. *Am. J. Psychiatry* 128:51.

Buchsbaum, M., and Silverman, J. 1968. Stimulus intensity control and the cortical evoked response. *Psychosom. Med.* 30:12.

Callaway, E., Jones, R.T., and Layne, R.S. 1965. Evoked responses and segmental set of schizophrenia. *Arch. Gen. Psychiatry* 12:83.

Chapman, L.F., and Walter, R.D. 1965. Action of lysergic acid diethylamide on averaged human cortical evoked responses to light flash. In J. Wortis (ed.), *Recent Advances in Biological Psychiatry*, vol. 7, p. 23. New York: Plenum Press.

Cohen, R. 1973. The influence of task-irrelevant stimulus variations on the reliability of auditory evoked responses in schizophrenia. In A. Fessard and G. Lelord (eds.), *Human Neurophysiology, Psychology, Psychiatry: Average Evoked Responses and Their Conditioning in Normal Subjects and Psychiatric Patients*, p. 373. Paris: Inserm.

Corby, J.C., and Kopell, B.S. 1972. Differential contributions of blinks and vertical eye movements as artifacts in EEG recording. *Psychophysiology* 9:640.

Corssen, G., and Domino, E.F. 1964. Visually evoked responses in man: A method for measuring cerebral effects of preanesthetic medications. *Anesthesiology* 25:330.

Crighel, E., and Ciurea, E. 1966. Flash-evoked potentials in man. Variability of the evoked responses. *Electroencephalogr. Clin. Neurophysiol.* 21:99.

Dolce, G., and Kaemmerer, E. 1967. Effect of the Benzodiazepin adumbran on the resting and sleep EEG, and on the visual evoked potential in adult man. *Med. Welt* 67:510.

Domino, E.F., Corssen, G., and Sweet, R.G. 1963. Effects of various anesthetics on the visually evoked responses in man. *Anesth. Analges.* 42:735.

Dongier, M., Dubrovsky, B., and Garcia-Rill, E. 1973. Event related slow potentials in psychosis. Presented at *Annual Meeting of Society of Biological Psychiatry* in Montreal, Canada.

Dongier, M., and Bostem, M.F. 1967. Essais d'application en psychiatrie de la variation contingente négative. *Acta Neurol. Belg.* 67:640.

Eason, R.G., Groves, P., White, C.T., and Oden, D. 1967. Evoked cortical potentials: Relation to visual field and handedness. *Science* 156:1643.

Ebe, M., Meier-Ewart, K., and Broughton, R. 1967. Further studies of i.v. diazepam (Valium) and evoked potentials of photosensitive epileptic subjects and normal controls. *Electroencephalogr. Clin. Neurophysiol.* 23:491.

Emde, J. 1964. A time locked low level calibrator. *Electroencephalogr. Clin. Neurophysiol.* 16:616.

Ertl, J.P., and Schafer, E.W.P. 1969. Brain response correlates of psychometric intelligence. *Nature* 223:421.

Floris, V., Morocutti, C., Amabile, G., Bernardi, G., Rizzo, P.A., and Vasconetto, C. 1967. Recovery cycle of visual evoked potentials in normal and schizophrenic subjects. *Electroencephalogr. Clin. Neurophysiol.* suppl. 26:74.

Floris, V., Morocutti, C., Amabile, G., Bernardi, G., and Rizzo, P.A. 1968. Recovery cycle of visual evoked potentials in normal, schizophrenic and neurotic patients. In N.S. Kline and E. Laska (eds.), *Computers and Electronic Devices in Psychiatry*, p. 194. New York: Grune and Stratton.

Floris, V., Morocutti, C., Amabile, G., Bernardi, G., and Rizzo, P.A. 1969. Cerebral reactivity in psychiatric and epileptic patients. *Electroencephalogr. Clin. Neurophysiol.* 27:680.

Gartside, I.B., Lippold, O.C.J., and Meldrum, B.S. 1966. The evoked cortical somatosensory response in normal man and its modification by oral lithium carbonate. *Electroencephalogr. Clin. Neurophysiol.* 20:382.

Gross, M.M., Begleiter, H., Tobin, M., and Kissin, B. 1966. Changes in auditory evoked response induced by alcohol. *J. Nerv. Ment. Dis.* 143:152.

Hall, R.A., Rappaport, M., Hopkins, H.K., and Griffin, R. 1973. Tobacco and evoked potential. *Science* 180:212.

Helmchen, H., and Kunkel, M. 1964. Befunde zur rhythmischen Nachschwankung bei optisch ausgelösten Reizantworten (evoked responses) im EEG des Menschen. *Arch. Psychiat. Zeitschr. ges. Neurol.* 205:397.

Heninger, G.R. 1969. Lithium effects on cerebral cortical function in manic depressive patients. *Electroencephalogr. Clin. Neurophysiol.* 27:670.

Heninger, G.R., McDonald, R.K., Goff, W.R., and Sollberger, A. 1969. Diurnal variations in the cerebral evoked response and EEG: Relations to 17-hydroxycorticosteroid levels. *Arch. Neurol.* 21:330.

Heninger, G.R., and Speck, L. 1966. Visual evoked responses and mental state of schizophrenics. *Arch. Gen. Psychiatry* 15:419.

Hillyard, S.A. 1969. The CNV and the vertex evoked potential during signal detection: A preliminary report. In E. Donchin and D. Lindsley (eds.), *Average Evoked Potentials— Methods, Results, and Evaluations*, p. 349. Washington, D.C.: National Aeronautics and Space Administration.

Ishikawa, K. 1968. Studies on the visual evoked responses to paired light flashes in schizophrenics. *Kurume Medical Journal* 15:153.

Jewett, D.L., Romano, M.N., and Williston, J.S. 1970. Human auditory evoked potentials: Possible brain stem components detected on the scalp. *Science* 167:1517.

Jones, R.T., Blacker, K.H., and Callaway, E. 1966. Perceptual dysfunction in schizophrenia: Clinical and auditory evoked response findings. *Am. J. Psychiatry* 123:639.

Jones, R.T., Blacker, K.H., Callaway, E., and Layne, R.S. 1965. The auditory evoked response as a diagnostic and prognostic measure in schizophrenia. *Am. J. Psychiatry* 122:33.

Jones, R.T., and Callaway, E. 1970. Auditory evoked responses in schizophrenia: A reassessment. *Biol. Psychiatry* 2:291.

Kornhuber, H.H., and Deecke, L. 1965. Cerebral potential changes in voluntary and passive movements in man: Readiness potential and reafferent potential. *Pflügers Arch. Ges. Physiol.* 284:1.

Lewis, E.G., Dustman, R.E., and Beck, E.C. 1970. The effects of alcohol on visual and somatosensory evoked responses. *Electroencephalogr. Clin. Neurophysiol.* 28:202.

Lewis, E.G., Dustman, R.E., Peters, B.A., Straight, R.C., and Beck, E.C. 1973. The effects of varying doses of Δ9-tetrahydrocannabinol on the human visual and somatosensory evoked response. *Electroencephalogr. Clin. Neurophysiol.* 35:347.

Lifshitz, K. 1969. An examination of evoked potentials as indicators of information processing in normal and schizophrenic subjects. In E. Donchin and D.B. Lindsley (eds.), *Average Evoked Potentials: Methods, Results, and Evaluations*, p. 318 and p. 357. Washington, D.C.: National Aeronautics and Space Administration.

Malerstein, A.J., and Callaway, E. 1969. Two-tone average evoked response in Korsakoff patients. *J. Psychiatr. Res.* 6:253.

Mayfield, D., and Brown, R.G. 1966. The clinical laboratory and electroencephalographic effects of lithium. *J. Psychiatr. Res.* 4:207.

McCallum, C. 1969. The contingent negative variation as a cortical sign of attention in man. In C.R. Evans and T.B. Mulholland (eds.), *Attention in Neurophysiology*, p. 40. London: Butterworths.

McCallum, C. 1973. Some psychological, psychiatric and neurological aspects of the CNV. In A. Fessard and G. Lelord (eds.), *Human Neurophysiology, Psychology, Psychiatry: Average Evoked Responses and Their Conditioning in Normal Subjects and Psychiatric Patients*, p. 295. Paris: Inserm.

McCallum, W.C., and Walter, W.G. 1968. The effects of attention and distraction on the contingent negative variation in normal and neurotic subjects. *Electroencephalogr. Clin. Neurophysiol.* 25:319.

Overall, J.E., and Gorham, D.R. 1962. "The Brief Psychiatric Rating Scale." *Psychol. Rep.* 10:799.

Overton, D.A., and Shagass, C. 1969. Distribution of eye movement and eye-blink potentials over the scalp. *Electroencephalogr. Clin. Neurophysiol.* 27:546.

Perry, N.W., and Childers, D.G. 1969. *The Human Visual Evoked Response. Method and Theory.* Springfield, Ill.: Charles C Thomas.

Petrie, A. 1967. *Individuality in Pain and Suffering.* Chicago: University of Chicago Press.

Picton, T.W., and Hillyard, S.A. 1972. Cephalic skin potentials in electroencephalography. *Electroencephalogr. Clin. Neurophysiol.* 33:419.

Poire, R., Tassinari, C.A., Regis, H., and Gastaut, H. 1967. Effects of diazepam (Valium) on the responses evoked by light stimuli in man (lambda waves, occipital "driving" and average visual evoked potentials). *Electroencephalogr. Clin. Neurophysiol.* 23:383.

Prieto, S., Villar, J.I., and Bachini, O. 1965. Influencias farmacologicas sobre la respuesta visual provocada en el hombre. *Acta Neurol. Latinoamer.* 11:295.

Regan, D. 1972. *Evoked Potentials in Psychology, Sensory Physiology and Clinical Medicine.* London: Chapman and Hall, Ltd.

Rhodes, L.E., Dustman, R.E., and Beck, E.C. 1969. The visual evoked response: A comparison of bright and dull children. *Electroencephalogr. Clin. Neurophysiol.* 27:364.

Ritter, W., and Vaughan, H.G. 1969. Averaged evoked responses in vigilance and discrimination: A reassessment. *Science* 164:326.

Rodin, E.A., Domino, E.F., and Porzak, J.P. 1970. The marihuana-induced "social high." *JAMA* 213:1300.

Rodin, E.A., and Luby, E.D. 1965. The effects of some psychotomimetic agents on visually evoked responses and background EEG. *Electroencephalogr. Clin. Neurophysiol.* 19:319.

Rodin, E., Grisell, J., and Gottlieb, J. 1968. Some electrographic differences between chronic schizophrenic patients and normal subjects. In J. Wortis (ed.), *Recent Advances in Biological Psychiatry*, vol. 10, p. 194. New York: Plenum Press.

Rodin, E., Zacharopoulos, G., Beckett, P., and Frohman, C. 1964. Characteristics of visually evoked responses in normal subjects and schizophrenic patients. *Electroencephalogr. Clin. Neurophysiol.* 17:458.

Roth, W.T., and Cannon, E.H. 1972. Some features of the auditory evoked response in schizophrenics. *Arch. Gen. Psychiatry* 27:466.

Rynearson, R.R., Wilson, M.R., and Bickford, R.G. 1968. Psilocybin-induced changes in psychologic function, electroencephalogram, and light-evoked potentials in human subjects. *Mayo Clinic Proceedings* 43:191.

Saletu, B., Itil, T.M., and Saletu, M. 1971. Auditory evoked response, EEG, and thought process in schizophrenics. *Am. J. Psychiatry* 128:336.

Saletu, B., Saletu, M., and Itil, T. 1972. Effect of minor and major tranquilizers on somatosensory evoked potentials. *Psychopharmacologia* 24:347.

Saletu, B., Saletu, M., and Itil, T.M. 1973. The relationships between psychopathology and evoked responses before, during and after psychotropic drug treatment. *Biol. Psychiatry* 6:45.

Saletu, B., Saletu, M., Itil, T., and Coffin, C. 1972. Effect of stimulatory drugs on the somatosensory evoked potential in man. *Pharmakopsychiat.* 5:129.

Saletu, B., Saletu, M., Itil, T.M., and Hsu, W. 1971a. Changes in somatosensory evoked potentials during fluphenazine treatment. *Pharmakopsychiat. Neuropsychopharmakol.* 4:158.

Saletu, B., Saletu, M., Itil, T. and Jones, J. 1971b. Somatosensory evoked potential changes during thiothixene treatment in schizophrenic patients. *Psychopharmacologia* (Berl.) 20:242.

Saletu, B., Saletu, M., Itil, T.M., and Marasa, J. 1971c. Somatosensory-evoked potential changes during haloperidol treatment of chronic schizophrenics. *Biol. Psychiatry* 3:299.

Satterfield, J.H. 1972. Auditory evoked cortical response studies in depressed patients and normal control subjects. In T.A. Williams, M.M. Katz, and J.A. Shield, Jr. (eds.), *Recent Advances in the Psychobiology of the Depressive Illnesses*, p. 87. Washington, D.C.: U.S. Govt. Printing Office.

Shagass, C. 1967. Effects of LSD on somatosensory and visual evoked responses and on the EEG in man. In J. Wortis (ed.), *Recent Advances in Biological Psychiatry*, vol. 9, p. 209. New York: Plenum Press.

Shagass, C. 1968. Averaged somatosensory evoked responses in various psychiatric disorders. In J. Wortis (ed.), *Recent Advances in Biological Psychiatry*, vol. 10, p. 205. New York: Plenum Press.

Shagass, C. 1972. *Evoked Brain Potentials in Psychiatry.* New York: Plenum Press.

Shagass, C. 1973. Evoked response studies of central excitability in psychiatric disorders. In A. Fessard and G. Lelord (eds.), *Human Neurophysiology, Psychology, Psychiatry: Average Evoked Responses and Their Conditioning in Normal Subjects and Psychiatric Patients*, p. 223. Paris: Inserm.

Shagass, C., Overton, D.A., and Bartolucci, G. 1969. Evoked responses in schizophrenia. In D.V. Siva Sankar (ed.), *Schizophrenia: Current Concepts and Research*, p. 220. Hicksville, N.Y.: PJD Publications.

Shagass, C., Overton, D.A., and Straumanis, J.J. 1971. Evoked response findings in psychiatric illness related to drug abuse. *Biol. Psychiatry* 3:259.

Shagass, C., Overton, D.A., and Straumanis, J.J. 1972. Sex differences in somatosensory evoked responses related to psychiatric illness. *Biol. Psychiatry* 5:295.

Shagass, C., Overton, D.A., and Straumanis, J.J. 1974. Evoked potential studies in schizophrenia. In *Schizophrenia and Schizophrenia-Like Psychoses: Clinical Biologic Psychiatry Frontiers.* Tokyo: Igaku-Shoin Co., Ltd. (in press).

Shagass, C., and Schwartz, M. 1961. Reactivity cycle of somatosensory cortex in humans with and without psychiatric disorder. *Science* 134:1757.

Shagass, C., and Schwartz, M. 1962. Cerebral cortical reactivity in psychotic depressions. *Arch. Gen. Psychiatry* 6:235.

Shagass, C., and Schwartz, M. 1963a. Cerebral responsiveness in psychiatric patients. *Arch. Gen. Psychiatry* 8:177.

Shagass, C., and Schwartz, M. 1963b. Psychiatric disorder and deviant cerebral responsiveness to sensory stimulation. In J. Wortis (ed.), *Recent Advances in Biological Psychiatry*, vol. 5, p. 321. New York: Plenum Press.

Shagass, C., and Schwartz, M. 1963c. Psychiatric correlates of evoked cerebral cortical potentials. *Am. J. Psychiatry* 119:1055.

Shagass, C., and Schwartz, M. 1965. Visual cerebral evoked response characteristics in a psychiatric population. *Am. J. Psychiatry* 121:979.

Shagass, C., Schwartz, M., and Amadeo, M. 1962. Some drug effects on evoked cerebral potentials in man. *J. Neuropsychiatry* 3:S49.

Shagass, C., Schwartz, M., and Krishnamoorti, S.R. 1965. Some psychological correlates of cerebral responses evoked by light flash. *J. Psychosom. Res.* 9:223.

Shagass, C., Straumanis, J.J., and Overton, D.A. 1973. Effects of lithium and amitriptyline therapy on somatosensory evoked response "excitability" measurements. *Psychopharmacologia* 29:185.

Silverman, J. 1972. Stimulus intensity modulation and psychological Dis-Ease. *Psychopharmacologia* 24:42.

Small, J.G., and Small, I.F. 1971. Contingent negative variation (CNV) correlations with psychiatric diagnosis. *Arch. Gen. Psychiatry* 25:550.

Soskis, D.A., and Shagass, C. 1974. Evoked potential tests of augmenting-reducing. *Psychophysiology* 11:175.

Speck, L.B., Dim, B., and Mercer, M. 1966. Visual evoked responses of psychiatric patients. *Arch. Gen. Psychiatry* 15:59.

Spilker, B., and Callaway, E. 1969. "Augmenting" and "reducing" in averaged visual evoked responses to sine wave light. *Psychophysiology* 6:49.

Straumanis, J.J. 1964. Somatosensory and visual cerebral evoked response changes associated with chronic brain syndrome and aging. Unpublished M.S. thesis, University of Iowa, Iowa City.

Straumanis, J.J., Shagass, C., and Overton, D.A. 1969. Problems associated with application of the contingent negative variation to psychiatric illness. *J. Nerv. Ment. Dis.* 148:170.

Straumanis, J.J., Shagass, C., and Overton, D.A. 1973. Somatosensory evoked responses in Down syndrome. *Arch. Gen. Psychiatry* 29:544.

Straumanis, J.J., Shagass, C., and Schwartz, M. 1965. Visually evoked cerebral response changes associated with chronic brain syndrome and aging. *J. Gerontology* 20:498.

Sutton, S. 1969. The specification of psychological variables in an average evoked potential experiment. In E. Donchin and D. Lindsley (eds.), *Average Evoked Potentials— Methods, Results, and Evaluations*, p. 237. Washington, D.C.: National Aeronautics and Space Administration.

Sutton, S., Braren, M., and Zubin, J. 1965. Evoked potential correlates of stimulus uncertainty. *Science* 150:1187.

Sutton, S., Teuting, P., Zubin, J., and John, E.R. 1967. Information delivery and the sensory evoked potential. *Science* 155:1436.

Timsit-Berthier, M. 1973. Etude de la V.C.N. des potentiels lents evoqués et du potentiel moteur chez un groupe de sujets normaux et un groupe de malades psychiatriques. In A. Fessard and G. Lelord (eds.), *Human Neurophysiology, Psychology, Psychiatry: Average Evoked Responses and Their Conditioning in Normal Subjects and Psychiatric Patients,* p. 327. Paris: Inserm.

Timsit, M., Koninckx, N., Dargent, J., Fontaine, O., and Dongier, M. 1970. Variations contingentes négatives en psychiatrie. *Electroencephalogr. Clin. Neurophysiol.* 28:41.

Vaughan, H.G. 1969. The relationship of brain activity to scalp recordings of event-related potentials. In E. Donchin and D. Lindsley (eds.), *Average Evoked Potentials—Methods, Results, and Evaluations,* p. 45. Washington, D.C.: National Aeronautics and Space Administration.

Vaughan, H.G., Costa, L.D., and Ritter, W. 1968. Topography of the human motor potential. *Electroencephalogr. Clin. Neurophysiol.* 25:1.

Walter, W.G. 1966. Electrophysiologic contributions to psychiatric therapy. In *Current Psychiatric Therapies,* vol. 6, p. 13. New York: Grune and Stratton.

Walter, W.G. 1967. Slow potential changes in the human brain associated with expectancy, decision and intention. *Electroencephalogr. Clin. Neurophysiol.* suppl. 26:123.

Walter, W.G., Cooper, R., Aldridge, V.J., McCallum, W.C., and Winter, A.L. 1964. Contingent negative variation: An electric sign of sensorimotor association and expectancy in the human brain. *Nature* 203:380.

Wilson, R.E., and Shagass, C. 1964. Comparison of two drugs with psychotomimetic effects (LSD and Ditran). *J. Nerv. Ment. Dis.* 138:277.

research on violence: the ethical equation

Robert E. Litman, M.D., and
Louis Jolyon West, M.D.

University of California
Los Angeles, California

This symposium is generally concerned with the relationships between brain electrical activity and behavior observed in the laboratory. New and exciting methods for eliciting, storing, interpreting, and communicating information have been described. The application of these observations, methods, and models to the understanding of behaviors occurring outside the laboratory is inevitable. Yet, when we leave the animal model, and then we subsequently leave the laboratory, and finally when we leave the hospital to consider behavior as it occurs in other institutions and in the community, streets, and homes, we evoke a new set of methodological, procedural, and ethical considerations.

Unexpected sensitivities, and serious information and communication problems are encountered on a different level outside the laboratory, in clinical research and field research. We become increasingly concerned not only with what is new and true, but also with what is humane and just; not only with the need for knowledge, but with issues relating to the exercise and possible abuse of power. We enter those controversial interlocking areas of politics and morality called "social problems."

One of us (R.E.L.) once worked as an electroencephalographer for the Veterans Administration in Los Angeles. Several times a week he was asked to do brain wave studies on young veterans who had committed some type of antisocial action, and who claimed they had "blacked out" and could not remember the events. These events were variously described as: "beat up his wife and kids"; "killed a friend in a bar"; "impulsively robbed a market"; "was stopped while driving a stolen automobile toward Las Vegas." It was disappointing to learn that this type of behavior was unlikely to result from psychomotor epilepsy. In fact, spike-and-wave discharges were found in none of these patients, although there were a few cases with focal slow-wave activity.

Some years later he again came into contact with large numbers of people who were engaged in destructive behavior. These patients sought crisis intervention from the Los Angeles Suicide Prevention Center where he was chief psychiatrist. He was impressed by how difficult it was to understand, predict, or alter human behaviors by approaching the subject from only one point of view, whether it be bioelectrical or any other.

Nowhere is the need for holistic, multidisciplinary, comprehensive research more obvious than in approaching violence and aggression. Recent experiences at UCLA have provided the material for this report which focuses on ethical and political problems that must be considered.

UCLA Center for the Study and Reduction of Violence

For more than a year (August 1972-December 1973) in close association with many colleagues, the authors labored at the development of plans for a multidisciplinary Center for the Study and Reduction of Violence (CSRV) to be located at the UCLA Neuropsychiatric Institute. To our surprise, the concept of such a center was, from the time it was first announced, energetically opposed and bitterly attacked by a coalition of opponents over a variety of political and ethical issues. As a result of the controversy, funding of the Center, which had been scheduled to begin July 1, 1973, and for which more than $1,000,000 had been committed by state and federal sources, was delayed indefinitely by the California legislature. At present, the violence research program at UCLA (since reorganized) still cannot go forward without the approval of the legislature. Such action can only be expected after the concerned legislators review the complex equation represented by balancing the potential benefits of the CSRV's projected work against the possible dangers that carrying out such work might engender or even suggest.

What follows is a provisional report on the development of plans for the CSRV, with the reasons given by those who support it and those who oppose it. In effect, this will constitute a review of the principal political and ethical problems that we and other responsible researchers on violence can expect to encounter and, one hopes, to solve.

Moves toward the creation of a program to study life-threatening behavior were initiated by one of us (L.J.W.) during the summer and fall of 1972 through conversations and written communications with J.M. Stubblebine, then director of the California Department of Mental Hygiene (now part of a new amalgamated Department of Health). There was no difficulty in demonstrating the importance of violence as a subject of concern. For example, a UCLA coed had just been murdered on the campus in a parking structure. A public opinion poll had recently listed violence as the number one item of public concern in California. Spectacular murders in the state (for example, the assassination of Senator Robert Kennedy, the Zodiac murders, the Manson "family" murders) had been followed by a number of other frightening examples.

It was demonstrated that there existed at UCLA a substantial group of talented investigators working in areas related to human violence and aggression. The original concept projected two basic components. First, there would be support for specific research, training, and service projects, some already existing, others to be developed. Second, there would be a central core staff consisting not only of administrative and supportive personnel, but also of visiting and resident specialists in psychiatry, sociology, humanities, anthropology, program planning and evaluation, health education, police and correctional work, and especially experts in behavioral problems at the interface with law, ethics, and philosophy. After review in the Department of Health, the proposal was referred to the governor's office where it was approved and the center's establishment announced in the governor's "state of the state" address, January 11, 1973. During the next few months, a small group of part-time staff, including R.E.L. as director-designate, worked together to prepare a description of the overall project. These project plans were deliberately general and flexible, since the staff anticipated that there would be much planning, learning, and numerous changes during the first year of what was proposed as a continuing program. The introduction to the program description follows:

Purposes and Goals

Introduction: Violence is here defined as human behavior that seriously injures or destroys persons. The purpose of the new *Center for the Study and Reduction of Violence* (CSRV) is to study a variety of pathologically violent behaviors; their causes and precursors; conditions that foster or aggravate them; acceptable methods of preventing or diminishing such behaviors and pre-conditions; and techniques for treating or mitigating the harmful consequences.

The CSRV program will concentrate on violent behaviors that take place in an individual or small group setting; behaviors that are irrational, impulsive or uncontrolled; behaviors that are likely to bring perpetrators and/or victims into the sphere of responsibility of health-related professions, either directly or through consultation with other disciplines.

Elsewhere, a number of universities, government agencies and research facilities are independently sponsoring investigations of certain forms of violence. Specific studies by researchers in medicine, psychiatry, psychology, biology, ethology, sociology, anthropology, political science, history, philosophy, law, welfare, corrections, law enforcement, and other fields are concerned with particular aspects of the larger problem. However, the CSRV will undertake to develop a systematic and comprehensive body of knowledge concerning the entire range of individual and small group violent behaviors from the synoptic viewpoint of many disciplines. No other center in the world has a program of comparable scope in this particular area.

While the focus of the Center is on the violent behavior of individuals and small groups, the staff fully recognizes that by far the most important causes of violence are social. Violent behavior can only be studied properly within its social, political and economic context. In fact, the violent person must be viewed in the light of an entire array of social and cultural forces that impinge upon him.

However, the *interaction* between purely social forces and other forces must be studied, if maximal progress is to be made in the scientific understanding of violent behavior. Other forces arise from small group dynamics, from individual personality dynamics, and from psychobiological factors within the person under study. Plans by CSRV to approach the study of such forces and factors—always in relation to their social context, and always under the constraint of ethically acceptable methodology—are discussed below.

Scope

Sub-classes or categories of violent behavior that will come under scrutiny by CSRV include homicide, suicide, physical and sexual assault including that occurring within such institutions as hospitals and prisons, senseless or maniacal killing, neighborhood gang killings, assassination, the battering and abuse of children, and certain aspects of death and destruction on the highways and in the air.

It is difficult to estimate the total number of violent acts committed each year, since a great many such occurrences are never reported. During 1971, more than 100,000 crimes involving violence were reported in the State of California. However, the true total is undoubtedly much higher.

The magnitude and complexity of the problem of violent behavior requires that CSRV be a long-term undertaking, with an open-ended, flexible, and comprehensive program. As noted above, an understanding of violent behavior depends upon rigorous study of many different factors—some already known, others not yet identified—and the patterns of interaction among them. One way of classifying these factors would be under the general headings: social, psychological, and biological.

Social factors include problems within the family or group setting; educational or environmental deprivation; poverty; prejudices; racism; and cultural and social alienation.

Psychological factors include impaired maturation; character disorder; neurosis, psychosis; or situational reaction.

Biological factors include hormonal and metabolic processes; dysfunction, damage or disease to the central nervous system; and the use of various drugs, including alcohol.

Multiple factors are likely to co-exist, requiring complex formulations for the development of useful understanding of violent behavior; and, to repeat, the social context is an essential element in every case.

Next is an outline of the organization of the Center:

CSRV Organization

A. RESEARCH AND DEVELOPMENT
1. Violence Against Children
2. The Violent Adolescent in the Family
3. Normal Family Violence: Accommodation and Breakdown
4. Violence in the Schools
5. Sports as an Alternative to Violence
6. Epidemiology of Violence
7. Hormonal Aspects of Violence in Women
8. Hormonal Aspects of Passivity and Aggressiveness in Boys
9. The Sexually Violent Male
10. Chromosomal Factors and Violent Behavior
11. Violence and Minimal Brain Damage Syndrome in Children
12. Hemisphere Dominance Change and Self-Control
13. Drugs and Violence
14. Violence Among Heroin Addicts
15. Nutrition and Violence
16. Violent Behavior and Drug Use in Cross-Cultural Perspective
17. Victims of Violence

18. Estimation of Probability of Repetition or Continuation of Violence
19. Violence Among Veterans
20. Help for the Violent Sex Offender
21. Violence Prevention as a Community Crisis Service
22. Cultural Inhibitors of Violence

B. EDUCATION AND TRAINING: FELLOWSHIPS, BEHAVIORAL SCIENCES MEDIA LABORATORY

C. LAW AND ETHICS: PLANNING AND EVALUATION
   1. Ethics and the Law
   2. Planning and Evaluation

D. LIAISON

E. ADMINISTRATION AND EXTERNAL ACCOUNTABILITY

Criticism of the CSRV

The faculty members involved with the proposed new center repeatedly indicated that its interests were multidimensional, ranging broadly over the biological, psychological, and social fields. The material outlined above was made available to all who were interested. It was made clear that studies of the biological-physiological aspects of violence would comprise a minor part of the totality of the center's activities in terms of funds spent, number of projects, background and number of staff.

However, these statements, at press conferences and later at campus confrontations, received very little attention. Instead, dramatic media-directed announcements began to appear in the press. Some of these denounced the center as primarily a front for psychosurgery, under the dangerous leadership of Professor Frank R. Ervin.*

Actually Ervin was never involved with the CSRV and had no part in its planning or development. Nevertheless, a radical students organization called Students for a Democratic Society (SDS) pounced on the "UCLA psychosurgery project" in wildly accusatory articles in the *Daily Bruin* and

---

Ervin, a distinguished psychiatrist and scientist, had indeed recently joined the UCLA faculty, coming from Harvard where he had served as director of the Stanley Cobb Psychiatric Research Laboratory of the Massachusetts General Hospital. However, his first year at UCLA was spent largely abroad in primate studies, with the support of a Guggenheim fellowship. During this period he was under attack by a certain Dr. Peter Breggin of Washington, D.C., who was receiving much publicity for a "crusade" against psychosurgery. Ervin was one of Breggin's targets because he had previously been psychiatric consultant to a Harvard neurosurgical project involving treatment of psychomotor epilepsy in patients with temporal lobe brain disease; a few of these patients were violent; their treatment had been described in a controversial book by Harvard neurosurgeon Vernon H. Mark, co-authored by Ervin, entitled Violence and the Brain.

the underground press. Politically activist students suddenly began to picket with signs denouncing "A Clockwork Orange at UCLA," "Stop Psychosurgery at UCLA," "Fire Frank Ervin," "Drive West Into the Sea," and the like.

At first the staff assumed that the sudden hostile attack on the yet unfunded center was essentially political. The theme seemed to be, "If Governor Reagan is for it, we're against it." However, a small group of much more sophisticated political radicals, including two or three psychiatrists, took over leadership of the fight against establishment of the CSRV. They went to many community groups and organizations, ranging from the American Civil Liberties Union to the Black Panther Party, and persuaded them that the proposed center was in fact racist, fascist, sexist, and dangerous to human rights; in fact, nothing less than a government-sponsored program for mind control.

Many of these presentations were shrewd, sophisticated, and well tailored to the concerns of various liberal organizations. Most of these organizations accepted (even endorsed) the denunciatory statements without further ado, and without ever checking with UCLA to request the facts. Some of the arguments included the following:

1. *The Violence Center is a diversion and a delusion.* The causes for violence (and the reduction of violence) are related to vast social problems (for example, the class struggle) far beyond the scope of the UCLA project which will focus only on individuals. To offer hopes for psychiatric or medical solutions to such social problems is to waste time and money, and even worse, to shift attention from the true source of violence; in other words, to blame the individual offender rather than a repressive government, capitalistic economic system, institutionalized racism, brutal law enforcement policies, etc.

2. *Who are the violent people who would be studied?* They are mainly from low-income and ethnic-minority backgrounds, since these groups are over-represented in the crime statistics and in the prisons. "Racism is behind the whole UCLA program." A series of articles on psychosurgery directed against black people was published. Among more moderate critics, the charge of racism simply took the form of an accusation that this was another example of middle-class whites trying to study poor minorities who should instead be given the money to do something for themselves.

3. *The violence project intends to carry out unethical experimentation on prisoners.* Representatives of prisoners' groups stated that in fact it is impossible to do *any* research of *any* type involving prisoners, because there is no way for a prisoner to give free and informed consent. These strictures were said to apply also to persons on probation or parole. Proponents of the view that prisoners would surely be abused were able to cite a number of

incidents in which prisoners in fact had been subjected to dubious research or correctional practices involving drugs in California and other parts of the country. They said that the new center, creating a group of researchers in the university, would not provide more protection than would scattered individuals using unmonitored procedures elsewhere; rather, the CSRV would increase the danger of even more impropriety and exploitation because the university would dignify through its research the very processes by which prisoners are abused. Various groups expressed no trust in the university; instead, extreme distrust was the rule.

4. *The knowledge gained by the center will be abused, probably for the control and coercion of citizens who express dissent or deviation.* In any case, knowledge is power and this center would tend to increase the power of the state which already has too much power and a well-documented history of abusing power. Control mechanisms through which the general public is to be represented in monitoring the program will be ineffective.

5. *The whole concept of prevention through early recognition or diagnosis is unethical.* It leads toward preventive detention or involuntary treatment, probably with powerful chemical tranquilizers or other drugs. Increasing the accuracy of the prediction of dangerousness would actually help the repressive and brutal law-enforcement system.

Not all arguments against the center came from the political left. The right was also against it: The whole project will be a waste of effort, time and money. A group of professors studying violence has no connection with reduction of violence. The money should go for police equipment and other law-enforcement purposes. Giving funds to the university to study and reduce violence is ridiculous, since it is well known that in fact the university spawns and encourages violence.

Responses to Criticism

As applied specifically to the UCLA proposals, these criticisms were either grossly exaggerated or wholly irrelevant. Nevertheless, there are legitimate grounds for concern regarding the issues, both ethical and political, to which they appealed.

For one thing, these questions and criticisms reflected a wide-spread attitude, among professional persons and the public at large, that the present regulation of the research process where it involves experimentation on human beings is unsatisfactory. This current attitude has evolved gradually. A recent symposium concerned with nonscientific constraints on medical research (Merlis 1970) provides an example of medical researchers responding to the trend of public scrutiny.

Veatch and Sollitto (1973) reviewed biomedical research published since 1966 and found 43 questionable experiments that raised disturbing ethical questions. Disregarding the issue of informed consent, they listed the following issues: grave risks to subjects, risks to incompetent and incarcerated subjects, the rights of subjects in research with a placebo group, responsibility for harm to subjects. The authors recommended immediate establishment of a government committee to review informed consent and develop new mechanisms for research review. Since then Congressional hearings have been held, first by Senator Walter Mondale and more recently by Senator Edward Kennedy, on this issue. A tough regulatory bill has been drafted by Senator Kennedy's staff and approved by the Senate, although not yet by the House. The National Institutes of Health have also drafted a new statement on safeguards in research involving human subjects, now being circulated in the scientific community.

Physicians and scientists have responded to these new developments with some concern (Hussey 1973). It is feared that there will be restrictions on freedom of inquiry. Everyone agrees that experimental subjects need protection, but scientists feel that research investigators and their own professional societies and universities can solve this problem most effectively by voluntarily providing effective mechanisms for dealing with possible abuse. An editorial in *Science* (Etzioni 1973) suggests that there should be a step-by-step procedure of review, consisting first of local human-subjects committees. These would be composed of scientists, persons from other academic disciplines (such as humanities, law, and theology), and some representatives of the subjects themselves. The next step should involve regional and appeal boards. The highest step should be a nationwide board (having the same basic composition as the local ones but involving persons of national stature) to evolve review standards and clarify generic questions.

Other recent publications review the problems to be considered in future experiments with human beings (Torrey 1969, Katz 1972, Barber 1973) and related ethical issues (West 1969). The World Health Organization, professional organizations, universities, and the Department of Health, Education and Welfare, have all formulated a variety of regulations including creation of ethical review boards that can withhold prior approval of research involving human experimentation and disapprove of violators. With regard to the UCLA Center for the Study and Reduction of Violence, several review boards were proposed in addition to the already constituted human-subjects review committees of the department of psychiatry, the medical school, and the university.

The UCLA medical faculty generally agreed that there was urgent need for a program of studies on individual violent behavior. The medical faculty council (heads of all departments) unanimously endorsed the CSRV. So did the dean of the School of Medicine and the chancellor of UCLA. Such research had been recommended by the National Commission on the Causes and Prevention of Violence, by both American Psychiatric and Psychological Associations, and by many other individuals and groups who have studied the problems of human violence. However, in responding to the challenges regarding the new program, individual UCLA faculty members presented a variety of views concerning the definition of "violence," and different sets of priorities for what should be studied or what should be done first.

The postponement of the CSRV program at UCLA was, of course, a great disappointment. The opportunity was lost to conduct a thorough review, to discuss and comprehensively integrate background knowledge gathered from many individual studies, and to develop an overall conceptualization of what was meant by violence. The better part of a year could have been spent on definition, taxonomy, epidemiology, detailed examination of individual cases, and long-range planning. None of these activities has been possible beyond a rudimentary beginning.

In reviewing the ethical equation in research on violence, it is now clear that a major political mistake of omission occurred in our failure to communicate early and frequently with key California legislators on the objectives, methods, and significance of the proposed center. In retrospect it would have been politically wise also to have reviewed the proposal with representatives of various minority groups and of prisoners. On the other hand, scientists are not accustomed to involve the community *before* work begins; we are more inclined to wait until something of value has been accomplished, and then to report it.

Nobody is happy with the present system of criminal justice and corrections. Poor people, members of minority groups, and prisoners are the greatest victims of violence. But they also have the most to gain from new knowledge and from reforms including changes in existing institutions. We saw it as cruelly ironical that groups representing those who had the most to gain from the UCLA work had been so easily persuaded to oppose it, without finding out the truth of the matter for themselves.

The simple truth, as it happens, would have negated most of the arguments that were raised against the establishment of a Center for the Study and Reduction of Violence.

1. *Psychosurgery was a totally false issue.* The UCLA center never had any plans for research involving neurosurgical procedures or, for that matter, any type of surgery at all. Of nearly 40 faculty members involved in the project, not one was a surgeon. The issue was raised by certain individuals (like Breggin) who apparently wanted publicity. It was then used by SDS to alarm university students in an effort to mobilize their hostility toward the proposed center. We recognized and indeed emphasized that the use of brain surgery for behavioral modification requires moral decisions that can be

reached only after extremely careful review and thoughtful deliberation of the issues. In reviewing these issues, Mark and Neville (1973) make the following points: "Any medical procedure as drastic as neurosurgery should be used only when behavior is abnormal and bad, primarily because of an abnormality of the brain. Abnormal, violent behavior *not* associated with brain disease should be dealt with politically and socially, not medically." The same authors discuss the problems inherent in experimental treatments for persons in prisons, or in other conditions of diminished freedom, such as those persons who are committed to mental hospitals. The authors conclude that because freedom of consent is simply not practical for such persons, they should not be used as subjects for interventions which are drastic, irreversible, or experimental.

2. *The proposed program is not a waste of time and money; it is an approach that has proved its value many times at many universities.* Violence comprises a diverse and complex set of situations and behaviors. While some of the causes and solutions for human violence are indeed related to vast social problems, there is, in addition, a great deal of personal tragedy which results from individual violence of types that are not directly caused by major political or socioeconomic problems, and for which there may well be individual, psychological, psychiatric, or medical solutions or at least potentialities for help. Individual violence occurs in all social classes and at all economic levels. Very often the victim and the violent person are related through family or through friendship. Most of the domestic mass murders, assassinations, homicides, and assaults have individual psychopathological aspects which overshadow the general social theme. Seventy percent of homicides in America are not even crime-related, and extremely few are truly political.

Admittedly, the proposed center would approach only a part of the total problem of violence. However, our findings could certainly be integrated into larger social changes and improvements. At least psychiatry and related disciplines would make a beginning in studying life-threatening behaviors (and their consequences) by individuals and small groups under conditions traditionally considered to impinge on the sphere of our responsibility. Violence will not disappear no matter what we do, but that does not mean we should do nothing.

Individual violence occurs in all aspects of society. It would be wrong to focus on any one group, for that would miss the goal of the overall approach. The statistical facts of violence in ghettos do not make a concern for research on the subject automatically racist. In fact, much of the violence among poor and underprivileged urban groups is a consequence of institutionalized neglect. To postpone or avoid the challenge of this research opportunity would be the most racist of all the available options.

It is obvious that the time is long past for detached middle-class white scientists to be studying minority people. Many of the CSRV projects require that investigators possess appropriate ethnic backgrounds or personal experiences to give them a special insight or entrée into special subcultures, for example in certain central city urban neighborhoods, or in prisons. Of course, such helpers could not be hired until funding was obtained, and an argument against funding was that they had not been hired.

3. *The charge that the center would foster unethical experimentation on prisoners was totally without substance.* Opponents of the program were able to cite experiments in which prisoners and other underprivileged persons (for example, the untreated black syphilitics in the Tuscaloosa scandal) were abused, in various parts of the country as well as California. Yet, prisoners themselves need new approaches to problems of supervision, control, rehabilitation, and recidivism. New approaches to criminal justice and corrections in America are desperately needed.

One of the CSRV projects involved the designing and pilot staffing of a unique residential treatment facility and program in Los Angeles for sexual offenders, mostly rapists, released from the state's only hospital for mentally disturbed sex offenders, which is located at a great distance from any urban center. Among other things, this model therapeutic community (a sort of halfway house) featured considerable self-government, female therapists involved with male patients in appropriate settings, ex-convict and ex-inmate staff assistance, and extensive social re-education in participating in an urban environment.

As opposition to the CSRV grew, one of the developers and sponsors of this new program, himself an ex-prisoner, felt that he had to abandon it. He became persuaded that those volunteering for care in the new program would be technically parolees and thus unable to exercise free choice. Others have supported this view (Capron 1973). However, we feel that prisoners are not necessarily best served by safeguards that are so exaggerated as to prevent the most helpful new approach. As one prisoner put it, "These guys could protect us to death!"

Experiments on prisoners that expose them to significant risk or damage are certainly not permissible. There is still room, however, for discussion of ways and means to offer prisoners opportunities to participate in (or refuse to be part of) new and potentially valuable research programs involving no known risk and offering excellent possibilities for improving the quality of their own lives and that of others.

Unfortunately, at the present time, anyone who tries to mediate between prisoners and the penal establishment is suspect. And, of course, not everyone can do it. That is why the Neuropsychiatric Institute engaged a highly literate and gifted ex-prisoner as consultant to help devise methods by which experimental changes could be attempted in the correction system, using the prisoners as both subjects and co-investigators. Unfortunately, in the absence of the expected funding, this person could not be permanently retained.

We do need a system of safeguards for informed and truly free consent. To this end, experiments using prisoners might be devised and monitored by prisoners, acting individually and in committees, or by advocates for prisoners, in consultation with the sponsoring scientific group. A committee of prisoners, or at least a committee that included prisoner representation, should be responsible for reviewing any proposed projects that involve prisoners and any proposed volunteer subjects from a prison population. An example of a research program in which the support and cooperation of prisoners has been obtained is the project on prevention of individual violence located in Houston (Justice 1973).

4. *The argument that a successful Center for the Study and Reduction of Violence could produce knowledge that would eventually be used for nefarious purposes by the state is a subcategory of the entire issue of potential abuse of science.* With this in mind, we pledged ourselves to do no classified or secret work, and to make our findings public, not only to professionals, but to the general public as well, and also to the classes of persons who would be subjects of any research. Mechanisms were planned that would assure free access to the project's findings and insure that problems of special interest to all classes (for example, victims, minorities, both sexes, offenders, police) would be studied.

An advisory committee with public representation was to have been appointed by the chancellor of UCLA to help secure these goals. The larger problem of the eventual use of scientific knowledge is, of course, of ongoing concern to everyone because it involves all of us. Here again, as with the issues of human experimentation, scientists should employ review procedures and policy organizations to evaluate and plan for the eventual uses to be made of knowledge they generate. Nevertheless, all knowledge is potentially subject to abuse. Safeguards are the responsibility, not only of scientists, but of society as a whole.

5. *Evaluative, diagnostic, and predictive studies are not automatically unethical.* The idea that preventive detention is the only logical result of improved ability to predict dangerousness is to prejudge and preclude any new developments in diagnosis, treatment, remediation, and rehabilitation. The concept of clues (signs, symptoms, and history) that aid in prediction or diagnosis is vital for individualizing treatment approaches and providing a humane response to any individual's behavior. In fact, greater predictive power is much more likely to lead to earlier release of the less dangerous person, rather than longer confinement for the more violent one. Also,

unless there is some way of evaluating the persons receiving a certain treatment or involved in a certain rehabilitation approach, it is extremely difficult to measure the effectiveness of that particular modality.

There are great advantages in choosing relatively homogeneous populations for various treatment efforts (for instance, certain types of therapeutic communities). We acknowledge the problem inherent in labeling a person as potentially violent, but are constantly required to make such judgments as it is. Instead of dismissing the whole approach as unethical, we believe that this approach can be made to work to the advantage of the individuals at risk. In any case, society requires us to make our best prediction. And, if prediction is not improved, the most likely consequence is greater repression, more prolonged confinement for all offenders, and the restoration of the death penalty.

Summary

Proposals for research on human behavior today are likely to provoke controversy and hostility, especially if the experiments involve human subjects, and particularly if they have some relevant application to political-social life. Ethical standards for research on human subjects correctly demand free, competent, informed consent from subjects and great emphasis on protecting subjects from injury. In addition, the potential uses and abuses of research results must be considered. Public discussion of these issues is to be expected and should be encouraged. Scientists can expect to be misunderstood, at times heatedly opposed and confronted, and sometimes slandered, abused, or even attacked. Yet we should not retreat from the necessity to work on controversial problems.

Repeated, calm explanation and clarification of the issues and facts are an appropriate response to political criticism of valid scientific work. Sometimes opponents have interesting points to make, and their criticisms may well be constructively incorporated into the research plan. Because the problems of human violence are of great importance, and because science has much to contribute toward the amelioration of some of the harm done by violence, we continue to hope for long-term public support of research in this field. At the same time, great public suspicion of such research programs must also be expected.

Meanwhile, the scientist must continue to balance the vital equation. The potential risks inherent in all clinical research, human experimentation, or behavioral studies weigh on one side. Our responsibilities to develop new knowledge, to disseminate it, and to apply it for the good of mankind and for the improvement of the human condition, weigh on the other.

References

Barber, B., Lally, J., Makarushka, J.L., and Sullivan, D. 1973. *Research on Human Subjects*. New York: Russell Sage Foundation.

Capron, A.M. 1973. Medical research in prisons. *Hastings Center Report*, vol. 3, no. 3, p. 4.

Etzioni, A. 1973. Regulation of human experimentation. *Science* 182:1203.

Hussey, H.H. 1973. Human experimentation. *JAMA* 226:561.

Justice, B. 1973. *Reducing Violent Crime*. Houston: University of Texas.

Katz, J. 1972. *Experimentation with Human Beings*. New York: Russell Sage Foundation.

Mark, V.H., and Neville, R. 1973. Brain surgery in aggressive epileptics. *JAMA* 226:765.

Merlis, S. 1970. *Non-Scientific Constraints on Medical Research*. New York: Raven Press.

Torrey, E.F. 1969. *Ethical Issues in Medicine*. Boston: Little, Brown.

Veatch, R., and Sollitto, S. 1973. Human experimentation—the ethical questions persist. *Hastings Center Report*, vol. 3, no. 3, p. 1.

West, L.J. 1969. Ethical psychiatry and biosocial humanism. *Am. J. Psychiatry* 126:226.

violence and aggression: the state of the art

Richard D. Walter, M.D.

University of California-Los Angeles Medical School
The Neuropsychiatric Institute
Los Angeles, California

The focus of this review will be on the neurobiology of violence and aggression in man. Violence, in this context, will be considered as individual acts of pathologically aggressive behavior; thus war, revolution, race riots, and gang warfare will be excluded. This discussion, then, will be on a smaller subtopic, as opposed to a more global aspect of violence that would include the extensive areas of its social, economic, cultural, and psychological determinants. Still further, this review will not deal with animal studies, not because of any deprecatory feeling regarding their scientific merit, but because of a personal bias that they may be irrelevant. After all of these exclusionary clauses, is there any residue? The answer to this question appears to be the currently hot issue for debate—the magnitude, importance, and treatability of disorders of the brain resulting in violent behavior.

Is There a Lesion in Man that Results in Violence?

A vast amount of accumulated clinical experience and literature would certainly corroborate the statement that aggressive and violent behavior has been observed in patients with disorders of the central nervous system. Accepting this empiric evidence, and in keeping with the sometimes maligned medical model, the neurologist always asks, where is the lesion?

Violence and "Generalized" Brain Involvement

It is commonplace in neurology and psychiatry to observe violent behavior in the clinical context of the irascibility, striking out, the verbal and
physical threats and actions of the delirious and demented. The etiology of
the delirium may not be specific, as witnessed by the classical examples of
drunken aggressiveness, pathological intoxication, metabolic and pharmacologic encephalopathies, or the recovery phase from a recent, severe head
injury. Similarly, the type of dementia is not specific in that the same
behavior may be observed in the presenile and senile dementias, Huntington's chorea, postcerebral hypoxia, and encephalitic states. Surely if the
major contribution to the biology of violence consisted of this degree of
"brain damage," it would have long since been recognized even with the
crudities of clinical neurology. Perhaps, then, if there are these classical but
easily recognizable examples of brain disease and violence, there can be more
subtle forms that do not fall in the category of overt delirium or dementia.
Two proposals would indicate that this might indeed be the case.

Episodic dyscontrol syndrome. The recognition of this concept can be
roughly traced through the studies of Karl Menninger (1963) to the work of
Russel Monroe (1970) and the more recent publications of Lion (1972) and
Lion, Bach-y-Rita, and Ervin (1968 and 1969). The identifying features of
this syndrome are thought of as being "seizure-like" outbursts with a loss of
contact with the environment and symptoms that might be interpreted as
automatisms or aura. In the postviolent period there may be depression,
fatigue, or, rarely, relaxation or elation. Additional features might be found
in the character of the violent act, that is, a diffuse act with the target being
walls, furniture, other people, or the self. Pathological intoxication is a feature in many of these patients' histories.

Brain dysfunction has been proposed as the explanation for the episodic dyscontrol syndrome, based on the frequent histories of previous head
injuries, childhood seizure disorders, abnormal EEGs, and "soft" neurological signs. Mark and Ervin (1970) have developed the thesis further that
this syndrome represents not only brain dysfunction but probably a focal
disorder of the limbic system. They have made the analogy between this
syndrome and classical temporal lobe epilepsy, reasoning that dyscontrol
may be an example of limbic system pathology without the traditional
psychomotor seizure. A further discussion of this point will be carried out
under the heading of epilepsy.

Minimal brain dysfunction. The second notion, somewhat less force-
fully proposed, is that episodic dyscontrol is an adult extension of the pedi-
atric "minimal brain dysfunction" or "neurologically handicapped" child
syndrome.

In this context the argument is made that the two groups of patients have much in common, considering the history of perinatal and early childhood central nervous system traumas, the episodic symptomatology, the predominance of males, evidence of learning difficulties in the adult group, and "soft" neurological signs. The problem here, regarding neurological acceptability, is that the whole concept of "minimal brain dysfunction" in childhood is so nebulous and conceptually loose that the understanding of violence could not be advanced by this simple extension. One unknown cannot explain another unknown.

Violence and Hypothalamic Involvement

Neuropathology—that great arbiter of clinical judgment—should be expected to provide a crisp answer to the localization of a lesion in the human brain that results in violence. This, however, is not completely the case, since the correlation of neuropathological changes and violent clinical behavior does not have an extensive body of knowledge. There are probably a number of reasons for this paucity, the most obvious being the clinicians' low order of priority for violence or aggression over the traditional neurological signs or symptoms. A second reason is an old one: the absence of a discrete focus of many of nature's lesions.

The available reports, however, do indicate that bilateral lesions of the hypothalamus have been associated with rage and violent behavior. Alpers (1937) described a patient who complained of thirst and polyuria. (How much interesting behavioral information is frequently lost by neurologists' preoccupation with a classical problem of diabetes insipidus?) His wife, however, complained of her husband's fighting with friends. With the passage of time the patient became morose, coarse, abusive, and chased visitors from the house. Postmortem examination revealed a teratoma filling the third ventricle, with diffuse destruction of the hypothalamic nuclei from pressure.

Hypothalamic involvement is also the theme of the report by Reeves and Plum (1969) in which the patient exhibited uncooperative, overtly aggressive behavior with biting and scratching. More recently Killefer and Stern (1970) described episodic rage induced by slight provocation, and violent behavior directed toward hospital personnel and family members following removal of the patient's cystic craniopharyngioma. At autopsy the entire floor of the third ventricle from the lamina terminalis posteriorly to the mammillary bodies was found to be destroyed. Remnants of the mammillary bodies were present, but no other nuclei of the hypothalamus could be found.

Violence and Lesions in the Limbic System

The proposed localization for the expression of violent behavior in man, based on both clinical and electroencephalographic studies, is controversial. As an example, a heavily used, modern textbook of psychiatry (Kolb 1968) under the heading of psychomotor epilepsy has the following statements:

"Clinically the clouded state suggests a delirium with liberation of aggressive and occasionally, self destructive impulses. Acts of violence may be committed in these automatisms and may be of a strikingly brutal nature, the patient pursuing his crime to a most revolting extreme" (page 267). No reference is cited; no estimate of the frequency of this brutal activity is mentioned, but there is the authority of a textbook statement.

Several studies would indicate that the association of violent and aggressive acts with temporal lobe epilepsy in general is rare. Rodin (1973) studied 57 patients with a seizure disorder and with components of psychomotor epilepsy. In the process of the patients' diagnostic evaluation, the clinical seizure was activated in the laboratory with an intravenously administered convulsant. An electroencephalographic as well as a photographic recording was obtained of the ictal and postictal behavior. There were no instances of violent or aggressive acts. In addition, Rodin reviewed the history of 700 patients and found 34 who had committed aggressive acts. The profile that emerged in the study group was that of a young man of lower than average intelligence with a history of behavioral difficulties dating back to school age and without strong religious ties. The presence or absence of psychomotor epilepsy was not a relevant variable.

Ounstead (1969) examined 100 children with a variety of neurological problems including seizure disorders. A history of outbursts of rage was reported in 36 of these patients. Those patients who had "pure" psychomotor epilepsy were "uniformly intelligent and conforming children and none of them had rage outbursts at any time." A higher incidence of "aggressiveness"—38 percent—has been reported by Falconer (1973) in patients with temporal lobe epilepsy. Still another report on 666 cases of temporal lobe epilepsy by Currie et al. (1971) provides a different figure for aggressiveness. The psychiatric diagnoses were reported as 56 percent normal, 19 percent anxious, 11 percent depressed, 7 percent aggressive, 6 percent obsessional, and 6 percent with a severe disturbance of affect. Some patients showed more than one abnormal mental trait. Noteworthy in this report is the psychiatric evaluation of the nine patients with tumors confined to the temporal lobe. Two of these patients were aggressive-assaultive, two were suicidal and aggressive, one was depressed, one had uncontrollable fears, and two had unidentified psychiatric symptoms. A further comment on the relationship between neoplasms of the limbic system and violence is provided by the report of Malamud (1967). Eighteen patients are described who were found to have neoplasms on postmortem examination. All of these patients had received a psychiatric diagnosis, but only 3 of the 18 were described as having had violent outbursts, rage attacks, or "temper tantrums." The location of the tumors in these three patients were, third ventricle (one case), cingulate region (one case), and pole of the temporal lobe (one case).

There is, then, a considerable range in the various estimates of aggression or violence appearing in patients with lesions of the limbic system, either with temporal lobe epilepsy or with tumors of this region. This variation, as in all such clinical studies, might well be explained on the basis of difference in patient selection, or the variation in the meaning or significance of what is considered to be violent behavior.

Electroencephalographic Studies on Violence and Aggression

Considering the vast body of literature on electroencephalography, it is somewhat surprising to find so few studies specifically directed toward violence as opposed to other behavioral abnormalities. One of the earliest reports, which deserves to be replicated, was presented by Stafford-Clark and Taylor (1949). In the electroencephalographic examination of prisoners charged with murder, they found that the amount of electrical abnormality correlated directly with the degree of unpredictability of the crime. Only eight subjects were in the abnormal EEG and unmotivated crime category. In a more recent study (Sayed, Lewis, and Britain 1969), the incidence of EEG abnormality in 32 murderers judged to be "insane" was 65 percent, as opposed to nonpatient controls who had an incidence of 15 percent. The EEG abnormalities were not of the spike-wave type and the major finding was of the diffuse slow-wave type.

Many studies on patients diagnosed as having sociopathic behavior have revealed a high percentage of electrical abnormality (Hill and Watterson 1942, Hill 1944, Williams 1969). The reported rates of EEG abnormality in this group of patients have been remarkably consistent, at 50 to 60 percent, as compared to the rate for psychoneurotic individuals of 10 to 30 percent, or for a schizophrenic group at 30 percent. However, the type of electrical abnormality is not specific for sociopathy, and it is not confined to the temporal lobe.

It is conceivable that the technique most likely to supply information about violence and brain function is that of depth-electrode studies in man. EEG surface recordings rarely reflect all of the prominent electrical abnormalities that may be present in the deep structures, and there is, therefore, a better opportunity of observing the correlation of behavior and EEG events. In addition, the use of depth recordings in a chronic fashion permits activating procedures—pharmacological, electrical, or environmental manipulation —that would best provide this correlation.

Although this method might seem to be the most logical and profitable way to study the problem, there are serious disadvantages that have prevented the opportunity to study violence in man with this strategy. The disadvantages range from the formidable sampling problem with depth electrodes—only a limited number of sites within the brain can be recorded—to the more general problem of using such depth-electrode studies only in a clinical situation in which the results have a high probability of leading to a specific type of treatment, usually surgical.

The large body of literature covering the use of depth electrodes in man makes a convincing case for the localization of seizure foci, usually in, but not limited to, the temporal lobe in man. However, only a few observations have been reported that directly correlate EEG events and violent behavior. Mark and Ervin (1970) reported on one patient who demonstrated violent behavior (guitar smashing) on electrical stimulation of the amygdala, and another patient who exhibited hippocampal electrical abnormalities in response to hearing a recording of a baby cry, a stimulus of great emotional meaning to the patient. Another patient described by Heath (1955) demonstrated rage episodes on electrical stimulation of the amygdala; however, this was not a consistent finding.

The criticism has been made that these few cases stand out as rare and unique in contrast to the large number of patients who have been studied with chronically implanted depth electrodes. For example, in the 66 patients with temporal lobe epilepsy who were examined using depth electrodes at UCLA, no convincing examples of violent or aggressive behavior were observed during prolonged recording sessions or on electrical stimulation of the depth sites. There are a number of possible explanations for this apparent discrepancy; the first may well be the obvious difference in patient selection. At UCLA, the temporal-lobe seizure patients were more representative of the classical type, that is, those without a history of violence. The second difference may be that the format for the electrical-stimulation studies was different from that used by Mark and Ervin, not only in regard to the electrical parameters of the stimuli, but in the setting in which the study was undertaken. Third, no attempt was made to "activate" selectively such possible relationships by manipulating the patient's environment or providing nonelectrical stimuli that might be expected to evoke violence. That is, no attempt was made in the laboratory to provide a setting in which potentially violent acts would be more likely to occur.

Summary

Violence, as any other aspect of human behavior, is determined by a complex and interacting set of variables, although this statement has achieved the status of a platitude. However, the relative importance of disturbed brain function as a "cause" of violence in man, although currently debated, certainly has not been adequately studied. A review of the past reports on this subject indicates that the behavioral abnormality labeled violence has been observed in both diffuse and focal examples of brain disease, that there probably is a higher incidence of EEG abnormality in individuals exhibiting violent behavior, and that, though violent acts may occur, it is a rare feature of temporal lobe epilepsy.

The state of the art appears to be that there are suggestions for future research—the major one being the need for intensive, thorough, and meticulous studies of individuals who exhibit violent behavior, using all of the modalities of modern clinical and research techniques.

References

Alpers, B.J. 1937. Relation of the hypothalamus to disorders of personality. Report of a case. *Arch. Neurol. Psychiatry* 38:291.

Currie, S., Heathfield, K.W.G., Henson, R.A., and Scott, D.F. 1971. Clinical course and prognosis of temporal lobe epilepsy. *Brain* 94:173.

Falconer, M.A. 1973. Reversibility by temporal lobe resection of the behavioral abnormalities of temporal lobe epilepsy. *N. Engl. J. Med.* 289:451.

Heath, R.G., Monroe, R.R., and Mickle, W.A. 1955. Stimulation of the amygdaloid nucleus in a schizophrenic patient. *Am. J. Psychiatry* 111:862.

Hill, D. 1944. Cerebral dysrhythmia: Its significance in aggressive behavior. *Proc. R. Soc. Med.* 37:317.

Hill, D., and Watterson, D. 1942. Electro-encephalographic studies of psychopathic personalities. *J. Neurol. Psychiatry* 5:47.

Killefer, F.A., and Stern, W.E. 1970. Chronic effects of hypothalamic injury: Report of a case of near total hypothalamic destruction resulting from removal of a craniopharyngioma. *Arch. Neurol.* 22:419.

Kolb, L.C. 1968. *Noyes' Modern Clinical Psychiatry*, Seventh Ed. Philadelphia: W.B. Saunders.

Lion, J.R. 1972. *Evaluation and Management of the Violent Patient*. Springfield, Ill.: Charles C. Thomas.

Lion, J.R., Bach-y-Rita, G., and Ervin, F.R. 1968. The self-referred violent patient. *JAMA* 205:503.

Lion, J.R., Bach-y-Rita, G., and Ervin, F.R. 1969. Violent patients in the emergency room. *Am. J. Psychiatry* 125:1706.

Malamud, N. 1967. Psychiatric disorder with intracranial tumors of limbic system. *Arch. Neurol.* 17:113.

Mark, V.H., and Ervin, F.R. 1970. *Violence and the Brain.* New York: Harper & Row.

Menninger, K. 1963. *The Vital Balance.* New York: Viking Press.

Monroe, R.Q. 1970. *Episodic Behavioral Disorder: A Psychodynamic and Neurophysiological Analysis.* Cambridge, Mass.: Harvard University Press.

Ounstead, C. 1969. Aggression and epilepsy: Rage in children with temporal lobe epilepsy. *J. Psychosom. Res.* 13:237.

Reeves, A.G., and Plum, F. 1969. Hyperphagia, rage and dementia accompanying a ventromedial hypothalamic neoplasm. *Arch. Neurol.* 20:616.

Rodin, E.A. 1973. Psychomotor epilepsy and aggressive behavior. *Arch. Gen. Psychiatry* 28:210.

Sayed, Z.A., Lewis, S.A., and Britain, R.P. 1969. An electroencephalographic and psychiatric study of 32 insane murderers. *Electroencephalogr. Clin. Neurophysiol.* 27:335.

Stafford-Clark, D., and Taylor, F.H. 1949. Clinical and electro-encephalographic studies of prisoners charged with murder. *J. Neurol. Neurosurg. Psychiatry* 12:325.

Williams, D. 1969. Neural factors related to habitual aggression. *Brain* 92:503.

eeg findings in 73 persons accused of murder

John R. Knott, Ph.D.,
Romulo T. Lara, M.D.,
Jon F. Peters, M.S., and
Merl D. Robinson, M.D.

University of Iowa and
Iowa Security Medical Facility
Iowa City, Iowa

There have been previous reports of high incidences of anomalous EEG findings in persons charged with felonious assault or with murder (Hill and Parr, 1950, Hill and Pond, 1952). Gibbs, Bagchi, and Bloomberg (1945) have not, however, found impressive abnormalities in prisoners.

The present investigations were conducted on 73 prisoners referred for electroencephalograms by the Iowa Security Medical Facility between 1970 and mid-1974. All prisoners had been committed for evaluation because of charges of murder or attempted murder.

The EEGs utilized International electrode placements and bipolar and monopolar recordings in a series of seven selected montages. Both waking and sleeping records were obtained. All records were read (or reviewed) by one of us (J.R.K.). Most records were recorded by one of us (J.F.P.). Eye movement and EKG monitors were utilized throughout all recordings.

The basic findings are presented in Table 1. The classification of "normal" was used to include all "classical" normal EEGs, including "low voltage fast" (Gibbs and Gibbs, 1951). The classification of "normal limits EEG" included those who showed the minimal temporal slow and/or sharp activity described by Kooi et al. (1964) as well as the minimal temporal theta seen with physiological aging (one case). "Dysrhythmic or epileptiform" EEGs include those with clearly slower than normal, or focal, or epileptiform (spike) activity.

The findings in this group do not substantiate any claims that murderers as a group show excessive amounts of EEG abnormality. Only 4.1 per cent were clearly outside of normal limits. In fact, one had a history of seizures and multiple spikes; one had clear bilateral spiking in sleep but no seizures; and one had theta paroxysms awake, which could be activated by excessive alcohol, but no seizures. Since this latter patient's aggressive problems were primarily limited to states of intoxication, there may in this case be some tenuous relationship between the generation of theta and aggressiveness.

We do not feel that when all current data are evaluated, any generalizations concerning electrically-detectable (at scalp) abnormalities, representing some type of intrinsic cerebral dysfunction or pathology, can be supported.

TABLE 1. EEG Findings in Murderers

"Normal" EEG 61
"Normal limits" EEG 9
"Dysrhythmic or epileptiform" EEG 3

Total = 73

References

Gibbs, F., and Gibbs, E. 1951. *Atlas of Electroencephalography*, vol. I. Reading, Mass.: Addison-Wesley.

Gibbs, F., Bagchi, B., and Bloomberg, W. 1945. Electroencephalographic study of criminals. *Am. J. Psychiatry* 102:294.

Hill, D., and Parr, G. 1950. *Electroencephalography*, Ludgate Hill, England: MacDonald.

Hill, D., and Pond, D. 1952. Reflections on one hundred capital cases submitted to encephalography. *J. Ment. Sci.* 98:23.

Kooi, K., Guvener, A., Tupper, C., and Bagchi, B. 1964. Electroencephalographic patterns of the temporal region in normal adults. *Neurology* 14:1029.

the mind-brain dialectic: a commentary

Frank R. Ervin, M.D.

University of California-Los Angeles Center for the Health Sciences
Los Angeles, California

The time has come when the neglect of an exploration of our fundamental assumptions about the mind-brain relationship to behavior and,
therefore, to society must be made explicit. An undercurrent of confusion
about such issues impairs our clinical judgment and impedes our research
efforts. We give lip service to certain kinds of eclecticism without coming to
grips with the real issue, an ancient Cartesian dichotomy between mind and
brain.

There is a set of platitudes that we all use about multidisciplinary
research. The very concept of multidisciplinary research implies a dichotomy. Physics is the only scientific discipline which has developed a tradition
of examination of the axioms on which its major subdisciplines are based. In
biology we have made a strong and perhaps self-defeating attempt to cram
our experimental paradigms into those of nineteenth century physics, that is,
concepts of relatively linear, unicausal, single dependent and independent
variable experiments. We have done so with considerable success. However,
we have not learned to accept the obligation to clarify the rest of the
theoretical framework.

Medicine is even worse than biology, since medicine is to biology as
engineering is to physics. Medicine tries to make things work and doesn't
really care why. Unfortunately, it is medicine which has been the interface
between biology and the rest of the public. It is the practical interpreter for
society of what biology is doing. Medicine has not been a good interpreter

and has not fulfilled its role. This is not just an American peculiarity but relates to our general embarrassment about Sherrington's last work. We have never quite been able to come to terms with his greatness on the one hand and his own distress with the integration of the mechanics of the brain with the intricacies of the mind on the other hand. The heated discussions concerning violent behavior and the relevance of the neural mechanisms associated with "aggressive and violent" behavior in the laboratory have brought this issue into sharp focus. I quote from a recent letter in opposition to the proposed UCLA laboratory for the study of violence. "I am a neurophysiologist....It is clear to me that violent behavior is due to psychosocial frustrations and I wish that all the preoccupations about developing the Center would stop." While it is clearly true that "psychosocial frustration" is an important variable in influencing human behavior, to ascribe such a single cause to the complex problem of violent behavior is to embrace an explicitly reductionist philosophy. The implication is that an individual's act is merely the reflection of an abstract condition of the social surround. Reciprocally, my recent suggestion that some recurrently violent individuals have limbic system disruption as an important determinant of their impaired impulse control has been interpreted by both critics and supporters as a reductionist statement of mechanistic biology. The leap from that assumption to the expectation that surgical intervention is a logical consequence is a mechanistic extrapolation. For instance, Rodin recently reported that he had activated several hundred temporal lobe epilepsy (TLE) cases with megamide in the EEG laboratory and had never seen an episode of aggressive behavior. He argued that the relationship suggested between TLE and assaultive behavior was unjustified. Although he did misread the relationship, the important point is that the abnormal brain state *alone* is not sufficient to induce violent behavior. It must be present in an appropriate psychosocial context. For example, Huntsberger implanted electrodes into the cat hypothalamus and demonstrated that the cat will attack if offered an appropriate target during hypothalamic stimulation. If the animal is offered an escape route, it is as likely to choose to escape as to attack. If there is no target available, it is unlikely that anything will occur except the characteristic defensive posturing. A more elaborate study by Elliot Valenstein focused on other stereotyped behaviors induced by self-stimulation of the hypothalamus of both cats and rats. He showed that whether the animal is stimulated to drink, to gnaw wood, to eat, and so on is dependent on a variety of factors including the availability of various environmental objects and variables in his internal state. This phenomenon is particularly true in man.

The interaction of brain state and environment is quite striking. In attempting to understand the processes underlying recurrent episodic discontrol in the self-referred patients we studied, we concluded that clinical recognition of the syndrome was difficult because the doctor was distracted by the absence of the external stimulus trigger which is usually present in these cases. In our laboratory studies of TLE cases who had indwelling electrodes, we, like Revine, almost never elicited attack behavior. However, using telestimulation with the patient back in a hospital ward setting, using exactly the same anatomic and physical stimulus parameters, the clinically characteristic patterns of attack behavior could be elicited by stimulating in the presence of a socially significant setting or other individuals. This interaction of internal and external disequilibrium states is obviously not just of theoretical nor diagnostic significance, but expands the spectrum of potentially useful therapeutic tactics, since these two variables are interactive at all times.

It should be clear, then, that I am suggesting a view of the brain which has it imbedded at all times in a social matrix of both present and past stimuli. There are increasing numbers of experimental paradigms to support this point. The early study of Lasagna determining the LD50 of amphetamines in mice was a striking example. He pointed out that the minimum lethal dose for amphetamines in mice is quite variable depending on whether the mouse is housed in isolation or with other mice. That is to say, the social matrix in which the animal exists is a variable determining how sensitive the animal is to a pill. More recently, Redmond et al. have pointed out that the use of reserpine for the pharmacological induction of a model of depression in the stump-tailed macaque can only be seen in the context of the relationship of the animal to its social troop. In fact, the quality of the behavioral disruption induced by depleting the animal of as many catecholamines as possible depends not only on the animal's presence in the troop, but indeed its existing position in the troop's social hierarchy. This demonstration that the interaction between the habitual and social matrices of an animal can serve as an amplifier of the effect and a determinant of the phenomenon suggests the necessity for defining and utilizing a socio-biological paradigm even when studying the effects of drugs, hormones, and certainly brain lesions on behavior. With such a paradigm it becomes possible to begin to evolve a kind of topography of the violent state as one looks at an individual. Indeed, one could begin to deal with precisely the equation which Dr. Walter presented and to begin to think of ways to formulate the proper weighting constants.

The same need for clarity arises in regard to etiology as exists in the area of brain-environment interactions. This is true not only in regard to the present social surround and the response to it, but also in terms of the past. I was delighted with Dr. Kellaway's thoughtful paper because it illustrated two points: The tremendous neglect apparent in American science of developmental brain studies and the lack of interest in the autogenesis of either brain or behavior. This is so not just because it is a difficult topic but because of a kind of blind spot implicit in the kind of atheoretical biases that I mentioned earlier. To be specific, Dr. Kellaway's review of the visual system made it clear that the very structural development of the brain is dependent upon its sensory experience. Indeed, our recent studies have shown that the whole infrastracture of the visual system can be made to disappear under certain conditions. One would think these structures are so phylogenetically predetermined and so built into the system that they were not to be disposed of by simple environmental manipulation. However, in 1918 H.A. Carlson did the first study which suggested this environmental determinant of structural things. More recently Dr. James Prescott, primarily on the basis of theoretical and inferential issues, has pursued that thinking, attempting to account for certain behavioral changes seen in infants or children who had been subjected to early isolation. The study by Heath on monkeys subjected to maternal and social deprivation according to the Harlow model showed abnormal EEGs recorded from depth structures. Prescott has suggested that this early childhood deprivation of proprioceptive and vestibular inputs from lack of handling leads to a developmental failure or deterioration of important central proprioceptive pathways, including cerebellar and perhaps limbic ones. This failure is reflected in later life by certain inabilities to control impulses. Whether or not Prescott is correct in this conceptualization, attempts in later life to modify behavior make the whole set of understandings about causation, therapy, and prevention more interesting and more complex than the spirit in which most recent conversations have taken place.

Relevant to this general argument is the kind of issue raised by Adey. Adey's work has attracted as much fire from his colleagues, although somewhat more quietly, esoterically and intellectually, as other studies have attracted socially. The whole field he is trying to develop has been neglected historically and under-funded currently. This is not just accidental but because he has, in fact, stepped on one of those sensitive philosophical points.

Underlying some of this is a major scientific issue. The issue is essentially: Is it possible to make any sense out of studying organized brain tissue, or must one wait for full understanding of cellular interactions and synaptic structure and detail? Then, after a century of studying these elements and having come to understand then, simply add those elements together and one has a brain! The argument further states that, although one may be clinically impatient and want to rush in with the EEGs and evoked potentials and similar tests, they are simply a way of keeping out of trouble until the "real scientists" understand how to put a brain together. This also has clear philosophical roots, and Adey has violated them by suggesting that it is not only necessary to look at the emergent properties of aggregate elements but that, in fact, those very emergent properties have a dialectic feedback on the rest of the system. That is a very interesting step into a quantum-mechanical understanding of how the brain is put together instead of a linear, binary approach and is not only heretical but dangerous.

The way of thinking about the brain that I have been suggesting begins to edge logically in to the same kind of argument that I have made previously, that the brain and its surround are not to be separated one from another. There is a way of looking at the brain as simply an improbable decrease of entropy in a certain region; that it is a nexus of a lot of past history and current surround; that this little spatio-temporal matrix is terribly important at the moment, but cannot be usefully or fruitfully treated entirely in isolation if we are to think about it as the organ of behavior.

Now, am I raising these topics to suggest a resolution by committee that we all be in favor of one philosophical view of the brain? I am suggesting that we had better start being explicit about what our assumptions are and what their implications are when we present our data. Then, perhaps, we can begin to converge on those areas in which we disagree because of assumptions and those in which we disagree because of data.

Let us come back to the theme at hand to make the point that I am appalled by the current form of controversy around this issue and its intellectual degeneracy. It absolutely amazes me to find otherwise sensible scientists or, indeed, active radical critics of the social system willing to reduce the whole issue of "violence" to a simple construct, and thereby to embrace an idealist metaphysics, which, in the heat of the arguments, leads to statements or implications that say "there is no brain" or "the presence of the brain is irrelevant." This is destroying the intellectual caliber of scientific discourse in the last part of the twentieth century.

In closing, we might ask, "What is the state of our society, especially the subsociety of biology and medicine?" What we see around us is an increasing preoccupation with getting away from dealing with pieces of the real world, be it biological, social, or physical, and embracing what are more clearly idealist metaphysical causes such as scientology, astrology and others which one finds infiltrating every level of discourse in medicine, science, and politics.

index